THE COMPLETE IDIOT'S GUIDE® TO

Massage

By Joan Budilovsky
and Eve Adamson

alpha books

A Division of Macmillan General Reference
A Simon & Schuster Macmillan Company
1633 Broadway, New York, NY 10019-6785

Macmillan Publishing books may be purchased for business or sales promotional use. For information please write: Special Markets Department, Macmillan Publishing USA, 1633 Broadway, New York, NY 10019.

International Standard Book Number: 0-02862708-3
Library of Congress Catalog Card Number: 98-87303

00 99 98 8 7 6 5 4 3 2 1

Interpretation of the printing code: the rightmost number of the first series of numbers is the year of the book's printing; the rightmost number of the second series of numbers is the number of the book's printing. For example, a printing code of 98-1 shows that the first printing occurred in 1998.

Printed in the United States of America

Alpha Development Team

Publisher
Kathy Nebenhaus

Editorial Director
Gary M. Krebs

Managing Editor
Bob Shuman

Marketing Brand Manager
Felice Primeau

Senior Editor
Nancy Mikhail

Development Editors
Phil Kitchel
Jennifer Perillo
Amy Zavatto

Assistant Editor
Maureen Horn

Production Team

Book Producer
Lee Ann Chearney, Amaranth

Production Editor
Christina Van Camp

Cover Designer
Mike Freeland

Cartoonist
Jody P. Schaeffer

Photograher
Ann Censotti

Illustrator
Wendy Frost

Designer
Kevin Spear

Indexers
Cheryl Jackson
Lisa Stumpf

Layout/Proofreading
Angela Calvert
Megan Wade

Contents at a Glance

Appendices

Contents

Part 3: Massage Basics 105

Appendices

Foreword

If this were heaven, or the afterlife, or the spirit realm, and if we all existed as little bits of conscious brilliance radiating from that great source of universal love, we wouldn't need to touch each other. Communication would be an effortless undertaking, instantaneous and spiritual.

Temporarily waylaid as we are in our seemingly inconvenient physical bodies, however, touch means a great deal to our very existence. Unfortunately, society tends to forget the importance of touch as it develops more (or less) sophisticated means of communication. Touch is something reserved for intimate relationships...isn't it? Massage and bodywork are just therapies for pulled muscles...aren't they? Touching can get you in big trouble these days so we're better off avoiding it...right?

No, no, and no! For those of us currently engaged in the physical stage of our spiritual evolution, touch, massage, and bodywork are more than occasional indulgences or even profound modes of communication. They're life skills. They should be taught in the primary schools (and not just to students of massage therapy)!

Whether you're a massage therapist, an eager amateur, or a first-time recipient of a massage, for you now, in this special book, massage and bodywork are taught with love and humor. Joan and Eve clearly see massage and bodywork as more than an occupation, a technique, or a method of stress management. For these authors, touch is an important part of a journey towards self-actualization and a deeper knowledge of our fellow human beings.

Massage and bodywork involve certain specific techniques and knowing something about the physical structures of the body. But the authors never forget that bodywork also involves the interrelationship of body, movement, stillness, energy, mind, mindfulness, and spirit. Through touch we can communicate with each other to reach a deeper understanding of our place in the universe. Joan and Eve show us how touch can relax, loosen, and free our whole selves.

In childhood, we took ourselves for granted. We moved, we played, we wondered, and we understood at some basic level how to be a part of the universe. Life's vicissitudes tend to obscure our innocent sense of self, but this truly holistic book teaches us how to know ourselves again, and how to know each other as fellow human beings. Read this book, enjoy its amiable humor and affectionate guidance, use what makes sense to you and speaks to you, and learn to get back in touch.

Bernie Siegel, M.D.

Bernard S. Siegel, M.D., a New Haven surgeon, is the author of the best-selling Love, Medicine and Miracles; Peace, Love and Healing; *and other books.*

Introduction

Imagine what it would be like to live *in* your body. If you're like many people, you just live *with* your body: tolerating it, complaining about it, sometimes pleased with it for looking good or performing the way you expect. To truly live *in* your body is to integrate body and mind to such an extent that your mind and muscle, sense and sensibility, feeling and movement work in perfect concert. To live in your body is to know your body, to trust it and relish it and communicate with it and care for it, allowing it to be an integral part of your self-concept.

Now imagine what it would be like to communicate with your loved ones on a level far exceeding speech. Imagine transmitting healing and loving energy to your partner, your children, to all the rest of the human race—even to all living creatures. How would your family evolve? How would our world evolve?

Many of us tend to live in our minds. We are defined by our minds, or so we think. We are what we know, what we've experienced, what we remember, what we learn, and what we perceive. We know each other through communication, by sharing thoughts and feelings and by talking and learning about each other.

But the body knows, too. The body experiences and remembers, learns and perceives. It stores knowledge in its tissues; it transmits information to the brain and receives signals back again. It radiates communicative energy, and it determines our health, which in turn has a profound effect on our mental, emotional, and spiritual processes.

What does all this have to do with massage? Everything. To experience massage, either as giver or receiver, is to activate the body-mind. Communication with others becomes both physical and spiritual. We touch and are touched, as energy flows between two souls. When we are touched, our bodies respond as if they are finally receiving what they've needed all along. Indeed, they are. Massage activates the systems of the body to work at their most efficient and most productive. It turns the mind toward the positive, the joyful, the healthy, and the loving. It reintroduces us to our fellow human beings. "Hello! Here we are, in this life together!"

Although we can only begin to explain how important massage and the healing power of touch has been for our lives, we hope this book can help you craft a similar journey. Touch has the power to bring you health, strength, and vitality. It has the power to heal your body, your mind, and your relationships. Touch can wake you up, tune you in, and teach you to love with more strength and wisdom. For without touch, we are alone. With it, we are life.

How to Use This Book

This book is divided into six parts, each bringing massage into your life in a different way. Part 1, "Can You Feel It?" introduces you to the healing, stress-relieving, and confidence-boosting power of massage. We help you determine your personal massage needs, fill you in on the history of this ancient healing art, and elaborate on the many physical, mental, emotional, and even spiritual benefits of massage, from relieving your backache to the benefits of truly connecting with another human being through touch.

Part 2, "Getting in Touch with Your Body-Mind," helps you get to know your own body a little better. What does your body know and remember? What do your senses tell you? How do your various systems work, from your nervous system to your digestive system? How do muscles work, and what can massage do for your muscles? We also offer a brief lesson in the Oriental concept of the body, including energy meridians and pressure points, and end with a brief discussion of your brain, the brain-body conversation, and how you can integrate body and mind for a more self-actualized you.

Part 3, "Massage Basics," tells you everything you always wanted to know about getting, or giving, a massage, including how to set up a massage center at home, how to choose a great massage therapist, and what the differences are between the many types of bodywork out there, from Swedish massage and sports massage to energy therapy, psychophysical therapies, and Oriental techniques.

Part 4, "Different Strokes for Different Folks," goes into more detail about the technical aspects of giving a Swedish massage. We explain how to do the basic strokes: effleurage, petrissage, compression, percussion, friction, vibration, and range of motion.

Part 5, "Massage the Senses," is your self-indulgent section. We'll teach you how to be your own best friend by learning the fine art of self-massage. We'll give you lots of information about the powerful and "scentsual" world of aromatherapy, and we'll give you the skinny on the spa experience, whether you'd like to take a spa vacation or create a spa in your own home.

Part 6, "Massage for Your Life," makes massage just a little more personal. If you suffer from minor or major health problems, whether insomnia or cancer, indigestion or heart disease, we'll tell you how massage can help you. If touch is an emotional issue for you, we'll show you how massage can help you to overcome your fears by giving you what you need. We'll tell you all about sports massage, the special ways massage can help women, men, infants, kids, and seniors, and we'll even show you how to give your beloved pet a wonderful massage. Whoever you are and whatever you do, we'll show you how massage is right for you!

Touching Tidbits

Throughout this book are four types of extra information in boxes for your touch enlightenment:

Massage Minute

These boxes are full of fun anecdotes, trivia, and factoids about the fascinating world of massage and bodywork.

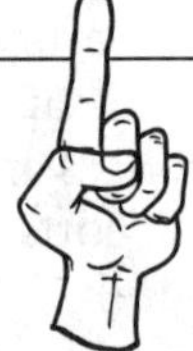

Touch Talk

These boxes give definitions for massage-related terms, so you'll be fluent in the language of touch.

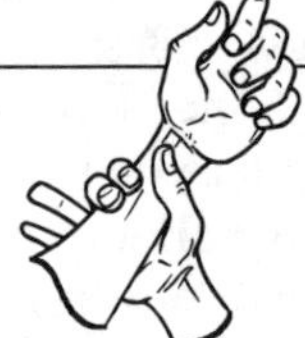

Your Finger on the Pulse

These special boxes offer you tips and advice for making the most of your massage and your health in general, too.

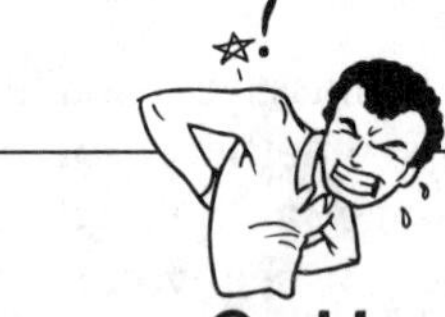

Ouch!

These cautionary boxes contain information about how to avoid potential problems.

Acknowledgments

Many were involved in the process of writing this book, for this book is about touch. Both our lives have been touched by more people than we could possibly name, but they are each in our thoughts and hearts. We can't help but name a few, however.

Thank you to Steve Lux, who was Joan's very first massage teacher at "Mother Sunshine" in DeKalb, Illinois back in 1978. Thank you to all the many wonderful massage teachers Joan has had through the years and to the many massage therapists who have worked their healing ways upon us both. Thank you to Joan's pals, Kathie Huddleston (her incredible Webmaster for **www.yoyoga.com**), Chuck Reiter (graphic artist extraordinaire), Jack Pantaleo (wonder-writer), Maureen Brutto (earthbound angel), and Mary Humphrey (Reiki healer), whose dear friendship and professional expertise have helped Joan significantly through her ever-expanding careers.

Thank you to all the people responsible for putting this book together: Lee Ann Chearney, our faithful and diligent book producer; all the people at Macmillan, including our excellent editorial director Gary Krebs, our nifty development editor Jennifer Perillo, our cool managing editor Bob Shuman, our smiling cartoonist Jody Schaeffer, our sensitive production editor Chris Van Camp, and the many people in production, publishing, and marketing, who are directly responsible for getting this glorious book together and into your healing hands. Thanks also to Wendy Frost, our beautiful illustrator; Ann Censotti, our classy and hip photographer; Paul Davenport, our wise Tech Editor, who so carefully assured our accuracy and edited out our "toxic waste products"; and the other helpful folks at the Florida School of Massage, especially Mike Loomis, sports-massage expert. Thank you to the Touch Research Institute for providing us with such a complete body of research proving the benefits of touch. Thanks to Val Linn, for a super pregnancy massage that proved to Eve how well those aches and pains really can be relieved, and our beautiful models, Melanie Heifetz (who happily posed for a majority of the photos in this book and also for our classy front cover photo, shot by our photographer, Ann Censotti, Bob Rumba, John and Leona Budilovsky, and Joan's cat, Mufasa.

A big thank you to Dr. Bernie Siegel, the foreword writer for our book, whose own books have impacted our lives in incredibly healing ways; thank you to our parents, John and Leona Budilovsky (Joan's) and Richard and Penny Watson (Eve's), who have always encouraged us in creative growth and experimentation, who inadvertently raised us to resist having employers, and whose own creative spirits led the way to our respective and inevitable careers.

Thank you to Joan's twin sister, Jane, and brother, John, who continue to teach her profound lessons in love, and thank you to all Joan's massage clients and students throughout the years who have brought so much light into her life.

Thank you to Eve's husband, Todd, who was a selfless martyr when it came to being a guinea pig for this or that massage technique ("Honey, let me see how this one works"), to Eve's son, Angus, whose toddler spirit was inspirational, and to Eve's gestating son-to-be, who considerately continued to gestate until this book was finished (and it was close!). Thank you to Eve's sisters: Micki, who is getting lots of lectures on infant massage these days, and Elisabeth, who has known for years that Eve can give a great (if not professionally trained) massage, and to Eve's dogs, The Chewdog, Whiskey, and Zeke, who were happy to oblige when it came to testing out our dog massage techniques.

Thank you to the many who have blessed us with their touch, and the many who have honored us by letting us touch them. And thank you, dear reader, for as your hands hold this book, we are truly touched.

Special Thanks from the Publisher to the Technical Editor

The Complete Idiot's Guide® to Massage was reviewed by an expert who not only checked the accuracy of what you'll learn in this book, but also provided valuable insight to help ensure that this book tells you everything you need to know about massage and its effects on the body. Our special thanks are extended to Paul Davenport.

Paul Davenport, LMT, is regarded as one of the nation's most innovative thinkers in the field of massage and massage education. He is director and owner of the Florida School of Massage in Gainesville, Florida. He has been responsible for the creation of comprehensive awareness-oriented massage therapy training and experiential anatomy and physiology courses for massage schools throughout the United States.

Mr. Davenport shared the task of providing editorial guidance for this book with many of the staff members of the Florida School of Massage (FSM). FSM has 25 years of experience providing massage education as a vehicle for personal growth and empowerment, cultivating compassionate touch in a nurturing community experience. FSM can be reached on the Internet at www.massageonline.com or at (352) 378-7891.

Part 1
Can You Feel It?

Massage is not only good for busting stress, it's also good for gaining and maintaining whole-body fitness and for healing. Massage is also a vital way to maintain the human connection. You'll learn about these and other massage benefits in Chapter 1.

In Chapter 2, we'll give you some massage history. You may be surprised to learn how long massage has been around. We'll also answer that nagging question in the backs of so many minds: What about that whole massage parlor business? Is massage, well, respectable? And you'll find out why giving a massage is as good as getting one!

Part 1 ends with a self-examination to help you determine your personal massage needs. What bad body habits do you have? How much stress are you under? We'll even provide a quiz so you can take a good look at your lifestyle, and then learn how massage can help you. We'll also explain how massage can be as relaxing to your mind as it is to your muscles.

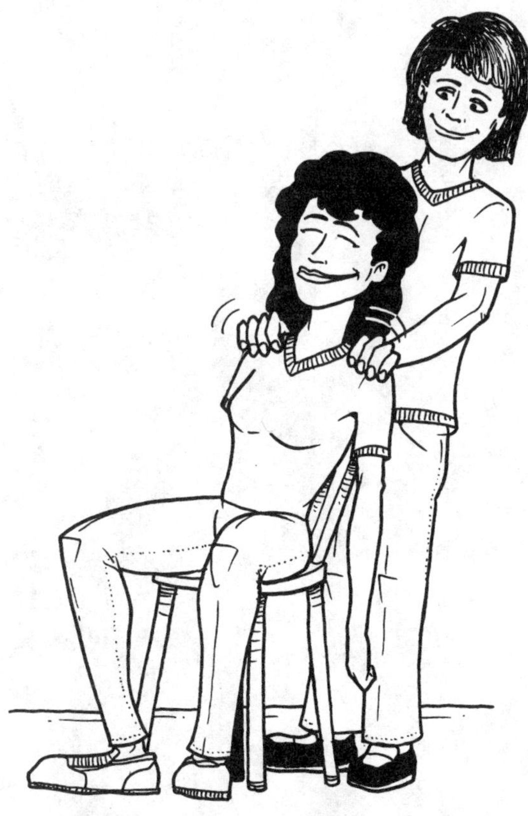

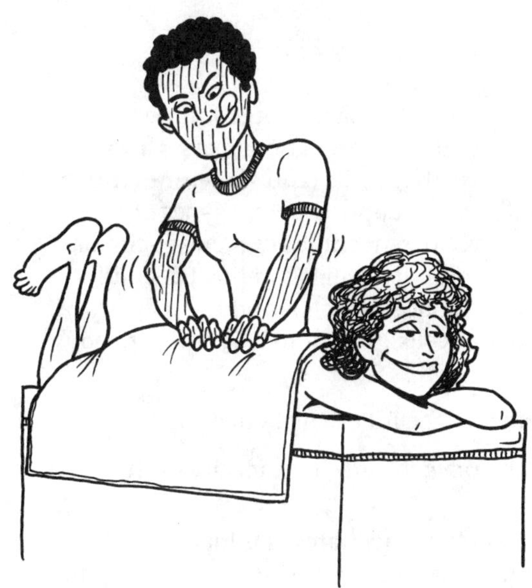

Chapter 1

What's So Great About Massage?

In This Chapter

- Why humans require touch
- How massage relieves stress
- How massage keeps you healthy
- How massage can give you a better life

Who doesn't love a good backrub? We all know that backrubs feel great, but do you know why? Sure, they relax your muscles, but they do more than that—they bring us into physical contact with another human being, and that, in itself, is a powerful experience. Add to that experience the trained, therapeutic touch of a massage therapist, and you have a potent tool for improving your physical, mental, and spiritual health: *massage.*

And it's been that way since the beginning of medical care—probably since the beginning of human existence! For example, ancient Egyptian drawings from as early as 2500 B.C. show medical practitioners treating the hands and feet of patients. These drawings are considered by many to represent an early form of a type of massage called *reflexology*.

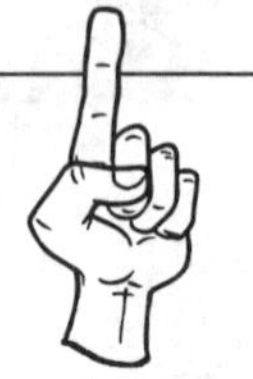

Touch Talk

Massage is the systematic and manual manipulation of the soft tissues of the body. **Reflexology** is a system of massage based on the concept that the stimulation of certain areas of the body (typically the feet, hands, and ears) can affect the health and function of other areas, systems, or organs in the body.

What exactly is massage? Massage is much more than a backrub that feels good. The term encompasses a variety of techniques that use the hands (and sometimes the arms, elbows, and feet) to apply different types of pressure to the body. These techniques increase circulation of blood and lymph (lymph is a yellowish bodily fluid that assists in cell nourishment and the delivery of waste products out of cells), which helps the entire body to be healthier.

Massage also provides the following benefits:

- Increases the oxygen-carrying capacity of the blood
- Helps break up and facilitates elimination of the waste products or harmful toxins that build up in overworked muscle tissue
- Loosens contracted muscles and stimulates sluggish muscles
- Balances the nervous system
- Improves circulation to, and condition of, the skin
- Improves circulation to, and condition of, internal organs

Massage is powerful healing touch that results in increased physical and mental health for both the receiver and, surprisingly, the giver! Massage comes in many shapes and forms, but all types of massage or *bodywork,* to use a more encompassing term, have one thing in common: the human touch.

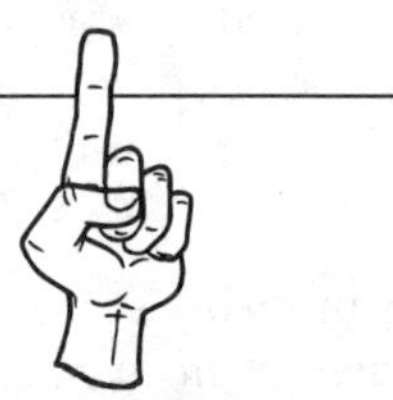

Touch Talk

Bodywork is the systematic manipulation of the body through massage, movement, energy work, or other manual therapies.

Touching: The Human Connection

It's instinctive to touch. Touching makes real the connection between one living being and another, and all the intricate communications systems in the world can't duplicate the satisfying nature of touch. Unfortunately, in our technically oriented world, touch is becoming less and less common. For example, doctors once relied on touch as a crucial diagnostic tool, but today, touch has been largely replaced by high-tech equipment. You're more likely to feel metal or plastic on skin than skin on skin!

Fax machines, multiline telephone systems, e-mail, and the Internet make it possible to reach virtually anyone without seeing them face-to-face, let alone touching them. Many people today have just as many (if not more) "personal" relationships with people via the Internet, phones, or television than with those they see and touch. Our society has yet to witness the full effect that this touch-free society has on human growth, health, and potential, but considering the dramatic benefits of touch, we will most certainly notice a change eventually—and it may not be a welcome one.

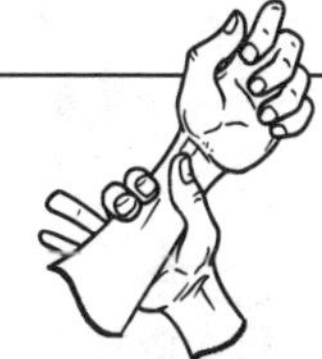

Your Finger on the Pulse

Do you find yourself slumping at your desk or slouching in your chair? Do you hunch over as you rush to catch the train or the bus? Try a massage! Massage helps maintain good posture and keeps your body more balanced so you'll be less likely to slouch. Massage also increases the flow of nutrients to your bones, making them stronger and healthier.

People have become uncomfortable with touch, and because touch has often been abused by the unscrupulous, people are also (often justifiably) afraid of it. Doctors must be very careful how they touch their patients. Expensive lawsuits may result from a misunderstanding. Teachers, coaches, baby-sitters, and neighbors have to be careful how they touch children, and a whole generation of kids is growing up untouched. Some school districts have even instituted "no-touch" policies. Sure, that may be safer. But is it better?

A Massage Minute

One study compared animals isolated from one another with animals housed together. The isolated animals consumed more food and weighed more, but they had smaller brains than the animals housed together in close physical contact with each other.

In another study, the metabolism of baby rats whose mothers were taken away shut down, and the rats stopped growing, even though they were kept warm and given food. When researchers stroked the rat pups with a brush to mimic the mother's licking, however, the rats quickly regained full health.

Research has proven time and again that infants need to be touched, held, and cuddled to thrive. Infants who are never touched often die. If they don't die, they grow up with severe emotional problems. Premature infants who receive infant massage

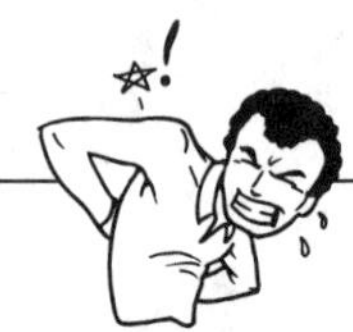

Ouch!

When you first receive a professional massage, you may be surprised at the multiple effects. Relaxation and pain relief are great, but massage can have a psychological effect as well, releasing repressed emotions you may have buried. Don't be surprised if during or after a massage, you feel particularly emotional, even weepy. You may also find yourself ready to deal with a sensitive issue you've been avoiding.

typically gain more weight faster than premature infants who don't receive massage but otherwise receive adequate care. Even animals thrive on touch. Many studies have demonstrated that mice, rats, rabbits, puppies, and kittens all gain more weight and thrive best when they're touched frequently. Touch is part of the human modus operandi—or it should be. What better way to touch effectively, inoffensively, and lovingly, than through massage?

Massage Is a Great Stress Buster

Massage goes beyond fulfilling the simple human need to be touched. (A couple of good hugs a day may satisfy that need.) Massage has overall health benefits, not the least of which is relieving stress in "sense-ational" fashion.

Stress acts on your body like a traffic jam in your nervous system. Your muscles tense, your brow furrows, your nervous habits come out. You feel blocked. You're stiffer, both mentally and physically. Have you ever noticed how your memory doesn't seem to work as well when you're under a lot of stress? You may forget to make an important phone call, miss an appointment, or breeze right past the dry cleaners on your way home, where the suit you require for tomorrow's presentation hangs waiting.

Stress is insidious because you can't exactly diagnose it with a test, but its effects can be extreme. Too many hours, days, and weeks spent with your shoulders hiked up around your ears and your face contorted into an expression of aggravation can be physically and emotionally devastating. Here are just a few of the physical and psychological effects of stress:

- Blood vessels shrink in response to hormones commonly released when your body is under stress. The result is less efficient circulation.
- The flow of nutrients and removal of waste products is reduced.
- Your heart has to work harder.
- Your digestion slows down.
- Your breathing becomes shallow.
- You may develop migraines, ulcers, anxiety attacks, or depression.

In other words, you just don't feel good.

A massage can bring you back to yourself. The physical touch of massage can help bring you out of your problematic past and back from your uncertain future to concentrate on the present moment. Living in the moment isn't easy in this complex society, but at least for awhile, at least during a massage, it becomes possible.

As we've already mentioned, massage increases circulation, which means everything in your body begins to work more efficiently. Tense muscles are kneaded into a relaxed state again. *Connective tissue* fibers (composed chiefly of *collagen*) around joints are stroked into a healthier and more elastic or free relationship.

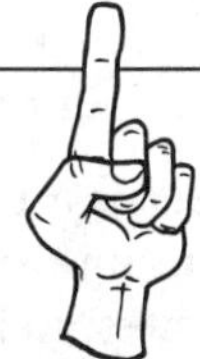

Touch Talk

Connective tissue consists of a matrix of tough, fibrous material that provides a support system for the entire body and lubrication for joints. **Collagen** (from the Greek word *kolla*, meaning glue) is a gelatinous substance found in connective tissue, bones, and tendons.

Even your emotional "circulation" is improved. Often the cause of stress is obvious—too much to do, too little time and money! But sometimes the reasons are trickier, and regular massages can help to free up your psychological state, setting loose buried feelings and conflicts. Massage helps your body to work the way it was meant to work. A smoothly running system handles everyday stress better. You'll control your stress instead of letting it control you.

Researchers have estimated that up to 80 percent of disease is stress-related. Stress accumulates over time, blocking the natural healing processes within the body. The equation is simple: Too much stress equals dis-ease.

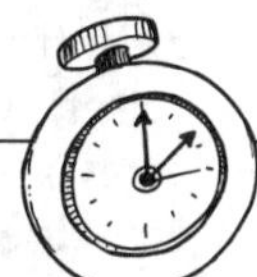

A Massage Minute

In a University of Miami Touch Research Institute study, 26 people were given chair massages in their offices twice a week for five weeks. During these five weeks, the people experienced reduced job stress, were less depressed, had higher alertness, and could solve math problems more quickly and with fewer errors than before they had massages.

Massage Promotes Whole-Body Fitness

It's easy to get excited about becoming fit and neglect the big picture. Whole-body fitness involves a complete, start-to-finish approach. It doesn't mean dashing from a four-hour stint at the computer to a quick hour of high-impact aerobics and then back to the office where your fitness attempts are quickly forgotten as you reach for a candy bar and slump back into your chair. Whole-body fitness means taking on a fit lifestyle, perhaps a little at a time, that includes stress management, a healthy diet, mental preparation, and an adequate warm-up and cool-down before and after a workout. Perhaps most importantly, whole-body fitness should include pre- and post-workout body care, and that means noticing and nurturing your body all the time, not just during your obligatory workout.

Massage is an important part of nurturing the fit or getting-fit body because it keeps everything fine-tuned, circulating well, and eliminating properly. It also increases body awareness, helping you to remember where you live. If you own a house, you take good care of it so it doesn't break down or lose its resale value. Shouldn't you be even more attentive to your body? If you neglect your body's needs, you just may break down early on in your fitness attempts. Frustrated by pain, injury, or lack of energy and endurance, you may give up. A well-cared-for body is bound to last longer and stay healthier.

Athletes love massages, for good reason. Massage reduces fatigue and increases energy by activating and balancing the entire body. After an intense workout, massage can play an important part in the body's recovery process by speeding elimination of accumulated wastes that make muscles sore and by stimulating overworked areas to heal themselves. This process enables athletes to train more effectively and for longer amounts of time without injury.

When you exercise regularly, your capillaries multiply in response to the body's demands for more oxygen and better elimination. Until this process takes place, however (in the new or irregular exerciser), you may work your muscles past the point where they can get enough oxygen. They'll also be unable to eliminate waste as efficiently. The result is pain, but fitness does not necessitate pain. Frequent massage as an integral part of a fitness program can increase circulation to the point where your muscles will already work like those of a more experienced athlete. A pain-free athlete can continue to work out, which is a preferable alternative to sitting on the sidelines with ice packs and heating pads.

When a previously sedentary person begins a vigorous exercise program, or even when an experienced athlete pushes a little too hard, more can be injured than muscles. *Tendons* and *ligaments* are subject to pulls and tears. Joints are also easily injured and tend to atrophy when they aren't used regularly. Sudden movement can then damage the connective tissue within and around the joint. Massage stimulates this connective tissue, keeping it vital and flexible.

Athletes know that injury is an unwelcome side effect of an active life. Massage is great help when sprains and strains are a problem because it stimulates the injured area, helping it to heal faster (although a sprain or strain shouldn't be massaged while still inflamed). Especially good for minor injuries that don't require medical attention, massage can often speed healing and prevent the injury from becoming a chronic problem.

If you're committed to whole body fitness, make massage part of your plan, and you'll keep your body working better. You'll also enjoy your workout a lot more if you know your reward is an hour of massage!

Massage Is Healing Power

Sometimes illnesses or injuries occur beyond the normal strains and sprains common in an active life. When that happens, massage transforms effortlessly from fitness component to physician's assistant. Massage, just like many other forms of alternative health care, is based on the concept of *vis medicatrix naturae*, or the body's ability to heal itself. This concept has been interpreted in various ways by Eastern and Western medical practitioners. Many massage therapists subscribe to the traditionally Eastern idea that the body contains energy channels through which a "life force" flows. When these channels become blocked, physical problems result. Massage frees these blocked areas, allowing the body's life force to flow freely and unimpaired.

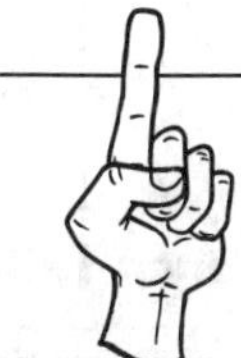

Touch Talk

Tendons are the tough connective tissues connecting muscle to bone; **ligaments** are tough connective tissues that hold bones to bones.

Even if this Eastern concept of recuperation sounds a little far out to you, be aware that massage isn't some fringe version of health care considered not quite respectable by your local doctor. Plenty of doctors here in the West prescribe massage as part of a treatment plan for a wide range of problems, and Swedish massage, the type of massage most common in the United States, is based on a Western view of anatomy. Massage therapy has the distinction of being increasingly embraced by both alternative and mainstream medical circles—probably because virtually no one can deny its benefits.

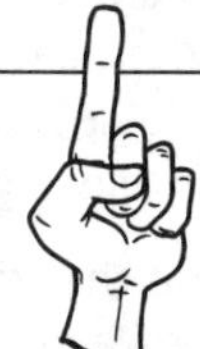

Touch Talk

Vis medicatrix naturae is a term coined by Greek physician Hippocrates (460 to 377 B.C.), who is considered the "Father of Medicine." This term refers to the body's natural ability to heal itself.

Massage can be an effective way to relieve pain without drugs or in conjunction with certain drug therapies, and it is particularly helpful for maladies such as the following:

- Headaches, jaw and neck pain
- Asthma
- Arthritis
- Digestive problems
- Insomnia
- Minor aches and pains

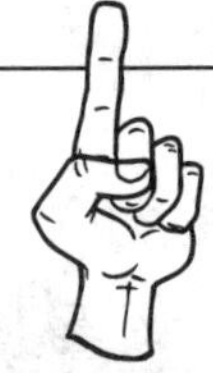

Touch Talk

Essential oils are aromatic oils distilled from organic plant sources, including flowers, leaves, and bark. Different essential oils are thought to have different, potent effects on body, mind, and spirit.

Massage can certainly be, and frequently is, practiced as a healing art. The soft tissue manipulation massage employs works therapeutic wonders on the body, not only by improving circulation but by lowering blood pressure and heart rate, alleviating pain and swelling, and bolstering the immune system. It may stimulate or calm the nervous system depending on what techniques are used. It may improve breathing and relieve a number of respiratory difficulties. It may improve liver and kidney function and all processes of elimination. It flushes the body with oxygen and nutrients that the stressed, sick, or injured system may not be circulating effectively.

Because massage therapists are highly trained in anatomy (whether they take a Western or Eastern approach), certain massage techniques involve "picking up" and manipulating particular muscles, directly stimulating certain organs, or applying pressure to particular points associated with problem areas. When these areas are injured or are the cause of illness, massage can be a quick and effective way to aid and speed up healing.

Beyond the traditional Swedish massage, there are many other branches of bodywork. Here are a few examples:

- **Aromatherapy massage** uses *essential oils* to take advantage of the healing power of scent. Aromatherapy massage is particularly effective for chronic conditions such as stress, digestive problems, hypertension, joint stiffness, fatigue, insomnia, and menstrual problems. (See Chapter 19.)
- **Craniosacral therapy** manipulates the skull bones, spinal cord, sacrum (the large, flat, triangular bone near the base of the spine), and related tissues to treat chronic pain, such as migraine headaches and TMJ. (See Chapter 11.)
- **Reflexology** involves applying pressure to certain areas of the feet, hands, or ears, which are considered reflexes to other areas of the body, including specific organs, tissues, and joints. (See Chapter 11.)

- **Reiki** involves light hand placements to channel energy. It is commonly used to treat many physical, mental, and emotional problems and to help achieve spiritual focus. (See Chapter 12.)
- **Shiatsu** and other forms of **acupressure** apply pressure to certain points along the body's energy channels to stimulate the life force, helping the body to heal itself. (See Chapter 12.)
- **Trigger point therapy** or **myotherapy** uses applied pressure to certain points in the body to relieve pain. Although similar to shiatsu and acupressure, these therapies are based on a more Western conception of anatomy. (See Chapter 11.)

Love Thy Body, Love Thyself

Massage's effects go even deeper than healing the physical body. When you choose to receive a massage, you're sending yourself a message: I'm worth this level of care. In addition to (or quite possibly because of) massage's physical benefits, massage makes you feel darned good about yourself! How can you help but feel good about living in a body that's been so carefully and purposefully renewed? Massage makes you feel fantastic both inside and out. No matter what your level of self-esteem, it'll be improved after a great massage experience. You'll feel even better if you receive massages regularly.

Unfortunately, however, our culture sometimes has a problem with people who're good to themselves in such a wonderful way. A lot of people can't help but feel a little bit guilty when they get a massage. "Shouldn't I be getting some work done?" "I could've used this money to buy something for the kids." "This is *so* self-indulgent!" This type of thinking assumes a false premise: that getting a massage is selfish. On the contrary, caring for your body in this way is ultimately *un*selfish. You'll be healthier, so you'll be more available and more effective, not to mention less of a burden on those who would have to care for you if you became sick. You'll be less stressed, so you'll accomplish more. You'll love yourself, allowing you to truly love others. The fact that massage also feels really, really good is just a side benefit!

Loving yourself enough to get (and give) regular massages is an important step to having a joyfully energetic and ultimately fulfilling life. A healthy body contributes to a happy state of mind. Don't waste another minute wallowing in low energy, chronic pain, and disappointment with your lack of willpower. Get a massage, and everything will look easier, better, and brighter.

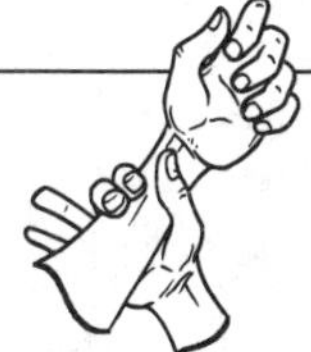

Your Finger on the Pulse

Many massage therapists admit that giving a massage is as therapeutic and spiritually uplifting as getting a massage. Just think: If you get a massage for every massage you give, you'll be getting twice the benefit!

The Least You Need to Know

- Humans are meant to touch and be touched.
- Massage relieves stress by relaxing tight muscles, improving circulation, and releasing repressed emotions.
- Massage is a great part of a fitness program because it improves endurance, flexibility, and speed of healing.
- Massage is a great therapeutic tool for many injuries and illnesses because it improves circulation of blood, oxygen, and nutrients to all parts of the body, helping the body to heal itself.
- Getting a massage is a great way to improve your self-esteem, making you a more effective and happier person.

Chapter 2

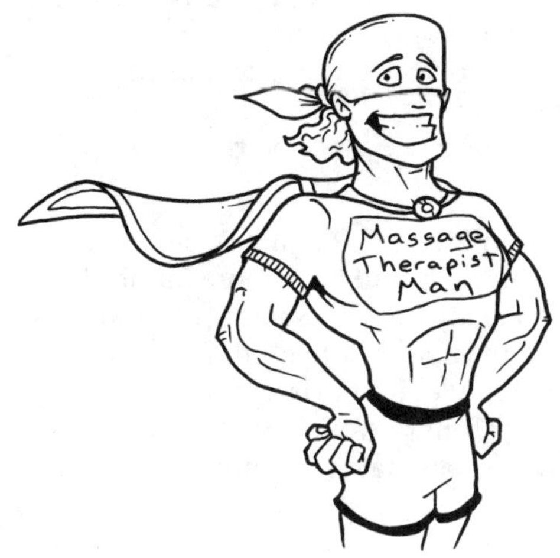

Massage Power: Beyond Backrubs

In This Chapter

- Why you "knead" a massage
- How massage therapy is good for your health
- The illustrious history of massage
- Are you qualified to give a massage?

We've already talked a little about why massage is so much more than a backrub. But you still might think that you aren't quite justified in getting one. Maybe you think you can't afford it, or worse, don't really deserve it. But massage needn't be expensive, and it's certainly a pleasure with very utilitarian effects, improving performance, attitude, and even happiness.

Ah, happiness. That elusive feeling that comes and goes. Just when you think you've mastered it, it slides away again. But can massage really increase your happiness? Massage helps you to stay focused on where you are and how you feel in the moment by highlighting and emphasizing that intimate connection of the mind to the body via the senses. Imagine your mind listening to your body, and nothing else, for one full hour. What luxury. What intensity. And ultimately (often immediately), what joy!

You Knead a Massage

Whether you're a tax accountant, a 9-to-5'er, a professional athlete, a stay-at-home parent, or a massage therapist, you "knead" a massage. Oh, sure, you're not going to drop dead without one. You'll probably be able to get along just fine—if you can ignore that nagging headache, that lingering depression, that crick in your neck, that lower back pain. You'll be all right, sitting there at your computer hour after hour, or carrying those heavy boxes around all day, or bending over the stove, or hoisting your toddler around, or sitting behind that steering wheel, or lugging that pregnant belly from home to work to home, or handling the problems of a host of people who depend on you (you get the picture).

But wouldn't it be wonderful to do all those things and feel great at the same time? You just might be able to work (and play!) more effectively and have more fun in the process with the help of massage. Whether you feel ready to collapse under the stresses of everyday existence or whether you're feeling pretty good about yourself, a massage can make you feel better than you feel at this moment. Because massage has such favorable effects on the body and the mind, helping them to work better and more efficiently, anyone, no matter what his or her physical, mental, and emotional state, can benefit.

How can you tell if massage is right for you?

- If you don't feel good about your body,
- If you love your body,
- If you sometimes get depressed,
- If your job is stressful,
- If your life is stressful,
- If you find it difficult to exercise,
- If you exercise a lot or are very active,
- If you want to maximize your athletic performance,
- If the demands on your time are sometimes overwhelming,
- If you feel low on energy,
- If you frequently perform the same few movements over and over,
- If you always seem to be coming down with one minor illness after another,
- If your marriage or relationships could use some improvement,
- If you sometimes feel isolated from others,
- If you often go through the day untouched by another human being,
- If you feel like you rarely have time for yourself,
- If you've lost touch with the joy life can offer,
- If you like to do everything you can to embrace the joy in life,

Then massage is right for you!

Therapy Versus Fun

There are all kinds of reasons to get a massage. A doctor may prescribe massage for therapeutic purposes, or you may get a massage regularly to deal with chronic pain, an injury, or low energy. Maybe you're interested in learning more about using bodywork to help improve your posture and alignment, improve your attitude, help you to move efficiently and easily, or even release repressed emotion.

But massage can be fun, too. Even if you can't think of one single physical problem you have that might be helped by massage, don't think you aren't justified in getting one—or many! Unlike double hot fudge sundaes, massage is one of those precious things in life that feels good *and* is truly good for you!

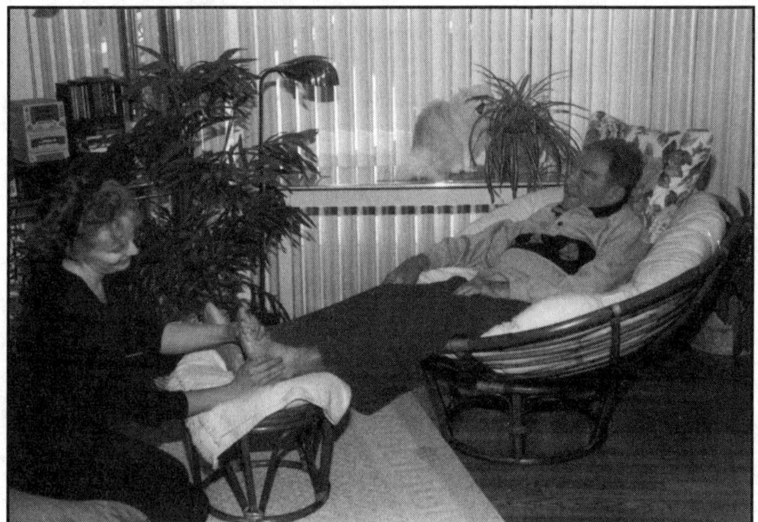

Joan gives John a relaxing foot reflexology session.

A Massage Minute

According to the National Institutes of Health, approximately 20 million Americans receive some form of massage or bodywork every year. Do you think 20 million Americans would do anything of their own free will if it weren't lots of fun?

Head to Toe Heaven

Massage can feel like heaven—or as close to it as earthbound humans can get! During a massage, the following transformations may take place within your body:

- Your metabolism increases, energizing you
- Your muscles relax
- Your blood and lymph circulation improves, delivering more oxygen to your internal organs and your skin—you'll leave the massage table with a healthy glow
- Tension, anxiety, and fatigue are reduced
- Your blood pressure lowers
- Your heart rate slows
- Your body releases *endorphins* (chemicals that relieve pain)

Many people report feelings of euphoria or a heightened sense of awareness after a massage. At the very least, you'll feel deliciously relaxed and refreshed. All that, and it's still good for your health? Believe it!

No More Parlor Games

Maybe you still feel a bit hesitant about massage. Isn't "massage" a word from the realm of red light districts, 900 numbers, and heavily made-up Madams ("So you want a *massage,*" wink wink)? In fact, massage has been around for thousands of years, enjoying respectability and frequent use. Aside from a lapse in the Dark Ages (when many wonderful things were temporarily stifled), massage has always been practiced to enhance people's health. It wasn't until the end of the 19th century that massage developed its somewhat seedy, overtly sexual reputation, which has lingered through much of the 20th century—even as physicians and athletes continued to use it as a form of physical therapy.

Indeed, massage became so popular in the 19th century that practitioners begin to pop up everywhere, hoping to cash in on the trend. In 1894, the British Medical Association investigated the practice of massage and uncovered much in the way of unscrupulous conduct, from practitioners without any training to houses of prostitution hiding under the guise of massage "parlors." The reputation of the profession suffered, and fewer and fewer people sought out massage. Add to that the 19th-century idea that touching was considered a sinful, bodily pleasure. Even piano legs were modestly covered because displaying them was thought to be too suggestive. Touch, decadence, massage, sin, the body, prostitution: the words all began to be used together.

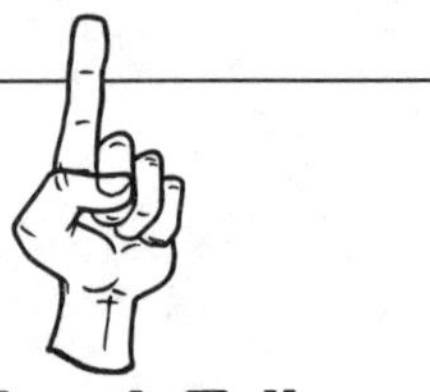

Touch Talk

Endorphins are neuropeptides that work within the brain to relieve pain, affect emotions, and contribute to feelings of euphoria after intense physical activity. Similar to morphine, endorphins are the brain's "homemade" painkillers.

As the 20th century progressed, a few persistent believers in massage developed systems that began to earn respect. But, because of massage's still-questionable reputation and other advances in technological means of rehabilitation, massage remained largely behind the scenes in the world of medicine, athletics, and health maintenance. It wasn't until the 1960s, when interest in natural health enjoyed a resurgence, that people rediscovered the therapeutic benefits of massage. As holistic health practices continue to gain in popularity and the cost of traditional medical care continues to skyrocket, people are seeking more affordable, natural, intuitive, and preventative types of body care.

Your Finger on the Pulse

Take advantage of the benefits of touch whenever you can. Hug and kiss your loved ones, hold hands with your partner in public, make a point to "snuggle" more often with your partner in a nonsexual way. It's good for you!

In the 1970s and 1980s, professional associations for massage and other forms of bodywork began to appear, and massage schools enjoyed dramatic gains in popularity as well as respect. The Federation of Bodywork Organizations formed in 1991 to develop standards in the field, and in 1992, the National Certification for Therapeutic Massage and Bodywork exams became available. Many states now require that massage therapists be licensed. Massage is once again a respected and highly valued form of body care.

Of course, there are a few massage parlors here and there whose employees aren't, shall we say...licensed. But legitimate massage therapy centers are proliferating and massage is steadily regaining its reputation as a superior therapy and method of stress relief. Now that the concept of massage therapy is losing its stigma, people can enjoy the many advantages of touch, including nonsexual intimacy and the touch-bond with another human being, without having to worry that their reputations will be ruined.

A Massage Minute

The ever-increasing respectability of massage is no accident. In many states, practitioners must be licensed, and licenses may be revoked, suspended, or canceled if practitioners have been convicted of a felony, have engaged in any act of prostitution, are addicted to narcotics, alcohol, or other substances that might interfere with job performance, or are guilty of deceptive advertising.

A Brief History of Massage

Thousands of years ago, when Ugh and his mate, Ooga, lived in a cozy cave, Ooga massaged Ugh's shoulders after a long day of game hunting, and he, in turn, rubbed her back, which was achy from tedious hours stooping to dig up roots and tubers. When their son, Ugh Jr., would trip over a rock while practicing with his new spear, he would instinctively rub and massage his bruises and scrapes.

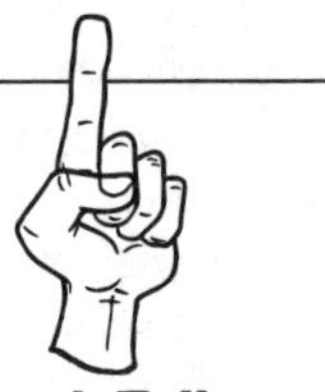

Touch Talk

Amma is an ancient Chinese form of massage. It incorporates centuries of experience gained by Chinese health practitioners on the effects of stimulating certain points on the body in various ways. **Tui-na**, which literally means push-pull, is the term for modern Chinese massage.

All right, maybe we're only imagining the details of massage in the days of the cave dwellers, but cave paintings in the Pyrenees dating as far back as 15,000 B.C. demonstrate the use of touch as a method of healing. Other prehistoric artifacts suggest that ancient cultures made a practice of rubbing herbs on the body. Touch is certainly a primal human instinct, beginning with the moment a new baby latches on to its mother's breast. Mother and baby know, at least roughly, what to do, and the human species would never have survived as long as it has without knowing that touch nurtures, replenishes, and heals the human body.

From China to Sweden to America

Although massage has probably existed in rudimentary form as long as humans have, the Chinese were the first to systematize it. Back in 3000 B.C., the Chinese used a combination of herbs, exercise, and massage of particular points on the body (this type of massage was known as *amma*) to treat illness and maintain health. *Amma* was described in an ancient book called the *Cong Fau of Tao Tsu*. Even today, massage is an important part of health maintenance in China, although it's now known as *tui-na*.

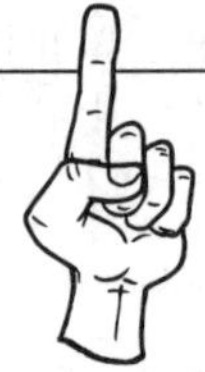

Touch Talk

Ayur-Veda is a sacred Hindu text and also a native Indian system of health care. The word is often translated as "science of living" or "art of life." **Ayur-Vedic** practices include massage, often practiced in conjunction with bathing.

Massage has been well known in India for over 3,000 years, and the *Ayur-Veda,* a sacred Hindu text written around 1800 B.C., listed massage as one of its principles of hygiene. Other Hindu texts also contain descriptions of hygiene that include *tshanpau,* or massage at the bath. Tshanpau included kneading, tapping, and applying friction to the body, as well as anointing the body with perfume and cracking the finger, toe, and neck joints.

The Japanese began to practice and develop their own form of amma in approximately the 6th century A.D., naming the points on the body delineated by amma as *tsubo*. The Japanese further developed massage to manipulate *chi*, or the life force, within the body. They also developed a method of finger pressure on particular points of the body called *shiatsu*, still popular today (see Chapter 12 for more on shiatsu).

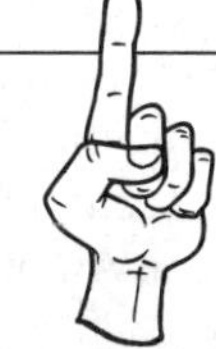

Touch Talk

Tsubo is the Japanese name for the specific points on the body that can be pressed or rubbed to stimulate chi. **Chi**, also known as qi or ki, is the energy of the life force that flows through the body. **Shiatsu** is a specific method of massage that uses finger pressure on tsubos to manipulate chi.

Although massage is firmly rooted in Eastern tradition, we Westerners certainly weren't about to be left out of the loop! The buzz about massage spread from the East, eventually influencing the modern system of Swedish massage.

Even though Swedish massage is rooted in the Eastern tradition, the Greeks also developed notions of the health benefits of massage before 300 B.C. Aesculapius, a Greek priest and physician, developed the concept of gymnastics, which was a combination of exercise and massage. The first gymnasium, which he founded, was a place of learning, healing, exercising, and philosophical discourse. Greek women, too, used massage for health and beauty, and Hippocrates, known as the Father of Medicine, believed all physicians should be trained in the proper use of massage for healing. The famous Greek baths were a place where philosophy was discussed, tensions were eased away, and massage was frequently practiced.

Like many other aspects of Greek culture, the Romans procured the art of massage, using it as an integral part of hygiene and as a medical treatment for many conditions. But the fall of the Roman Empire resulted in a decline in all the arts and sciences, including the practice of massage. The magnificent public baths soon came to ruin, and massage became suspect because of its emphasis on the physical body, something considered evil during this time of religious fervor. A few midwives and natural healers continued the practice, but they were often persecuted for doing "Satan's work." This period is appropriately known as the Dark Ages. The art and science of massage persisted throughout the Middle Ages largely because of an Islamic Persian philosopher, physician, and writer known as Rhazes (or Razi), who was a dedicated follower of Hippocrates. He wrote an encyclopedia of Arabic, Roman, and Greek medical practices that refers to massage as a means to treat and prevent disease.

Massage resurfaced in Europe with the Renaissance, as all the arts and sciences were revived. Mercurialis, a professor of medicine at the University of Padua in Italy, wrote a book on gymnastics and massage, recommending the latter as part of a complete mind-body treatment. Sixteenth-century physicians began to use massage in the treatment of their patients, and a French barber/surgeon, Ambroise Pare, supposedly restored the failing health of Mary, Queen of Scots through massage. The word *massage* comes from a French word, *masser*, meaning "to shampoo," and the word *shampoo* comes from a Hindu word meaning "to press." (The root of the word probably came from the Arabian word *mass* or *mash*, meaning "to press softly.")

Massage continued to develop as a form of medical therapy and a method of folk healing throughout the centuries. Around the turn of the 19th century, Per Henrik Ling, a Swedish physiologist, developed a system of movements grounded in the latest knowledge of physiology as well as techniques practiced in China for thousands of years. He called his system Medical Gymnastics and based it on three types of movements: *active* (those performed by the patient), *duplicated* (those performed by the patient with the therapist's help), and *passive* (those performed on the patient by the therapist). The Ling System wasn't published until after Ling's death, but its popularity has been phenomenal. This system is the basis for Swedish massage, the most popular type of massage in the United States.

Sweden wasn't the only European center for massage. Dr. Johann Mezger of Holland coined much of modern massage terminology. Doctors in Germany, Denmark, and Norway also recommended, employed, and wrote about massage. In 1894, a group of women in England established The Society of Trained Masseuses (perhaps in response to the British Medical Association's investigation of abusers of the profession that same year), later registered as the Chartered Society of Physiotherapy in 1964.

Massage made its way to the United States from Europe through a New York physician, Charles Fayette Taylor, who learned the techniques of Swedish Movement Gymnastics in England. In 1870, Dr. S. Weir Mitchell of Philadelphia published a treatise on massage and good nutrition as important treatments for certain blood disorders. Massage was an important part of health care in the United States during and after World War I, where it was often used to treat soldiers.

After World War II, however, as more mechanical means of manipulation became popular (such as physical therapy), the popularity of massage began to decline. Postwar massage therapy usually focused on athletes and faded from the medical sphere. In mainstream society, where a general discomfort with touch existed (and still exists today), "taboo" overtones remained attached to the idea of massage in the minds of many Americans. Many people had (and still have) only experienced touch in the context of sex or violence.

By the 1960s, when massage therapy emerged once again as a holistic health discipline, it had become an integrated form of ancient Chinese, Japanese, Indian, Greek, Roman, Arabic, and European techniques, available in a variety of guises practiced by an ever-growing number of massage therapists and bodyworkers. Yet massage maintained the air of an "alternative therapy." Massage therapists were often employed as assistants to chiropractors.

East Meets West, Old Meets New

Massage is, as you can see, nothing new. It is, however, a continually evolving art/science that, in its present form, combines the wisdom of the East with the wisdom of the West, and ancient healing techniques with modern scientific knowledge. One of the wonderful things about massage therapy today is that it's more than a revival of the old or an exploration of a different culture or even simply "alternative medicine." It's all these things and more.

Depending on the type of massage or bodywork you intend to practice or receive, you can explore the intricacies of human muscles, bones, and joints or the equally intricate channels and passageways of the life force, chi. You can indulge your body through movement, through posture, through kneading and rubbing, through quick percussive movements, through the application of pressure to certain areas, or through gentle manipulation. You can cater to your body's needs solely through the avenue of your mind or through your other senses. Best of all, you can give or receive a massage secure in the knowledge that the techniques you are practicing have been tried, tested, and refined over thousands and thousands of years. Giving or receiving a massage is participating in an ancient and ever-evolving tradition.

Tradition Touches Science

Massage is certainly rooted in tradition, but today it is also firmly rooted in the latest scientific knowledge. Swedish massage (see Chapter 11) is based on a sound knowledge of *anatomy* and *physiology*. Sports massage (see Chapter 11) takes this concept further, specifically tailoring massage to the athlete's needs for high energy, flexibility, and muscle/joint regeneration after demanding activity. The concept of touch therapy has been and continues to be extensively studied by scientists at such prestigious institutions as the Touch Institute at the University of Miami. Massage is far from the fringe. It's a proven and legitimate method for maintaining and restoring health and vitality.

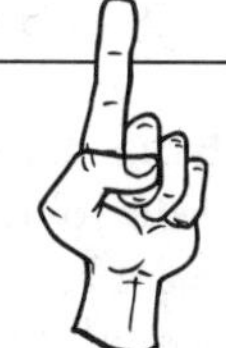

Touch Talk

Anatomy is the study of the structure of the body and the interaction of its parts. **Physiology** is the science of vital processes, mechanisms, and functions of organs and organ systems.

Massage Enters the 21st Century

After 5,000 years, we are only beginning to uncover massage's dramatic benefits and physical, mental, emotional, and social effects. Massage is the perfect personal and physiological therapy for the 21st century. As we move into a new era, people all over the world are becoming increasingly aware of the importance of integrating body and mind for the ultimate in total fitness and self-actualization.

The 21st century promises a new kind of social consciousness, wherein body/mind care translates to care of others and care of the world around us. Massage is the perfect system to ease us gently into such a mode of living, for by reconnecting with each other through the power of touch and learning more about our bodies and minds through the nurturing and strengthening that bodywork provides, we can connect to our inner selves and outer environments naturally and wholly.

Who Can Do a Massage?

"That may all be well and good," you might be thinking, "but there aren't any massage therapists in my neck of the woods!" Fear not, rural dwellers, denizens of small towns, and the budget-conscious among you. Although a professional massage from a trained therapist is a fantastic experience, it isn't the only option. Massage not only comes in many forms, but also can be practiced on many levels, and can even be accomplished effectively by you!

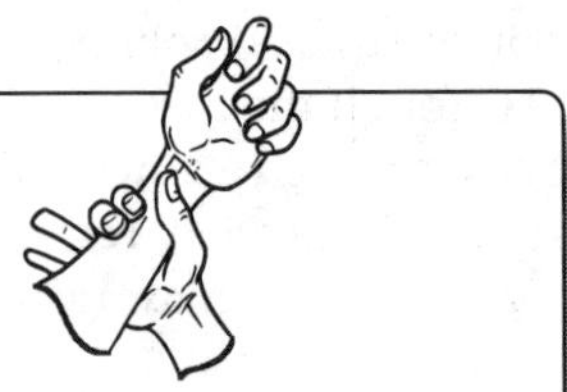

Your Finger on the Pulse

Self-massage is a great way to relieve tension, reduce stress, and alleviate muscle pain fast. Learning some basic pressure points or massage techniques to apply to yourself is a great stress-management technique. You'll feel so self-sufficient, too!

Yes, even without a license and intensive training, you can do massage on your loved ones, your friends, even on yourself. Sure, it would take lots of training to know everything there is to know about anatomy, life-force energy meridians, and all the various types of bodywork. But you don't have to be an expert to perform a great massage on someone else or even on yourself.

Is It Better to Receive than to Give?

Giving a massage can be as rewarding, relaxing, and energizing as getting one! Just ask any massage therapist. Giving a massage is communicating, skin on skin, with another human being. It's touching. It's more than therapy—it's a connection between two souls.

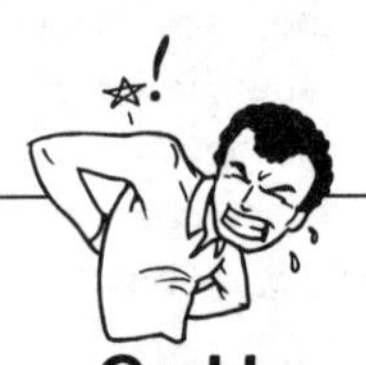

Ouch!

When giving a massage, always be aware of the person who is receiving the massage. Especially encourage them to tell you if something hurts. Even experienced massage therapists can't always tell when something is uncomfortable because each body is so different in its degree of sensitivity and pain tolerance.

Giving a massage also means giving yourself over to minute observation of the condition of someone else: Why are his shoulders so tight? Where is she feeling pain? Why is this muscle so much shorter on this side? Where is the pressure point that will relieve that headache? Focusing so completely on another person helps to remove you from your own body for awhile, and in doing so, you will come back more aware of it and more aware of the union between all bodies and all humanity.

Without the right awareness, concentration, and care, giving a massage can be tiring, tedious, or just plain boring. With the proper focus and commitment, however, it can be a spiritual experience. Plus, if your recipient has had a wonderful massage encounter, he or she will probably be glad to pay you back in kind. And that means you get the next one!

The Least You Need to Know

- Everyone can benefit from massage. Everyone!
- The practice of massage goes back 5,000 years or more.
- Modern massage is a combination of Eastern and Western traditions combined with the latest in scientific knowledge.
- Even you can give a great massage.
- Giving a great massage is as good for you as getting one!

Chapter 3

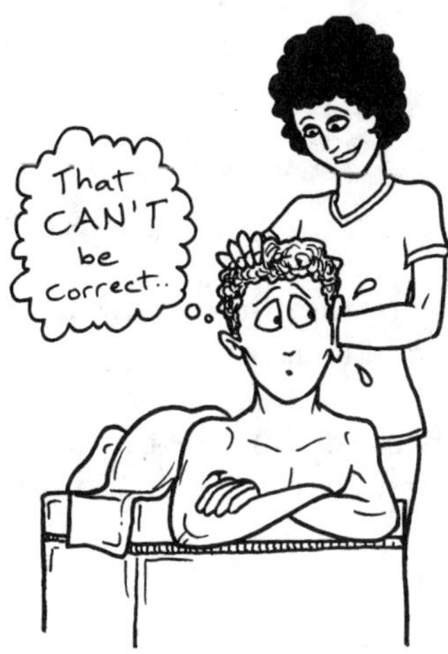

Working from the Outside In

In This Chapter

- What kind of massage could you use?
- Self-esteem: the key to body awareness
- How to live in your body-mind

Do you feel like your body reflects the inner you? Or is it just an often inconvenient container for the you that exists primarily, as you see it, in your brain? Unless your body is an integral part of your profession (if you happen to be, say, a professional athlete), you might consider your body merely a hanger for your business clothes, equipment for toting kids and groceries from here to there, or a relatively unreliable piece of machinery that runs down at the most inconvenient of times. Getting a massage is a great way to pay attention to your body, but it isn't the only way. A little attention to that vessel that carries you from birth through death, both before and certainly after you receive a massage, will help you to get even more out of the massage experience.

Start from the Body

Most of us go through life ignoring our bodies most of the time, but paying attention to your body has significant rewards. When you learn to acknowledge, notice, and nurture your body, you'll develop a whole new relationship with your physical container. You'll be more comfortable in your skin. You'll feel as though the outer you reflects the inner you. You'll also experience these benefits:

- Your body will be more likely to react the way you want it to, especially during times of stress.
- You'll feel better about your life in general and your place in the world.
- You'll have more energy.
- You'll look better.
- Perhaps most importantly, you'll develop a healthy relationship with your body. You'll learn to like the way your body looks, feels, and behaves.

Learning to be in tune with your body takes some practice and can only be accomplished by first examining your habits, your schedule, your environment, and your level of stress—in essence, your lifestyle.

Breaking Bad Habits

Just about everyone will acknowledge they've got a few bad habits: nail biting, hair twirling, an incurable chocolate chip cookie addiction. Bad body habits, on the other hand, are bad habits you might not even notice you have (another clue that you aren't paying enough attention to your body). Potential bad body habits are numerous; they include slumping, slouching, tending to twist towards one side, or overuse of certain muscles or joints.

Do you have bad body habits? The following are some common body transgressions:

- Slouching at your desk
- Always sloping your shoulders to one side
- Holding the telephone between your ear and your shoulder
- Crossing your legs (which can cut off circulation and can cause or aggravate varicose veins)
- Pulling your shoulders up slightly when under stress
- Locking your knees when standing
- Always sitting with one leg lifted, twisted, or turned

Bad body habits do more harm than you might realize, too. When your body becomes accustomed to certain positions or movements, those movements start to feel like the norm even though they're inhibiting your body from functioning correctly. Take the example of slouching at your desk, something many of us are prone to do. Sure, slouching looks bad; it makes you look heavier, clunkier, less graceful, even less happy. But slouching does damage to more than your appearance. It crunches all your internal organs together, compacting your lungs, your stomach, and your digestive tract. You can't breathe as deeply when you slouch. You can't digest your food as well. Your torso is built to be roomy, and when you slouch, you mess up your inner workings.

In addition, slouching is often caused by muscles contracting unnaturally. When you try to correct your slouch by forcing yourself to stand or sit in a more upright position, you may end up harmfully contracting other muscles, a not-necessarily-better option. Massage and other bodywork can help to correct slouching in a healthier way.

The same goes for habits such as hiking up your shoulders or always twisting to one side. When your muscles are continually tense or twisted, they can't receive oxygen or flush out toxins nearly as well. They won't work at optimum capacity. Such bad body habits are common side effects of too much stress. When you don't manage your stress, it runs rampant on your body, doing its dirty work. Eventually, you'll feel the effects, whether through muscle atrophy, frequent minor illnesses, or a general, overwhelming feeling of fatigue.

Stress Is a Form of Violence

When you allow stress to harm you, you're committing violence to yourself. Even if you consider yourself a gentle person who wouldn't hurt a fly, you are hurting yourself every time you don't manage your stress. Unfortunately, these days stress is a way of life for most of us. If stress is a part of your life, the best way to protect yourself from its harmful effects is to learn to manage it.

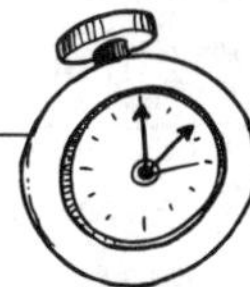

A Massage Minute

What happens, chemically, when you experience stress? A series of hormones signal your adrenal gland to release adrenaline and cortisol, which prepare your body to respond to stress. More blood is directed to your brain and muscles. Glucose and fat are released into your blood for energy, and a substance called fibrin is mobilized to combine with thrombocytes to assist blood clotting in case of injury. (You got that?!)

How are you supposed to manage stress? First, don't get all stressed thinking about how you'll manage your stress. We saw those shoulder muscles contracting, that brow furrowing! Take a deep breath, fearless reader, and read on. There are all sorts of options. Massage, of course, is one of the best options, but there are others, and the more of them you can implement, the better.

Mindful Meditation

A few minutes each day spent in quiet reflection, prayer, or whatever form of peaceful thought or non-thought you find works for you will do wonders for your stress level and ability to think clearly. You can learn meditation through a class, books, or even through on-line lessons on the Internet. Consider it mental health maintenance.

Heavy Breathing

Deep breathing renews you, fills your body with positive energy, and clears your mind. Most of us don't get enough oxygen, and deep breathing immediately delivers the oxygen our bodies crave. Take a break once or twice a day to step outside (preferably away from a polluted street) and take a few full, deep, fill-up-with-air-down-to-your-toes breaths. Breathe slowly, in through your nose and out through your nose or mouth. Try making your exhale twice as long as your inhale. Concentrate fully on your breath, forgetting everything else.

You may also consider learning a little bit about the structured deep breathing techniques, called *pranayama*, that yoga teaches. You'll be amazed at how such a simple, accessible, and absolutely free activity can make such a difference in the way you feel. Try the following pranayama exercise condensed from *The Complete Idiot's Guide to Yoga:*

1. Cover your right nostril with your right thumb.
2. Inhale through your left nostril.
3. Close your left nostril and hold the breath for a few seconds.
4. Uncover your right nostril and exhale through it.
5. Inhale through the right nostril, close it, and exhale through the left. Continue alternating nostrils.

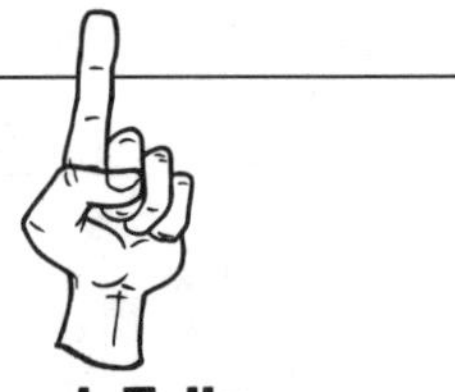

Touch Talk

Pranayama is the Hindu word for yoga breathing exercises designed to help you master control of the breath and, ultimately, your life force.

A combination of breathing, health-enhancing postures, and relaxation, yoga is a fantastic stress management technique, with lots of other great physical, mental, and emotional health benefits to boot!

Express Yourself

Sometimes, all you need to do to blow off steam is to talk about what's bugging you. The trick is finding a good audience. A friend, partner, or relative who will listen without offering advice or trying to fix your problem is the ideal. You might even be surprised to discover how you really feel about what's causing you stress. Sometimes putting things into words finally makes them clear.

If you don't have a good listener or if you just don't feel comfortable venting your problems out loud, try keeping a journal. A daily entry (it doesn't have to be long) in which you expound upon your day and how you felt about it can be great therapy. Like talking, sometimes writing about a problem can finally put it in perspective, and solutions will become apparent. As a great author (E.M. Forster) once said, "How can I tell what I think until I see what I say?"

Work It Out

A brisk walk, a brief run, a vigorous aerobics class, or a slamming game of racquetball can dissolve stress. And a massage afterwards spells pure relief!

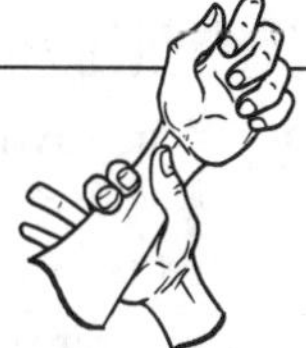

Your Finger on the Pulse

Uncover the way your lifestyle affects your body via an hourly body check. Try this today. Stop every hour or so and, without adjusting your position, examine how your body feels and what it is doing. You might be surprised at how seldom you find yourself in a good body position.

When Life Is a Real Pain in the Neck

Stress isn't the only way your lifestyle can damage your body. Almost any activity you do frequently, whether typing at a computer, loading packages onto a truck, carrying around an infant, or sitting all day in horrendously long meetings, will wear on your system. Maybe you love your job, your hobby, your lifestyle, but your body may not love what life does to it. Again, better body awareness will bring these work-related and lifestyle-related bad habits to light.

Could You Use a Massage? A Lifestyle Quiz

We'll admit it right now: No matter how you score on this quiz, we're going to say that you could certainly use a massage, because everyone can benefit from a massage. The purpose of this quiz isn't just to let you know you could use a massage, however. It's also to help you uncover some of the lifestyle factors that might be contributing to unhealthy body habits—or to let you know what you're doing right! We'll also analyze the ways in which massage can benefit you according to your lifestyle analysis.

1. I would describe myself as mostly:
   - A. Sedentary by choice. I don't move if I can help it, and there's nothing I hate more than exercise.
   - B. Sedentary out of necessity. My job doesn't allow me to get much exercise, and after work, I don't have the time, although I wish I could do more. Maybe someday I'll be able to make exercise a part of my life.
   - C. Active by choice. I love to be active whenever I can, and I'm in pretty good shape.
   - D. Active out of necessity. I have a physical job and/or a physical family, so I'm always moving, but I don't particularly enjoy it. I wish I could spend more time relaxing, but at least I'm physically fit.

2. At this moment, I can perceive tension:
   - A. Nowhere.
   - B. Everywhere.
   - C. In a few typical places: my neck, lower back, or legs.
   - D. In my neck, back, legs, joints, but it feels more like pain. I ache all over!

3. This is how I feel about my job:
   - A. It pays the bills for now, but I don't plan to be in this field forever.
   - B. Love it, love it, love it! It's my dream job.
   - C. Whenever I wake up in the morning and think about going to work, I get the most oppressive feeling and immediately feel stressed—but once I'm there, it's not always so bad.
   - D. If I could possibly get by with quitting, I would do so in a second—and boy would I love to tell off my boss!

4. My personal relationships are mostly:
   - A. Pretty satisfactory. I have lots of friends, although I wouldn't feel comfortable talking too personally to them. I get along well with most members of my family.
   - B. All give and no take. I'm the one everyone comes to with their problems, but I don't feel comfortable taking my problems to anyone. I'm supposed to be the "rock."
   - C. Very fulfilling. I have a few very close friends who are always willing to listen. My family is supportive and loving. I feel emotionally rich when I think about my friends and family.
   - D. Horrible. I often feel isolated. People aren't comfortable confiding in me, and I don't feel like I can confide in anyone. I have acquaintances but I wouldn't call them friends. People probably have no idea how lonely I am because I would never reveal my feelings.

5. When I am happy, my body:
   - A. Usually feels great. Feeling healthy and in-shape makes me feel happy.
   - B. Is the last thing on my mind! I'm happiest when I'm not thinking about my body—in fact, thinking too much about it is sure to bring me down!
   - C. Takes the day off. I'm happiest when I'm completely relaxing, pampering myself, taking it easy.
   - D. Is happy? Happiness sounds vaguely familiar…I think the last time I was really happy was when I was a kid. Back then, I was really "in" my body, but now my body is foreign and uncomfortable to me.

6. When I am stressed, my body:
   A. Tenses up in a few characteristic places, like my shoulders or my neck.
   B. Gets restless, telling me it needs to exercise to blow off steam.
   C. Gets sick.
   D. Wants nothing more than to curl up and go to sleep.

7. I probably touch other people:
   A. Multiple times per day. I have a very affectionate family.
   B. Several times per day. I kiss my partner good-bye and hug my kids before and after school. I shake hands or give little hugs to close friends when I happen to see them.
   C. Rarely. Touching makes me uncomfortable.
   D. Once or twice a day in a fairly formal manner, such as a handshake, a congratulatory slap on the back, ruffling the hair of a cute kid. But these days, you can't be too careful—touching can get you in trouble!

8. Strength-wise, I consider myself:
   A. Basically a big wimp, but most of the time, I don't mind too much.
   B. Pretty darned buff!
   C. I think I used to have muscles somewhere.
   D. About average, I guess. Not so weak that I feel impaired in any way, but I don't lift weights or anything.

9. When I look in the mirror, I usually think:
   A. "One of these days, I'm taking down all these mirrors so I don't have to inflict this kind of suffering on myself!"
   B. "Hmm, no movie star, but pretty good, considering!"
   C. Remember when Fonzie on Happy Days looked in the mirror to comb his hair, then put the comb away because he realized how perfect he already looked? That's me, baby!
   D. How on earth did I get to look so (old) (fat) (gray) (wrinkled) (dumpy)?

10. If I could go back in time and change one thing about my life, I would:
    A. Have chosen a career that makes a whole lot more money. I never have enough and it's my main source of stress.
    B. Take a risk to achieve my dreams. I've taken the easy and safe route most of my life, and I feel I've missed out on a lot of excitement and opportunity.
    C. Find my soul mate. My personal relationships aren't very fulfilling.
    D. Start the whole thing over again because I did it all wrong.
    E. Keep my past completely intact. I've had a good life, and I don't have any serious regrets.

Scoring:

Give yourself the appropriate number of points according to your answers:

1.	A. 4	B. 3	C. 1	D. 2	
2.	A. 1	B. 3	C. 2	D. 4	
3.	A. 2	B. 1	C. 3	D. 4	
4.	A. 2	B. 3	C. 1	D. 4	
5.	A. 1	B. 3	C. 2	D. 4	
6.	A. 2	B. 1	C. 4	D. 3	
7.	A. 1	B. 2	C. 4	D. 3	
8.	A. 3	B. 1	C. 4	D. 2	
9.	A. 4	B. 2	C. 1	D. 3	
10.	A. 3	B. 3	C. 3	D. 4	E. 1

What your score means:

If you scored between 10 and 20: Congratulations! You feel pretty good about yourself, your body, and your life. You're more self-aware and body-aware than average, and it pays off in good health and the ability to handle most stress that comes your way. To maintain a body (and an attitude) like yours takes work, but it's work you love. Adding massage to your body care routine is a great way to pamper and cherish the body that's obviously your friend.

If you scored between 21 and 30: You aren't perfect, and you know it. The good thing is, you don't mind much, either. Your health and body awareness could stand some improvement, but you don't tend to stress too much about the details, and that goes a long way towards good health. The key for you is to maintain your low-stress attitude while still striving to make positive changes in your body awareness. If you start to put too much pressure on yourself, you'll defeat the purpose!

Massage is a great way to improve your health and body awareness without adding stress to your life. Think of it as a well-deserved treat, a maintenance plan for your positive attitude. You don't need to worry too much about your health and your body, unless they start causing you problems, such as chronic illness, obesity, aches and pains, or depression. That's when your body is talking to you, and you should be prepared to listen.

If you scored between 31 and 40: Your body is calling, and you're not picking up the phone! But we've got news for you: Bodies will only take so much neglect before they turn on you. Yours may not have "turned" yet, but if you continue ignoring your body's needs, it won't be long.

It's time to sit down and engage in some serious self-reflection. Have a heart-to-heart with your body and try to discover what it's telling you it needs. A better diet? A little more exercise? Occasional pampering? You could certainly benefit from regular massage, not only because of the therapeutic effects on your health, but also as a way to get back in touch with the body you may have forgotten is yours, all yours.

Also, although it may be difficult, consider beginning massage therapy. If touch is a difficult issue for you, find a massage therapist who can progress at a rate you find comfortable. Massage will do wonders for your sense of self, re-introducing you to your body in a new way. Even if you don't believe it right now, you deserve to be happy, and your body deserves some TLC.

Go to the Heart of It

You might have noticed that a lot of the quiz had to do with gauging your self-esteem. When it comes to body awareness, self-esteem is at the heart of the issue. If you value yourself, you will value (and consequently pay attention to) your body.

Of course, you may have great self-esteem when it comes to your mind, even though you prefer not to think about your body more than you have to. You may be very proud of your intellectual abilities, your accomplishments, your career, your ability as a good parent or friend or partner. And even though you bought this book, we know you don't really consider yourself a complete idiot.

But until you can learn to esteem and value your body, you'll be missing a major piece of the self-esteem puzzle. Your body isn't separate from your mind, your emotions, or your "self." Mind, body, and spirit together equal the self, and they must be balanced if you, as a complete individual, want to be balanced. Along those lines, however, your mind and your emotions can help you with poor body esteem, because as we've said, they're all connected. If you can't quite accept your body for what it is, let the other parts of yourself offer their services.

Once More, with Emotion

One of the worst things you can do to your body and your self-esteem is to deny your emotions. What do emotions have to do with your body? Absolutely everything. When you repress your anger or sadness or disappointment, those feelings don't just disappear. They lodge in your body and slowly take their toll, tying muscles in knots, congesting the passage of blood and nutrients, blocking the flow of the life force.

How can you let your emotions out? There are many ways, including therapy and exercise, but bodywork is one of the best. When the body is manipulated in such a way that its physical processes are set free and circulation is enhanced, emotions buried in the body are also released.

A body-mind that holds stress inside will show it outwardly. Letting go of stress and negative emotions opens the body and the mind too!

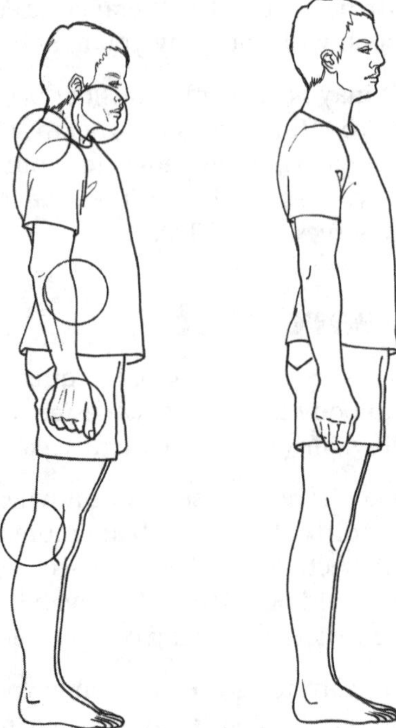

Learning to Live in Your Body-Mind

Once you've reacquainted yourself with your body, you can begin (or continue) the process of integrating your body, your mind, and your spirit. Our society teaches us, in many subtle ways, that body and mind are separate. Yet common sense reveals that they are, indeed, one: a body-mind. Body and mind can't be separated, and everything that affects one affects the other.

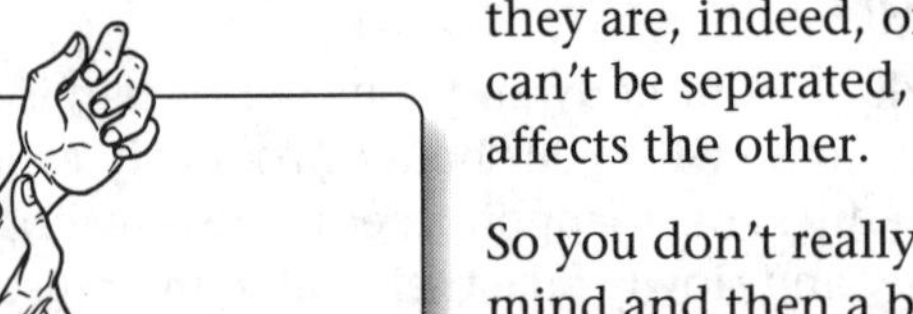

Your Finger on the Pulse

Many people find it extremely difficult to release their emotions. If you have trouble getting it all out, consider taking an acting class. Sometimes it's easier to purge your emotions when you are "in character" as someone else.

So you don't really have a body and then a mind or a mind and then a body. You have a body-mind. Learning to live in your body-mind means acknowledging the effects of everything you do, feel, and experience on your entire self. It's a holistic method of existence that makes sense and feels good. You'll soon discover that physical activity can heighten your spirituality, that spirituality can effect emotional release, that emotional release can enhance your physical health. You'll feel the way you look, you'll love the way you feel, and you'll become more whole. You'll literally be "pulling yourself together," and the result is sure to be something wonderful.

The Least You Need to Know

- Attaining body awareness means evaluating and breaking unhealthy body habits, reducing stress, and adjusting your lifestyle.
- How you feel about yourself can determine the best type of massage for you.
- Low self-esteem interferes with body awareness. Address your self-esteem issues by learning how to be calm, by practicing deep breathing, and by releasing your emotions.
- Living in your body-mind means integrating your body, mind, and spirit to achieve a whole self.

Part 2

Getting in Touch with Your Body-Mind

This part addresses an important but often-overlooked facet of massage: its power to heal, nurture, and integrate the body-mind. Don't worry, we'll explain what we mean by the body-mind. We'll also start out with a quiz to give you some insight into how well you know your body. Next, you'll learn about the knowledge your body holds inside it (beyond the stuff in your brain). We'll even help you plan your personal massage goals based on your body knowledge.

After that, we'll introduce you to your body. Even if you think you know your body pretty well, you may well learn a few new tidbits about your senses, your brain, and all the systems that make your body run. We'll also give you a massage-oriented lesson in body movement, muscles, posture, and muscle testing to help you determine which muscles are working pretty well and which ones prefer to clench up when you need them most.

Next, we'll expand our view of the body to include the Oriental perspective, including energy meridians, pressure points, and the causes of energy blockages and imbalances. We'll wrap up this part with an exploration of the brain-body relationship, which is at the heart of the body-mind.

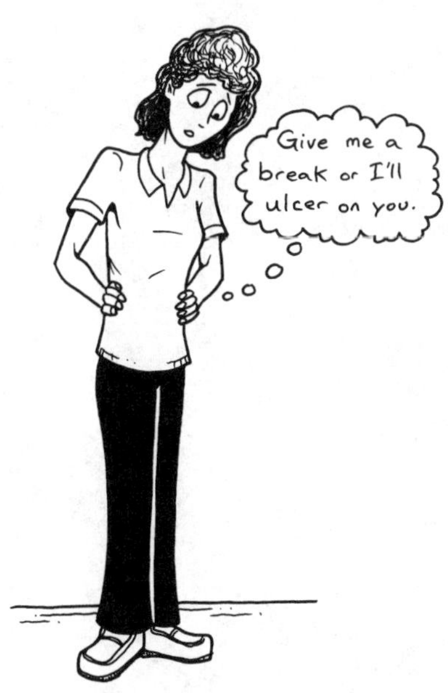

Chapter 4

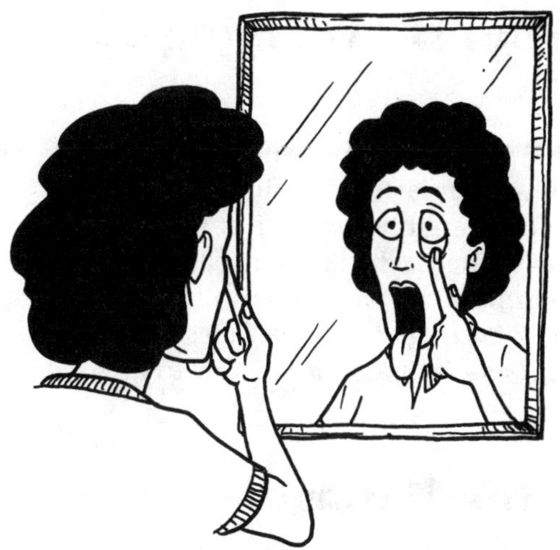

How Are You Feeling Today?

In This Chapter

- Your body's talking; are you listening?
- How to get in touch with your body memories
- Determine your personal massage goals
- Get back in touch with your senses

How are you feeling right at this very moment? Are you standing in a bookstore flipping through this book with one hip jutted out to the side, your spine a little bit bent, your head cocked? Maybe you're squinting because you don't have your glasses or the light in the store isn't very bright. Maybe you have a dull headache you barely notice because it's pretty much a part of your daily existence.

Or perhaps you're curled in a comfy chair as you read this page, sipping on a steaming cup of tea and nibbling on a sandwich. You might feel more relaxed than usual, just at the thought of getting a good massage, but what else do you feel? Are your wrists a little stiff after a long day at the keyboard? Is your back just a little achy because your chair doesn't let you sit straight? How's your stomach? Are you giving it room to process that snack? How's your energy level? Sure, it feels good to relax, but is that because you're so exhausted that you basically collapsed into that chair and couldn't summon the gusto to do anything other than turn the pages of a book? The point is, there are levels to how much you notice about how you feel. Are you ready, willing, and able to move beyond the level at which you normally exist? If you think so, keep reading!

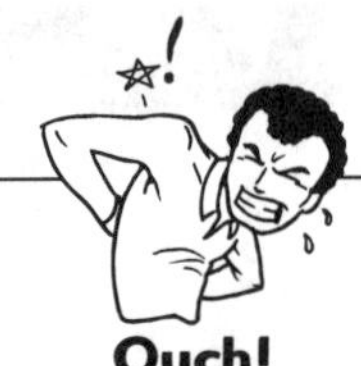

Ouch!

Are you stiff when you wake up in the morning, or are you refreshed and limber? Your sleeping position may be causing morning pain and stiffness. If you sleep on your stomach with your head on a pile of pillows, your back may be swayed unnaturally. Certain positions may also limit circulation. Examine your sleep habits and experiment with different positions.

What Is Your Body Trying to Tell You?

We've talked a lot about the importance of listening to your body. Once you've started listening, however, do you feel like you need an interpreter? Just because you recognize you have a headache or a sore elbow or stiff hip joints doesn't mean you'll automatically know what to do about it. Recognizing your body's messages is only the first step. Next, you've got to learn how to do some serious decoding.

A Quiz for the Massage-Challenged

How much do you know about your body? Do you get achy after exercise and know exactly which muscles you've pulled, or do you pop a few pain pills and hope for the best? Do you know the names of more than two or three of your bones? Do you know the difference between a tendon and a ligament? Try this quiz and test your body knowledge. The more you know about your body's massage-related mechanics, the more you'll benefit from massage (you'll give better massages, too!).

1. Which of the following wouldn't ever cause a headache?
   - A. Pulled muscles
   - B. Vision problems
   - C. Arthritis
   - D. Hormonal changes
   - E. Too much aspirin
   - F. Stress
   - G. Really loud kids
   - H. All of the above could cause a headache

2. Muscles benefit from massage, but skin doesn't receive any benefits.
   - A. True
   - B. False

3. Which of the following isn't a muscle?
   - A. Latissimus Dorsi
   - B. Biceps
   - C. Rectus Abdominis

D. Ilium
E. Tibialis Anterior
F. Satorius
G. Trapezius

4. What is the difference between a strain and a sprain?
   A. A strain is a torn or pulled muscle. A sprain is a joint injury resulting from a torn or stretched ligament.
   B. A strain is a pulled muscle. A sprain is a torn muscle.
   C. A strain is any muscle or joint injury, and various degrees of strains exist. A sprain is just another word for a very bad strain.
   D. They are the same thing.

5. What is muscle atrophy?
   A. A condition resulting from overuse of a muscle in which the tissues start to break down.
   B. A condition of muscle enlargement due to repeated activity, such as weight lifting, to the degree that flexibility and range of motion are severely inhibited.
   C. The wasting of muscle tissue due to lack of use.
   D. A degenerative muscle disease in which muscle fibers are gradually replaced with fat and connective tissue until the muscles become useless.
   E. The sense of pride you get when you beat somebody at arm wrestling.

6. What is connective tissue?
   A. The network of muscles throughout the body.
   B. A tough web-like framework of fluid and collagen fibers that supports and binds the various structures of the body.
   C. The fluid that cushions and supports the joints of the body.
   D. A blanket term for cartilage, tendons, and ligaments.
   E. What you need when you have a bad cold.

7. One important purpose of cartilage is
   A. To cushion bones and joints from each other and from external forces.
   B. To connect bones to bones.
   C. To cushion bones from muscles.
   D. To support injured or broken bones.
   E. To make you say, "Ewww!" when you bite into a hamburger and crunch a piece of it.

8. Condyle, Crest, Foramen, Fossa, Head, and Line are all words that describe what?
   A. Muscle types
   B. Joint types
   C. Intestinal irregularities
   D. Bone structures
   E. Massage therapists

9. Phalanges and metacarpals are
   A. Hand and finger bones
   B. Foot and toe bones
   C. Wrist and lower arm bones
   D. Ankle and lower foot bones
   E. Those strange metal parts left over after you assembled your child's new mountain bike all by yourself

10. About how many bones are found in the human body?
    A. 123
    B. 206
    C. 340
    D. 402
    E. Nobody ever bothered to count.

ANSWERS:

1. H. That was an easy one!
2. B. Your skin gets great benefits from massage; the increased circulation flushes your skin with nutrients and gives you a healthy glow.
3. D. Your ilium is your hip bone.
4. A.
5. C.
6. B.
7. A.
8. D.
9. A.
10. B.

Massaging the Data

How did you do? Are you feeling fairly proud, or are you feeling a little sheepish that you don't know more about your own internal workings? Fear not, most people aren't well-versed in the technical side of anatomy unless it's part of their job. But knowledge is always a good thing, and we're here to provide it. Check out the next two chapters for some serious body knowledge.

Releasing What Your Body Remembers

Body knowledge means more than knowing the name of the muscle you just pulled playing basketball or the joint that feels a little arthritic whenever it rains. Because mind, body, and spirit are all interconnected, being aware of the effect of all influences on the body is crucial for understanding the purely physical processes happening inside you. Just as an old sports injury might affect you for years afterward, so might an old emotional injury. Some massage therapists even specialize in treating the emotionally injured, working at a very gradual pace to earn their trust and re-familiarize them with the positive side of touch.

Although people differ in their opinions as to how much we can remember, some believe that the memory of being in the womb, massaged by the uterus and rocked by the amniotic fluid, is still within us. Others believe that the trauma of birth, especially when the birth was a difficult one, is still vividly imprinted on our bodies. Some bodyworkers specialize in infants and children, re-aligning and correcting small bodies that have been damaged in various ways by the birthing process.

Believe what you will, but your body remembers—not in the way your mind remembers, but by making you what you are, affecting how you feel, and influencing the way you stand, sit, or run. Your physical self is a product of the physical, emotional, and spiritual history of your whole self.

Respecting Body Knowledge

The fact that your body remembers is great news. If your first reaction is, "Oh no! My mother was in labor with me for three days, I was sick all the time as a kid, and then there was that skiing accident...," calm down. There's hope! The first step is to respect your body memories and what your body knows rather than denying or regretting your past's influence on your physical self.

What are your body memories? They may not be immediately easy to determine. Perhaps you have a particular penchant for or aversion to touch. Maybe you are fearful, nervous, or anxious "by nature." Maybe you love to give but have trouble receiving or vice versa. Maybe you can only sleep with your arms cradling your head. Maybe you always have to be with people, or prefer to be alone. Maybe you can't sit still for more than two minutes. Maybe you suffer from one or more phobias.

If you have a hard time analyzing your own personality, ask your family and friends how they see you. Then interpret your picture of yourself in terms of your body. Do your tense shoulders have anything to do with your fearfulness? Are your headaches linked to your isolation? Do you get irritable when you don't get enough hugs, or cuddling, or sex? Do you come down with a cold every time you know you'll be in a social situation with a lot of people?

Once you have an idea about where your body reactions come from (and you can't always know—maybe your headaches are due to some traumatic birth-canal experience, but maybe they are the result of your drinking too much coffee), you can tackle them from multiple perspectives, whether that means conscious behavioral modification, counseling, massage, or all of the above. Respect what your body knows about you. It is telling you not only where you've been, but also what you need to address about yourself. Your body is wise; learn from it.

C'mon Touch Me, Babe!

How do you feel about being touched? Some people just love it. You know them—they hug you and kiss you when they first meet you. Throughout your very first conversation, they put a hand on your shoulder to emphasize a point, pat your cheek affectionately, lightly rub your back to demonstrate their empathy with your point of view, and then give you another big hug when it's all over. Chances are, you could do with a little less touching, though you might not know how to tell them to leave you alone.

Then there are those people who back away as though you've got the plague if you stand too near to them. They may shake your hand, but from their withering touch, you can tell they're only doing it out of a sense of obligation or decorum. Don't even try to give them a friendly hug—they'd probably slug you.

Most of us fall somewhere in between these two extremes, enjoying hugs and caresses from loved ones but preferring to keep a distance from people we know less well. That's a smart way to be. When you allow yourself to be touched, you're putting your trust in the toucher, and in most cases, your trust is best placed in people you know well.

For some, that trust has nurtured and helped them along through life. For others, though, that trust has been betrayed. Their loved ones may have abused touch, either by touching violently or beyond appropriate boundaries or by withholding touch completely. The way you were touched as a child can profoundly influence your touch comfort level as an adult. Consider how you feel about touch, and then consider the reasons.

The Only Thing You Have to Fear Is Fear Itself (or Cold Hands!)

Are you fearful? Traumatic experiences can lead to rational and irrational fears. Examine your fears and their intensity. Are you profoundly terrified of closed spaces, or do you get just a little edgy as the elevator moves between floors? See whether you can link your fears to any experiences. Is your fear of water due to a near-drowning incident as a child? (Ask your parents; they may remember something you don't.) Maybe your big sister dunked you in the swimming pool one too many times, or maybe you just don't like to get your hair wet. Even if you don't know for sure, consider the options. You may suddenly find an answer to a mystery about yourself you never thought you'd solve.

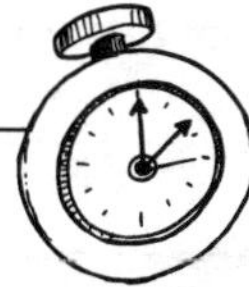

A Massage Minute

According to the Touch Research Institute, massage seems to stimulate a positive psychoneuroimmunological response in the body. What does that mean? It means that massage can improve your central nervous system's ability to deal with the repressed immune function resulting from negative emotions. It's also further evidence for the complex and inextricable relationship between the body and the mind.

Working It Out: Your Personal Massage Goals

The previous examples show you how to start examining your body knowledge and the links between your experiences, your personal history, and your physical condition. Whoever you are, you'll benefit from spending some purely personal and self-reflective time considering how you evolved physically, emotionally, and spiritually.

Follow up your introspection with the formation of some personal massage goals. Knowing what you need and want to get out of massage will make choosing the right type of massage easier. Plus, your massage will be more productive and more satisfying. Don't be afraid to share your personal massage goals with your massage therapist, so he or she can help you to reach them.

To help you define your goals, complete the following statements, preferably in writing:

1. The most crucial physical problems I'd like massage to address are

   ____

   ____

2. I expect the following benefits from massage:

   ____

   ____

3. I'm a little hesitant to get a massage because

   ____

   ____

4. Receiving a professional massage from someone I don't know makes me feel

    ____

    ____

5. In general, being touched makes me feel

    ____

    ____

6. This is how I don't like to be touched:

    ____

    ____

7. I would like guidance in the following areas (examples might be more graceful movement, proper posture, relaxation techniques, stress management, or pain relief):

    ____

    ____

8. Before I get a massage, I'd like to know more about

    ____

    ____

9. This is how I feel about my body:

    ____

    ____

10. This is how I feel about my health in general:

    ____

    ____

Opening Your Senses

Now that you have a clearer picture of who you are, what your body is doing, and why it's doing it, we've got another challenge for you. Your physical body is more than muscles, bones, joints, and skin. Your senses can be intense and enlightening avenues for increased body awareness, and getting in touch with them may help you to learn even more about who you are and where you've been. Although some bodywork (such as aromatherapy) is directly concerned with the senses, and almost all bodywork is intimately involved with the sense of touch, paying special attention to all your senses will heighten your massage experience—and your life experience.

A Massage Minute

When a baby is born, its brain connections are far from fully formed. Sensory input is required for the brain to fully develop. Without this input, a baby will stop growing and die. When sensory input is minimal, the child may develop irreversible intellectual and/or emotional disorders.

Listen Up

How often do you listen to your environment when no one is talking to you? You probably listen to music sometimes and to the television. Maybe you like to listen in on people's conversations at the mall or in crowded restaurants, just for fun. But what about those times when you are alone, or busy at work, or when you wake up in the middle of the night? Do you ever listen when you don't have to?

Try this exercise: Stop what you are doing right now and listen. Close your eyes, tune out your other senses, and hear what is going on around you. Try not to interpret the sounds; simply listen. Do you hear traffic noise? Voices? Birds? The whir of an air conditioner or central heat? A computer terminal's buzzing? Running water? Wind? Take some time now and then to tune in to what you hear.

Just like massage, listening is an art. The better we become at listening, the better we will become at giving (and receiving) massage. Being "in-tune" with oneself and the world around is an ever-evolving process. Developing attentiveness and keen listening skills help to make this process meaningful and enriching.

Taste It

Do you gulp down your food because you don't have much time for meals, or do you grab a candy bar from the vending machine to eat at your desk, or does your dinner usually consist of eating whatever your toddler didn't find appealing? Many of us don't ever take the time to savor our sense of taste, but noticing and appreciating taste is more than a nice experience. It also helps you to eat more slowly, to digest your food better, and to truly get the most from your meal. You'll be less likely to binge because every bite will be an experience. Better yet, almost any food, if it's thoroughly enjoyed, savored, and appreciated, will serve your body better. Nutrients will be absorbed more effectively, toxins won't be absorbed as well, and the food will be nourishing and strengthening.

Of course, basing your diet around whole, fresh, organic foods is not only better for you, but provides a more intense and pleasurable taste experience. You taste food the way it was meant to taste before it was altered, sprayed, preserved, shipped, dyed, waxed, canned, frozen, chopped, processed, mixed with more chemicals, sprayed again, and then consumed by you.

Smell It

You probably only notice your sense of smell when in the presence of a very strong odor, such as a sewage treatment plant, an apple pie just out of the oven, or someone who has overdosed on cologne. Just as your other senses become duller when they aren't used, your sense of smell may be pretty out-of-shape. Sometimes that's good—there are plenty of odors out there nobody wants or needs to smell. However, strong evidence exists that scent can be a powerful tool for influencing both your mood and your health.

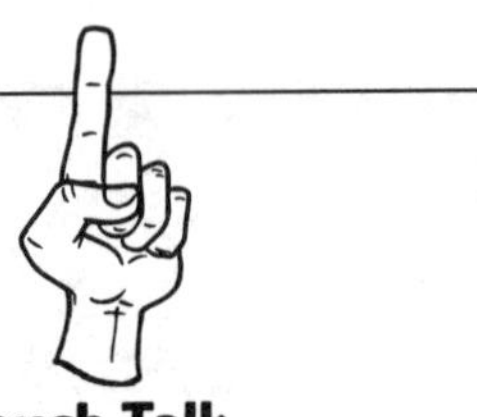

Touch Talk

Essential oils are the distilled essences of various plants that give those plants their fragrance. Only oils produced by steam distillation are technically pure essential oils. According to aromatherapists, the essential oil of a plant contains that plant's soul or life force, as well as its most valuable and concentrated healing properties.

Aromatherapy and aromatherapy massage are becoming increasingly popular (see Chapter 19) as people continue to discover how a fragrant bath of lavender, a slew of jasmine-scented candles, or an orange-oil massage can completely turn their mood around. To get back in touch with your sense of smell, take a little time each day to savor the smell of something wonderful—a steaming plate of spaghetti, a pot of lemon tea, a bouquet of roses. Or visit your local health food store and sample a few *essential oils* to see which scents appeal to you. You might be amazed at how much a brief "scent" session will relax and renew you.

See It

Sight is probably the sense we use the most and take for granted the most. You see the world around you, and that's how you get by. Right? A blind person would certainly disagree. Sight isn't an indispensable sense, but it's certainly a sense most of us rely on heavily.

One of the best ways to begin to truly appreciate and re-acquaint yourself with your sense of sight is to deprive yourself of it, even for just a few minutes. If you can, try this exercise outside: Sit comfortably and close your eyes. (Don't lie down, or you might fall asleep!) Try to tune out your other senses as well. You will certainly hear and perhaps smell things, but don't dwell on those impressions. Focus on the blackness or the swirls of color you see with your eyes closed. Don't even think about what you aren't seeing on the other side of your eyelids. When you feel thoroughly focused on the darkness or whatever else you "see" with your eyes closed, slowly open your eyes. Pretend you are seeing for the first time. Of course, you aren't, but your imagination is powerful and can assist you well in this exercise.

What do you see? First, notice the colors. Then notice textures, shapes, shades, shadows, light, dark, movement, and stillness. Notice tiny details you would never focus on: cobwebs in corners, the shapes of the tiniest leaves on a tree, the bristles on a toothbrush, or the curl and twitch of a squirrel's tail. Even if what you're looking at is as familiar as your own face in a mirror, try to see it for the first time, almost as if you didn't know what you were looking at, but were trying to form a primitive impression. This exercise is great for helping you to see all over again, increasing your body awareness one more notch. (Do it often enough, and you may decide to take up painting!)

Feel It

We've saved the sense of touch for last, partly because we've already said so much about it, but also because it may be the single most important sense in terms of maintaining or regaining whole-body health and a sense of well-being. You now know getting a massage is good for you, but you can certainly heighten your awareness of your sense of touch in many other aspects of your life.

Whenever you think of it, feel the texture of something nearby: your coffee mug, your bath towel, the refrigerator door, your child's cheek, or even your computer keyboard. Tune in to the differences in texture, temperature, weight, and even energy. Sensing energy is a fine art, but if you're paying attention, you can probably feel that your best friend's hand emanates more energy than your bath towel.

Also, try to touch those you love more often. No, that doesn't mean groping that cute guy or girl at the copy machine. It does mean embracing your family members whenever you possibly can (assuming they appreciate it). It means covering your kids with kisses, holding hands with your partner, and showing your support to close friends with a gentle pat on the back, an understanding squeeze of the hand, or a sympathetic hug. Try to go through life staying in touch with your loved ones. You'll all be a lot healthier, happier, and body-aware.

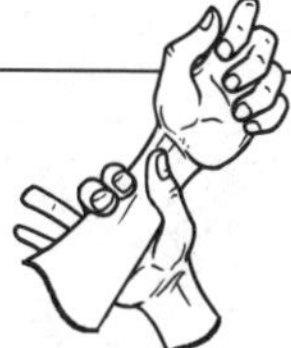

Your Finger on the Pulse

Consider scheduling a session in a sensory deprivation tank, if you can. (Call your local health club—if they don't have one, they may know someone who does.) These water-filled tanks allow you to float in darkness and silence, largely deprived of sensory stimulation. Although not for everyone (especially those made nervous by small spaces), some people find such sessions amazingly rejuvenating. A few progressive corporations even provide sessions in so-called "think tanks" so that executives can clear their minds.

The Least You Need to Know

- Listening to your body isn't enough—you also need to know how to interpret what it's saying.
- Your body retains the memory of all its physical, emotional, and spiritual experiences, influencing who you are today.
- Getting in touch with all your senses will increase your body awareness.
- Acknowledging your human nature and its needs and abilities will help you to live fully in your body-mind.

Chapter 5

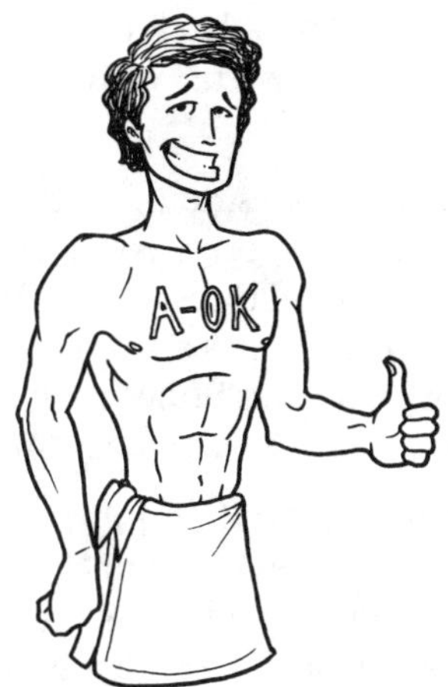

Massage Keeps All Systems Go

In This Chapter

- All about the systems that make your body work
- How massage benefits each body system
- How massage is more than skin deep

Even though, as we've said, you are more a body-mind than a body and a mind, it helps to understand a little about how the various body systems work before you can fully appreciate the effect your mind and your emotions have on those systems. For a massage therapist, especially, a thorough understanding of body systems and anatomy is crucial. Knowing how the machine of the body works allows the massage therapist to manipulate muscles, move joints, and redirect energy most effectively. Massage schools spend a good deal of time training their students in anatomy and the systems of the body. Even though you aren't a massage therapist (not yet!), you, too, can benefit from some basic body knowledge when you begin to learn how to give a massage.

'Dem Bones, 'Dem Bones...and Muscles, Too: The Musculoskeletal System

The most basic of all systems is the *musculoskeletal system.* Our skeletal systems are a little like the foundation and framework of a house. Our bones support our bodies and, to some extent, protect our organs. (How would your brain get through the day

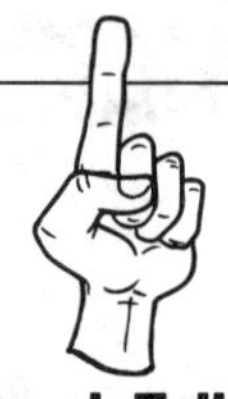

Touch Talk

Red **bone marrow** is a soft, spongy, blood-vessel-filled tissue in the center of bones. Yellow **bone marrow**, also at the center of some bones, stores fat. Red bone marrow manufactures the majority of red blood cells, which nourish bones and the rest of the body, and white blood cells, which protect against infection.

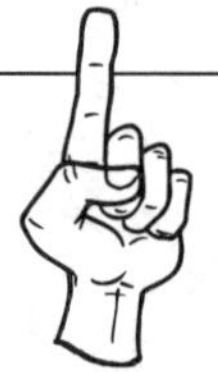

Touch Talk

Cartilage is a tough, elastic form of connective tissue, also known as gristle, with the primary function of cushioning and protecting bones and joints. **Ligaments** are bands of connective tissue that support joints and bind bones to other bones. **Bursae** are fluid-filled sacks that cushion muscles, tendons, and skin from bones in high-impact areas, such as shoulders or knees.

without that rock-hard skull?) Bones also serve as a foundation for the muscles that move us, which have to attach to something!

Unlike the structure of a house, bones do more than support us. Bones are filled with a spongy connective tissue called *marrow*, which manufactures blood cells and stores fats. The outer bone serves as a storehouse for minerals such as calcium, which gives bones their hardness and strength.

Bones are connected to each other at their joints, some of which are immovable, such as the joints of the skull (although some massage therapists would argue that even these joints can be manipulated). Some joints have various ranges of motion. All synovial joints are categorized as freely movable. Slightly movable joints are usually fibrous, such as those between the two bones of the lower leg, the tibia and fibula.

Cartilage, ligaments, and bursae all play their parts, too. *Cartilage* cushions joints and bones, as well as forming more movable external features, such as your ears and nose. *Ligaments* are bands of fibrous tissue that connect and support bones. *Bursae* are sacks that serve as cushions in high-pressure areas between bones and muscles, tendons, or skin.

What do bones have to do with massage? No, you can't loosen up a bone the way you can loosen up a muscle, but certain forms of bodywork can help to re-align bones that are slightly out of place or restore range of motion to stiff joints by manipulating the tissues that support the joints.

Also, when bones are broken or joints are dislocated or arthritic, massage can aid the natural healing process in several ways. Massage keeps circulation and elimination in the adjacent soft tissue at their peak, decreasing inflammation and facilitating the removal of waste materials. It also improves surrounding muscle tone and balance, which lessens stress on joints and bones.

A Massage Minute

Your body contains 206 bones: 8 in your skull; 14 in your face; 6 in your ear; 1 at the base of your tongue; 26 vertebrae (bones of the spine); 25 in your thorax (chest cavity); 64 in your upper extremities, including your shoulders, arms, and hands; and 62 in your lower extremities, including your hips, legs, knees, and feet.

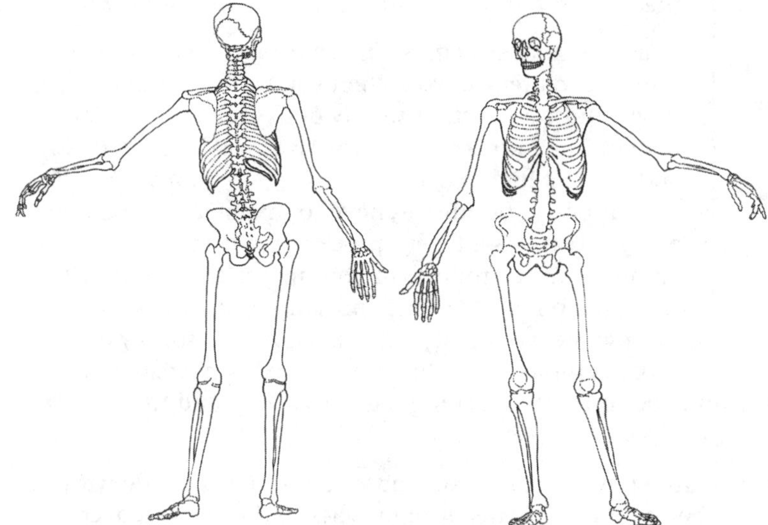

Getting down to the bare bones: the human skeleton, rear and front views.

Don't forget the darling of massage: the muscular system! Without muscles, you couldn't move. Your muscles are responsible for all movement in your body, both voluntary (such as when you lift a tennis racket) and involuntary (such as when your large intestine moves your dinner along).

Voluntary muscles, also known as *striated muscles* because they look striped when examined under a microscope, are attached to the skeleton. You influence the motion of these muscles on purpose. You decide to move your foot, or point your finger, or dance the tango. These are the muscles that can be massaged.

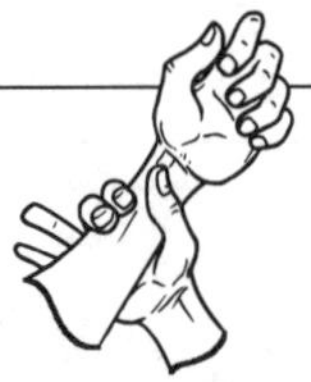

Your Finger on the Pulse

Lifting weights isn't the only way to increase muscle strength and improve muscle tone. If you'd like to increase your muscle strength but don't like weightlifting, try yoga, racquet sports, cycling, walking while holding light weights, or doing a few daily sets of sit-ups and push-ups. And remember, partially contracted muscles (often the result of overexertion) are functionally weaker because they have less capacity to do work. Massage can increase the functional strength of muscles by releasing muscle contractions.

Involuntary muscles, also known as *smooth* or *visceral muscles*, line the walls of your stomach, intestines, and blood vessels. These muscles don't attach to your bones and aren't influenced by your decision to digest that food or contract that blood vessel. They act on their own (with cues from your nervous system). Although these muscles aren't directly massaged, they can benefit from the increased circulation and better elimination the body experiences as a result of massage.

A third type of muscle exists only in your heart. Called your *cardiac muscle*, its cells are striated and grouped in bundles. They keep your heart beating and are involuntary (although some people claim to be able to slow their hearts almost to a stop purely by their own will).

Your muscular system is efficient, but it is certainly not immune to breakdown. When you work your muscles, they require a constant supply of oxygen and nutrients to continue functioning. If you overwork your muscles and create a higher demand for oxygen than your body can supply, your muscles have to manufacture their own energy. This less-efficient process results in the accumulation of waste products in your muscles. Soon, they'll reach the point of fatigue and simply stop working. Meanwhile, your body will keep trying to supply oxygen to the muscles and must also work to eliminate the build-up of toxins. Translation: You'll feel weak and tired, and your muscles are going to be very sore (and we don't just mean they'll be mad at you!).

Enter massage! Massage can loosen overly contracted muscles and speed the delivery of essential oxygen, but it also helps to flush toxins from muscles so they can recover more quickly. Because muscle soreness is an inflammatory reaction in response to tiny tears in the muscle, massage helps relieve soreness by moving fluid out of the tissue and reducing pressure on the tears (the cause of soreness). That's why so many professional athletes get massages after intense workouts: Massage speeds recovery and reduces post-workout pain. Getting a massage before a workout is a great idea, too. If your muscles are flushed with nutrients, loose, and flexible before your workout, you'll surely perform better because you'll have a muscular head start!

Pretty Nervy: The Brain and Nervous System

Consisting of your brain, spinal cord, and nerve tissue, your *nervous system* is command central, and without it, you'd be a house with a power outage—all that complex anatomy wouldn't work. Without your nervous system, you wouldn't have awareness. You wouldn't know who you are, where you are, or even that you exist. Not only that—without your nervous system, your heart wouldn't "know" to beat. Your lungs wouldn't "know" to breathe. Your nervous system does all the "knowing" for your body, plus all the coordinating. Your nervous system controls all your senses, movements, thoughts, and behaviors. Sounds like a system you'd better keep in good working order, doesn't it?

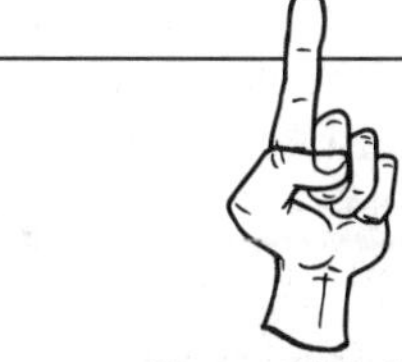

Touch Talk

Cerebrospinal fluid is the fluid that flows through and around the brain and down around the spinal cord. This fluid helps to bring nutrients to and carry waste from the brain and spinal cord, but it mainly serves as a shock absorber to protect these delicate and essential organs.

But what is the nervous system? Your *central nervous system* is your brain and spinal cord. It is protected by your skull and spinal vertebrae and covered with a tough connective tissue. For added protection, your brain and spinal cord "float" within the connective tissue in *cerebrospinal fluid.*

We could write an entire *Complete Idiot's Guide™* about your brain, but to simplify, this mass of nerve tissue contains over 10 billion neurons and consists of three main parts:

- The *cerebrum,* which is the front and top of the brain, controls speech, sensation, memory, reasoning, and emotions.
- The *cerebellum,* located under the cerebrum towards the back of the brain, maintains balance, muscle coordination, and muscle movement.
- The brain stem, at the base of the brain, connecting the brain to the top of the spinal cord, is a sort of air traffic control tower, helping to coordinate and transmit messages between the brain and the body, among other functions.

Within your brain, *neurons* are nerve cells that look a little like spiders. Each neuron has a *cell body,* nerve fibers called *dendrites* dangling from the body like spider legs, and one long nerve fiber, the *axon,* which looks like a bit of web extending from the neuron. Dendrites act like antennae, receiving signals from other neurons. These signals can move as fast as 225 miles per hour! They make us the movers and shakers that we are. After the dendrites receive these signals, they carry them back to the cell body. When enough signals are received, the neuron generates an electrical impulse, which is transmitted to other nerve cells.

Unlike many other cells in the body, brain cells can't reproduce. Plus, they need a continual supply of oxygen and glucose to function correctly—without these nutrients, they quickly die. Breathing deeply and improving circulation through massage are two ways to enhance the flow of oxygen and nutrients to the brain.

Your spinal cord extends from the brain down through the spinal column. Its job is to serve as a sort of superhighway for nerve impulses to and from the brain, as well as a central meeting point for peripheral nerves throughout the body that send and receive impulses, including nerves from the heart, blood vessels, other organs, and muscles.

You've got nerves all over your body. The next time someone says to you, "You've got a lot of nerve!," you'll know they are right! Most of these nerves send their impulses to the brain where they're sorted out and interpreted into action or thought, either voluntary—"I'm going to run one more mile; go legs, go!"—or involuntary—"I shouldn't have run that extra mile! My heart is racing and I can't catch my breath!"

Some involuntary impulses, such as muscle contractions, occur without reaching the brain, but massage can help re-establish the "brain connection," allowing you to regain control of some of these involuntary functions. For example, you can sometimes voluntarily relax your muscles, keeping them from involuntarily contracting.

How can massage benefit your central nervous system? When your muscles are relaxed and your circulation is primed, your nervous system sends the message to the brain: "Everything's A-OK down here!" Your brain will respond by making you feel that everything's OK. In other words, you'll feel less stressed. Massage also keeps circulation functioning at its optimum so that it can properly supply the brain and the rest of the nervous system with the nutrients they need, which makes the nervous system work more efficiently.

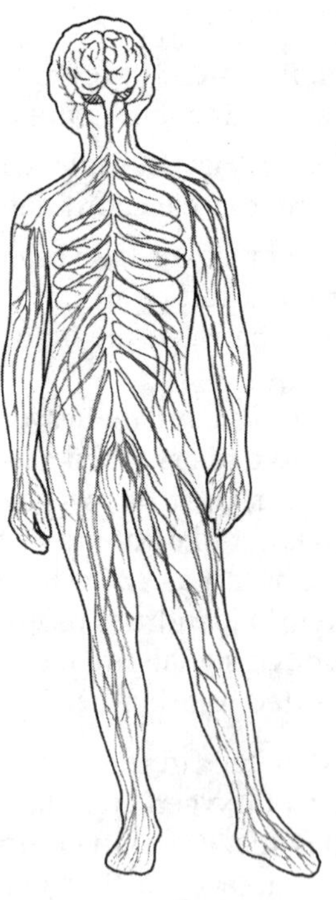

The nervous system consists of a network of pathways for the brain to send and receive messages throughout the body.

Deep Breath, Strong Heart, Strong Body

A few paragraphs earlier, we mentioned that deep breathing can benefit the brain by delivering more oxygen. Deep breathing does more than help the brain, however. It nourishes your blood via your *circulatory system,* which, as you probably know, travels everywhere in your body, from your scalp to the tips of your toes. Breathing is the way we keep the blood oxygen-rich and pure, and breathing depends on your *respiratory system.*

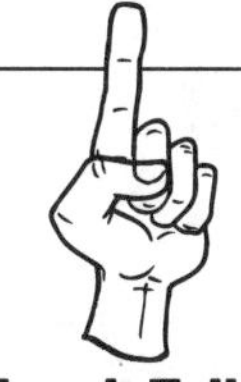

Touch Talk

The **larynx** is a box of cartilage at the back of your throat containing your vocal cords; it's your voice box. The **trachea** is the passageway between your larynx and your bronchial tubes; it's your windpipe. **Bronchial tubes** are a subdivision of the trachea, which are part of the lungs. Your **lungs** are the primary organ of respiration in which the exchange of oxygen and carbon dioxide takes place.

The Respiratory System

The respiratory system is basically a system of energy exchange: oxygen for carbon dioxide and water. Our bodies need oxygen to combine with nutrients and extract energy. The principal waste products of this process are carbon dioxide and water. Through the respiratory system, we breathe in oxygen from the air, and then breathe out carbon dioxide and water in exchange. We get what we need, and we eliminate what we don't need.

Just as we breathe in oxygen and breathe out carbon dioxide, plants of the earth breathe in carbon dioxide and breathe out oxygen. It's a perfect symbiotic relationship, and one more good reason to keep our homes, yards, and the entire earth abundantly supplied with plant life.

Your respiratory system consists of your nose, nasal cavity, *larynx, trachea,* and lungs (which contain the *bronchial tubes*). All these parts work together to bring air from your nose to your lungs, where it comes in contact with your blood through a network of ultra-fine blood vessels called *capillaries.* When you breathe, oxygen enters the blood and is delivered to the far reaches of the body. Meanwhile, the air in your lungs becomes rich in carbon dioxide. You exhale to get rid of it.

Certain massage techniques can relieve congested lungs. Massage also helps to loosen and relax the muscles around the ribcage, giving your lungs more room to breathe.

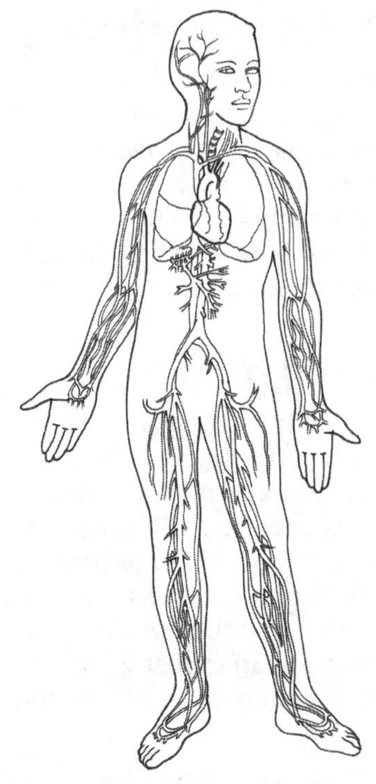

The cardiovascular, respiratory, and circulatory systems work together to deliver oxygen to the body.

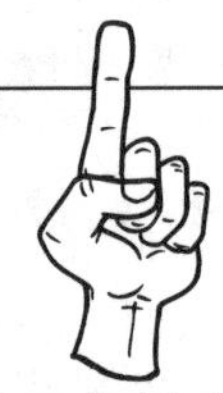

Touch Talk

Arteries are blood vessels that transport blood away from the heart. **Veins** are blood vessels that carry blood to the heart, where it follows a circular passage to the lungs, picks up oxygen and drops off carbon dioxide and water, and then returns to the heart. **Capillaries** are tiny, semi-permeable blood vessels that branch out between the smallest arteries and veins, helping in the distribution of oxygen and nutrients and the removal of waste materials.

The Circulatory System

The heart of your anatomy is the *circulatory system*, which consists of two parts: the *cardiovascular system* and the *lymphatic system*. The cardiovascular system consists of your heart, blood, and blood vessels, including *arteries, veins,* and *capillaries*. The lymphatic system consists of your *lymph, lymphatic vessels*, and *lymph nodes*.

The purpose of your cardiovascular system is to keep blood moving through your body, and the entire system is powered by your heart. Your heart, which is more pear-shaped than heart-shaped, is about the size of your fist and contains four inner chambers separated by valves (among other things). The heart doesn't need any external nerve fibers to keep it beating; its rhythmic pulse is internally generated.

Every day, an average heart beats 100,000 times, pumping more than 2,000 gallons of blood. If you live to be 70 years old, your heart will probably beat more than

2.5 billion times. So the length of our lives could be more accurately stated by the number of heartbeats than years (but who's counting?).

The purpose of the lymphatic system is to work in conjunction with the cardiovascular system as a sort of storm sewer system to deal with excess fluids. It works like this: the liquid part of blood (plasma) leaks out of the capillaries, delivering oxygen and nutrients to tissues. About two-thirds of the plasma leaks back into the capillaries, draining the tissues of waste materials. What is left is drained by the lymphatic system and returned to the blood.

To keep your entire body properly nourished and functioning, your circulatory system must be in good working order, providing your tissues with oxygen and nutrients, and eliminating pesky waste products that might gum up the works. How does massage help? Think of massage as the ultimate hostess, making sure all the party guests (blood cells) circulate and mingle—it's the Martha Stewart of your circulatory system!

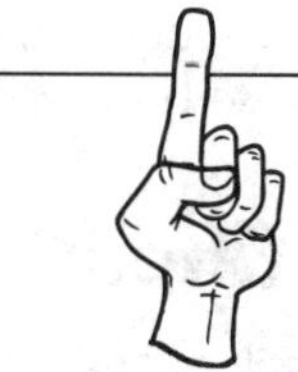

Touch Talk

Lymph is a clear fluid derived from blood that helps to provide cells with nutrients and to drain away waste products. **Lymphatic vessels** are vessels that serve as passageways for lymph. **Lymph nodes** are bundles of tissue along the lymphatic vessels that produce substances to purify toxic substances within lymph.

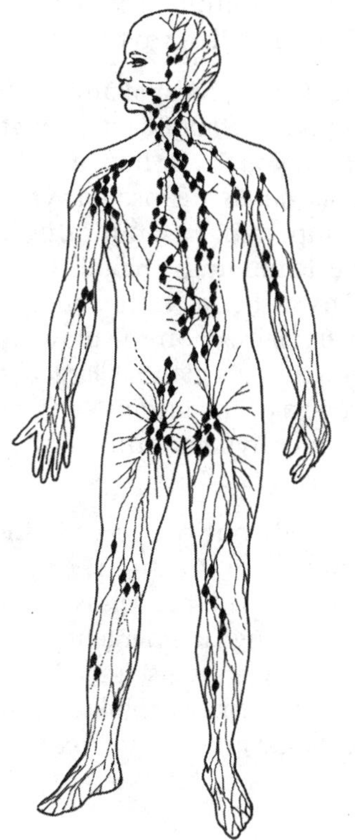

Massage helps the lymphatic system more effectively do its job of purifying the body.

Massage's manipulation of soft tissue directly affects the efficiency of your circulation, encouraging lymph formation, flow, and movement through the lymphatic vessels. Massage also has a dramatic effect on your cardiovascular system. Massage increases blood circulation, lowers blood pressure, increases heart volume, and dilates blood vessels so they work more efficiently.

What Chemistry! The Endocrine System

The *endocrine system* is probably one of the least understood systems, at least by the average person on the street. It consists of a group of *endocrine glands* that manufacture *hormones*. Hormones are powerful substances that influence a wide range of bodily functions having to do with your growth, health, and sexuality.

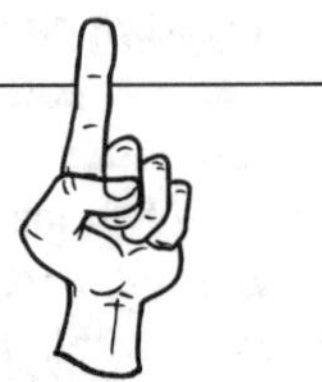

Touch Talk

Endocrine glands are organs that manufacture hormones. **Hormones** are chemical substances manufactured and secreted by endocrine glands that act on the body in many ways.

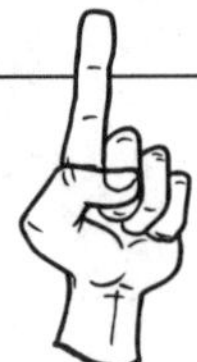

Touch Talk

Adrenaline, also called *epinephrine*, is a hormone released by the adrenal glands. It stimulates the heart and initiates other bodily processes, readying the body for quick action.

The most influential gland is probably the *pituitary gland*, because its hormones stimulate the release of so many other hormones in so many other glands. This tiny gland, about the size of a marble, hangs from the underside of the brain and is responsible for a huge array of bodily processes, from how tall you'll be to the development of sexual organs to the aging process. The *pineal gland* is located deep within the brain and secretes the hormone melatonin over a 24-hour cycle. Melatonin is thought to contribute to synchronizing biorhythms, such as the circadian rhythm or body clock.

The *thyroid gland*, located around the trachea, is responsible for your metabolic rate, which is how fast you burn up the food you eat or how much energy you use. The *parathyroid glands* are located very close to the thyroid and are important in monitoring and maintaining the level of calcium in the blood. The *thymus gland* is a small mass of tissue between the lungs, above the heart. (This gland is not shown on the drawing.) Active until puberty, the thymus gland is largely responsible for the effectiveness of the immune response in children. After puberty, the thymus shrinks and glandular tissues are replaced with fat.

Adrenal glands, one over each kidney, are responsible for your reactions to stress—they release *adrenaline* into your system when the brain sends them the message that you are experiencing an emergency, whether that be rage or fear. Adrenal glands also secrete corticosteroids, which perform such tasks as regulating the sodium/potassium levels in blood and enhancing tissue healing.

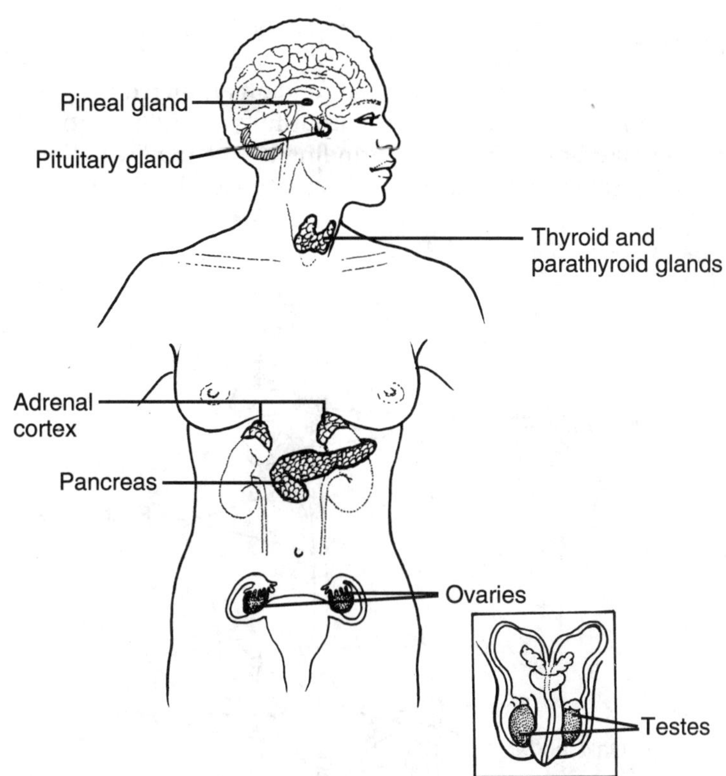

The endocrine system consists of a group of endocrine glands that manufacture hormones.

The *pancreas* figures into the successful functioning of both the digestive and the endocrine systems. For the digestive system, the pancreas releases enzymes that help break down substances such as carbohydrates and proteins. The pancreas aids the endocrine system by secreting the hormones insulin and glucagon, which control the level of glucose in the blood. The most common disease associated with the pancreas is diabetes mellitus, in which insulin-producing cells of the pancreas are destroyed. See Chapter 21 for more on diabetes and massage. The female ovaries and male testes are a part of the endocrine system too. For more on these glands, see the section that follows on the female and male reproductive systems.

A Matter of Processing and Elimination

It would be convenient if we could get all of our nutrients from breathing, but then we would miss the fun experience of food! Our bodies have to do something with the food we put into them, however. Enter digestion, exit elimination!

The Digestive System

You make the most of the food you eat by sending that food on an incredible journey through the *digestive system.* Imagine you are eating a beautiful salad filled with nutritious veggies. First, you take a bite. You chew, grinding up the food with your teeth and tongue and creating saliva, which begins to digest the food right there in your mouth.

Massage aids in the functioning of all your internal organs, such as the liver, gallbladder, and those of the digestive system.

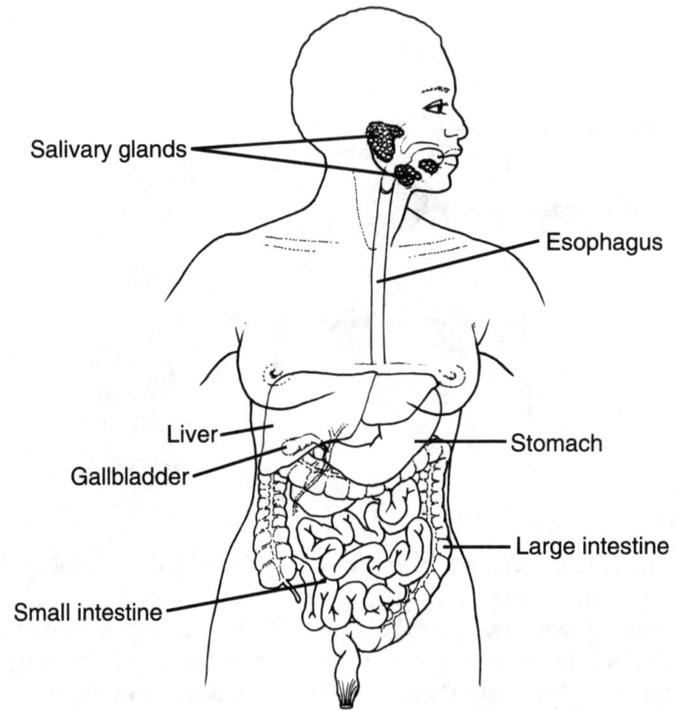

Next, you swallow. Your bite of salad, already bearing little resemblance to its original form, moves down your throat, through your esophagus, and then lands in your stomach. Here, *gastric juices* digest the food further. Then it's off to the small intestine, where nutrients from the vegetables are absorbed and shuttled to other parts of your body.

By the time your salad—if we can still call it that—gets to your large intestine, all the goodies have been digested, and all that's left is the stuff your body can't use. Your large intestine transforms this waste material into feces, which are then expelled.

A Massage Minute

The liver is the body's chemical laboratory. One of the body's largest internal organs, the liver controls and regulates the levels of many types of substances in the blood. Bile, the liver's waste product, is transported to the gallbladder. The digestive system uses bile to emulsify fats contained in food.

The Excretory System

Waste matter—like it or not, we're all full of it. Although the lymphatic system does a bang-up job of eliminating waste matter from the blood, the body has other excretory processes, too.

The actions and functions of all your cells produce waste products, and these waste products are excreted by your body in a number of ways. The digestive system breaks down food into substances that the body can use and then separates what we need from what we don't need. What we need is absorbed, what we don't passes through. Also, your kidneys and skin both secrete water and waste materials, via urination and sweating, respectively, and your lungs excrete carbon dioxide and water whenever you exhale.

You needn't move your bowels every day—many people don't, and that's normal. If you suffer from uncomfortable constipation, however, try addressing your digestion by eating more natural fiber in the form of fresh fruits and vegetables and whole grains and upping your fluid intake. In rare cases, constipation could signal a spastic colon, an obstruction, or other medical problems. If constipation isn't relieved by dietary changes, see your doctor.

Gender-Specific Systems

So far, all the anatomy we've talked about belongs to everyone. But as you know, we aren't all the same anatomy-wise. Men and women have distinctly different anatomies, for the very good reason of keeping the species alive. Unlike some simpler life forms who can reproduce all by themselves, we need each other for socialization, for touch, for affection, and to reproduce.

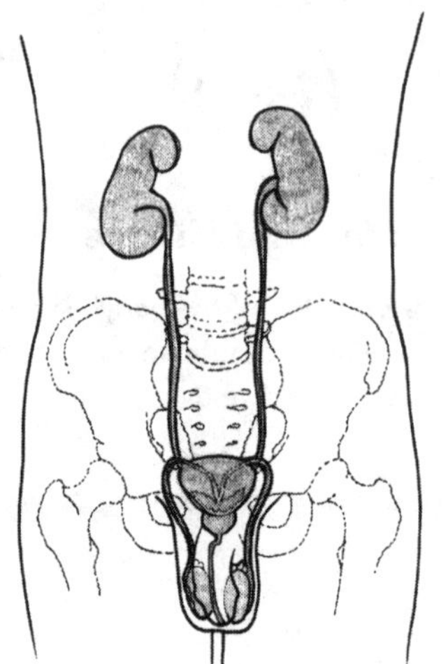

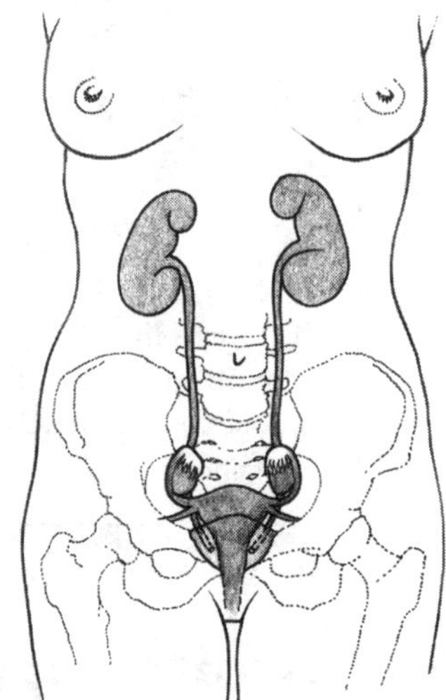

The male and female reproductive systems, shown in relation to the kidneys, organs of the excretory system located just above the waistline.

The Female Reproductive System

What do gals have that guys don't have? Plenty! Among other things unique to women are ovaries, a uterus, a vagina, and a vulva. (Stop smirking, guys—you're next.) *Ovaries* are glands that produce eggs for fertilization and secrete the hormones *estrogen* and *progesterone*. Estrogen helps to keep this cycle on schedule, and it is also responsible for making women look like women by triggering the development of breasts, hips, curves, and so on.

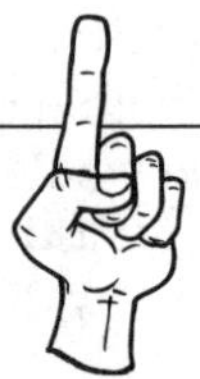

Touch Talk

The purpose of the **prostate gland** is to secrete a fluid that helps sperm to move and neutralizes the acidic environment in the vagina so more sperm can survive. The prostate surrounds a portion of the urethra and contains muscles that contract when semen (sperm plus fluids) is expelled.

We'll go into the benefits of massage unique to women in more depth in Chapter 24, but for now, know that massage can ease all the aches and pains that typically accompany menstruation, pre-menstrual syndrome (PMS), pregnancy, childbirth, post-partum healing, and menopause. Massage can help to make all these experiences easier and more joyful, too. (Well, maybe PMS won't be exactly joyful, but massage can certainly lessen the discomfort.)

The Male Reproductive System

What do guys have that girls don't? Men's reproductive systems include the testes, the notorious prostate gland, and the penis. The *testes* are glands that produce sperm and the hormone testosterone. Just as estrogen gives women their womanly appearance, *testosterone* makes men look like men: hairier, more muscular, and with lower voices than women. Testosterone also governs the manufacture of sperm within the testes.

Unlike women, who can only get pregnant for a few days each month, men are able to impregnate a female just about any time. They can also remain fertile much later in life than women because they manufacture sperm until they die, assuming testosterone levels remain adequate.

Can massage be helpful for the specific problems of manhood? Definitely. We'll go into the details in Chapter 25, but men can especially benefit from some of the psychological lessons massage teaches, such as the power of vulnerability and the pleasure of nonsexual touch. Massage can also keep you functioning at your peak capacity.

Skin Deep: The Integumentary System

Last but not least—for we wouldn't be a pretty sight without it—is the skin, also known as the *integumentary system*. Your skin does more than keep your innards in. It regulates your temperature, secretes waste products via sweat, absorbs nutrients, protects your internal organs from the onslaught of daily life, and breathes, too.

Most relevant for this book, your skin provides you with the sensation of touch. Your skin is crammed with nerve cells that allow you to feel differences in temperature, texture, and pressure. Your skin alerts you to pain so your nervous system can react accordingly. It also alerts you to the pleasurable sensation of human touch, to which your nervous system will also react, though in a much nicer manner.

Just like your other organs, your skin is nourished by blood and supported or sustained by lymph, so it makes sense that massage can be of great benefit. Not only does massage improve circulation to the skin so dramatically that you can see the healthy glow after a massage, but it also speeds the elimination of toxins and keeps the oil glands in your skin at peak performance so your skin stays better lubricated and more elastic. Because massage works directly on your skin, you may feel its benefits immediately and more dramatically on your skin than on any other part of your body. Beauty may only be skin deep, but you might as well keep that skin looking and feeling as good as possible.

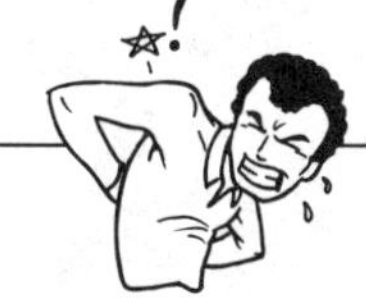

Ouch!

Some people have extremely sensitive skin. If massage is painful or uncomfortable to you because of the sensitive nature of your skin, always tell your massage therapist, who should adjust the pressure accordingly. Massage should never be uncomfortable and should never cause a rash, chafing, bruising, or any other type of uncomfortable skin reaction.

The Least You Need to Know

- Knowing a little about all the systems of the body will help you give better massages and will help you to understand your own body better before you receive a massage.
- Massage can improve the functioning and alignment of the musculoskeletal system.
- Massage can facilitate the smooth operation of the nervous system, and massage's stress-relieving effects can improve brain function.
- Massage can make circulation more efficient, relieve lung congestion, and generally improve the workings of the respiratory and circulatory systems.
- Massage can improve digestion and elimination.

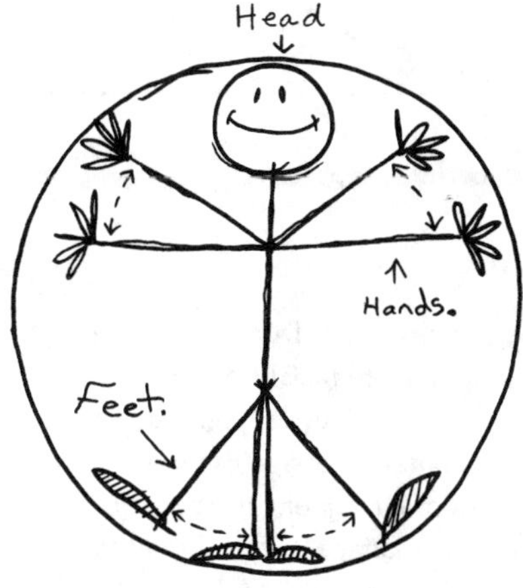

Chapter 6

The Body Made Easy

In This Chapter

- How do your muscles help you move?
- What is a muscle, anyway?
- Which muscles need massage the most?
- What is *homeostasis* and what does it have to do with your posture?

Now that you've got a little background on the various systems of the body and how massage can help them work better, let's check out your muscles—specifically, how your muscles move. After all, muscles are what massage does best!

When you receive a massage, you probably aren't thinking, "Boy, that feels great on my integumentary system!" or "The best thing about that experience was its positive effects on my systems of elimination!" Chances are, you're thinking, "There's nothing like a good foot massage," or "Hallelujah! My back pain is gone!" What you're primarily noticing are the changes massage has wrought in your musculoskeletal system.

Massage works chiefly on your muscles, so in this chapter, we'll be looking at the specific muscles treated by massage. First, though, let's look briefly at how your muscles make your body move, in order to shed a little light on the various massage techniques you'll learn later.

A Massage Minute

One of the most common types of muscle dysfunction is the muscle spasm. During a muscle spasm, the muscle involuntarily contracts. Examples of muscle spasms are facial tics, charley horses (cramps in the calf muscle), hiccups, convulsions, and stuttering. Muscle spasms can be caused by physical stress on a muscle, emotional stress, injury, or illness. Massage can work directly on muscle spasms to relax the contraction. Certain types of movement re-education, such as the Alexander technique (see Chapter 12, "More Kinds of Massage"), can also address certain types of muscle spasm.

The Body in Motion

You might think you can move in all sorts of ways, especially when you're coaxed onto the dance floor to cut loose. But technically, you only move in three ways: *flexion/extension, abduction/adduction,* and *rotation.*

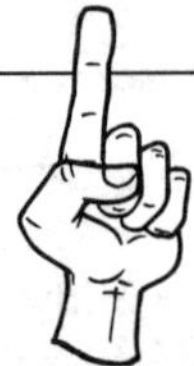

Touch Talk

Flexion is any movement that decreases the angle of a joint. The opposite movement is **extension**, any movement that increases the angle of a joint. **Abduction** is any movement that moves a body part away from the body's midline. **Adduction** is any movement that brings a body part toward the body's midline. **Rotation** is any movement that revolves a body part around an axis.

- Flexion occurs when you decrease the angle of a joint, like when you bend your elbow to show off your chiseled biceps muscle.
- Extension occurs when you increase the angle of a joint, like when your jaw drops open at the sight of someone's far larger chiseled biceps.
- Abduction involves moving a body part away from the center of your body, like when you lie on your side on the floor and raise your leg along with the leotard-clad aerobics instructor on your television. Adduction occurs when you lower your leg again.
- Rotation is when you revolve a body part around an axis, like when you turn your head to catch a second glance at a shiny new sports car—or its driver.

Another important thing to remember about movement is that for every muscle action, another muscle moves in opposition. For example, when you flex your arm, your biceps contracts, but your triceps, the muscle along the back of your upper arm, extends. Remember that old physics formula from school: "For every action, there is a separate and equal reaction"? Muscles are no exception.

Massage and Muscles 101

Just what is a muscle, anyway? Muscles are the movement organs of the body. They are made from special cells that, unlike many other cells, can change their length. Muscles allow you to walk, raise your hand, and dance the tango. They also keep your lungs breathing, your heart beating, and all your other internal functions going.

But muscles don't do all that work for free. They take a lot of energy, mostly from the air you breathe and the food you consume. They also don't work alone. Muscles rely on your circulatory system to keep them nourished and to eliminate the by-products of their actions. They require the skeleton to hold them up, and they require the nervous system to tell them what to do.

What does a muscle look like? Different muscles have different appearances, but most muscles consist of muscle fibers arranged in bundles and held together by connective tissue. Muscle fibers and muscle bundles are bunched together in a parallel fashion, like a handful of sticks. In fact, each muscle fiber (or muscle cell) looks something like a stick, and muscle fibers typically extend the entire length of the muscle. To get even more microscopic, each muscle fiber contains thousands of mini-fibers, and each one of these contains thousands of muscle *filaments*. These filaments interact to help muscles contract.

The connective tissue that holds muscle fibers together also shapes and binds individual muscles and muscle groups, as well as attaching muscles to the skeleton. If you made an entire body disappear except for the connective tissue, you'd still be able to see pretty much all of the body's internal structures. At the ends of certain muscles, or in some cases all along the muscles, connective tissue turns into tough, elastic *tendons* that anchor muscles to bones, organs, or muscles. The place

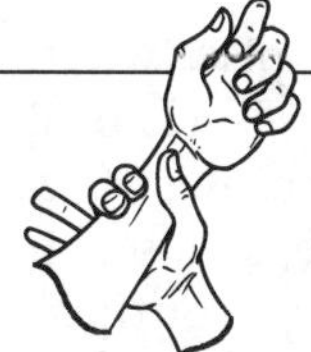

Your Finger on the Pulse

Different types of friction techniques work either in the direction of muscle fibers, called *longitudinal friction*, or perpendicular to muscle fibers, called *cross-fiber friction* (see Chapter 16, "Heat It Up and Shake It Out: Friction and Vibration"). Longitudinal friction stretches and straightens muscle fibers. Cross-fiber friction breaks up adhesions and helps injuries to heal.

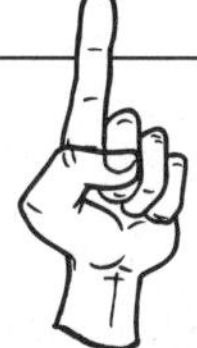

Touch Talk

The **muscle origin** is where a muscle attaches to a relatively immovable part of the skeleton, usually closer to the body's center. The **muscle insertion** is where the other end of the muscle attaches to the skeleton, a muscle, or deep skin layers and where movement takes place, usually further from the body's center than the origin. The **muscle belly** is the thicker, middle part of the muscle.

where a muscle is anchored to an immovable part of the skeleton is called the *muscle origin*. The origin is usually closer to the body's center and anchors the muscle. For example, the origin of the biceps muscle would be in the shoulder girdle.

The place where the other end of the muscle attaches to either bone, other muscles, or deep layers of skin is called the *muscle insertion*. The insertion is usually further from the center of the body and activates body movement. For example, the insertion of the biceps muscle is near the inside of the elbow, the joint that moves in response to a biceps contraction. The thicker, middle portion of the muscle is the *muscle belly*.

You've got 600 muscles in that body of yours, making up approximately half your weight, and each muscle can be massaged in a different way for different effects. That's a lot of massage! Muscles are layered and some are far deeper and more difficult to reach. By relaxing the outer layers of muscle, the deeper layers become more accessible.

Once the superficial muscles relax, it's easier to release tensions in deeper layers of muscle.

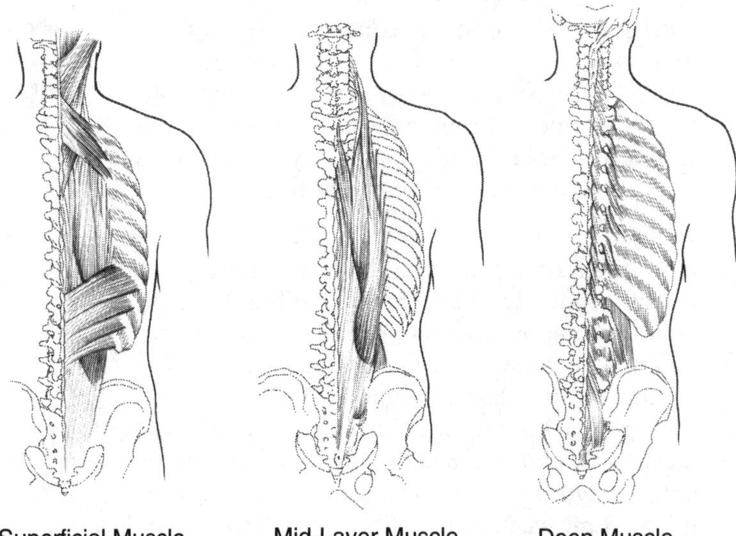

To help you determine which muscles are the most relevant for massage, let's work our way through the body on a little magical muscular tour. Our tour will be a necessarily broad look at muscles and muscle massage. As your massage expertise is refined, your massages can go deeper and explore smaller and more specific areas of muscle tension.

The Hip Bone's Connected to the...

Let's begin at the bottom. The muscles in your lower extremities tend to be larger and more powerful than those on top. They can get plenty sore, too, when your physical activity is too vigorous. Massage on the lower half should concentrate on the following muscles.

Let's Start with the Feet

You know your feet take a lot of abuse; you can tell by the way they feel at the end of a long day. A good foot massage can knead those tight, contracted foot muscles back to their original shapes, however. Concentrate on the *extensor muscles* on the front of the foot that extend the foot and the *flexor muscles* on the back of the foot that flex the foot (see the following figure). The *abductor hallucis* helps pad our feet and takes on a lot of the stress from walking, running, and so on. Massage can help to relieve the stress in this muscle, too.

Because the feet are farthest from the heart, poor circulation in them can be quite common. There are twenty-six bones in the foot with many extensor muscles on the front and flexor muscles on the back.

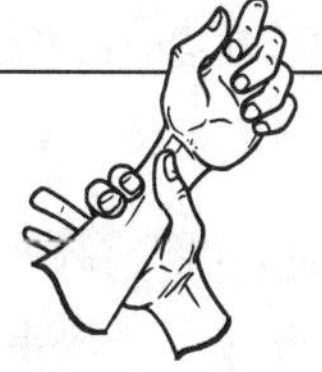

Your Finger on the Pulse

To strengthen your feet, take up dancing, walk barefoot around the house whenever you can, pick up small objects with your toes, flex and extend your feet when reading or watching television, and walk on your tiptoes.

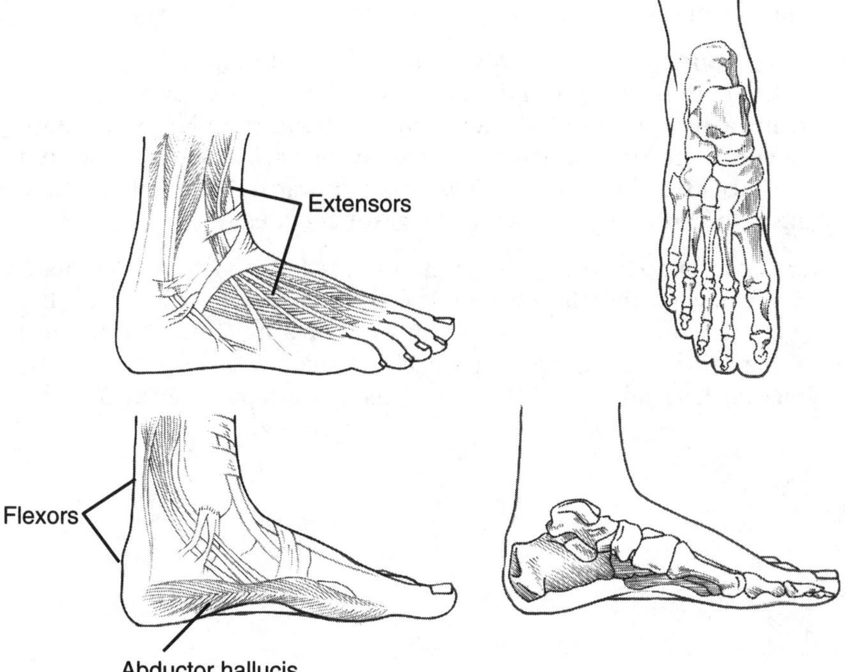

A Leg to Stand On

Your legs take as much abuse as your feet, but because the leg muscles and bones are bigger, they may not feel the stress as soon. Eventually, though, when you work too hard (or even sit for too long), your leg muscles will tighten and painfully contract. As we age, we lose a lot of strength in the leg muscles (perhaps because we do more sitting). It is therefore important to continue building leg strength (for example, through squats and lunges) so that you can continue to stand and walk comfortably into ripe old age.

The front of the thigh sports your *quadriceps*, four muscles that run from hip to knee and allow you to extend your leg at the knee. If you lift weights, you work your quadriceps when you do leg curls. These muscles are strong, but they can get pretty tight. Massage in this area can be deep and vigorous. Find the quadriceps muscles all along the front of the thigh from hip to knee.

The *hamstring muscles* (including the *biceps femoris* and the *semitendinosus* shown in the following figure) run along the back of your thigh from hip to knee. In many people, the quadriceps are stronger than the opposing hamstring muscles, causing the hamstring muscles to become strained. Tight hamstring muscles are also often the culprit when it comes to lower back pain. Massaging the back of the thigh can help loosen and relax strained and contracted hamstring muscles.

In your lower leg, concentrate on the *gastrocnemius* and *soleus* muscles. The gastrocnemius helps to flex both the knee and the foot, and the soleus flexes the foot. Walking, running, and any activity in which the ankle joint is frequently flexed can cause these muscles to become tight. Find the gastrocnemius at the back of the lower leg (your calf), from the knee extending about halfway down towards the foot. Find the soleus on the outside of the lower leg, just below the gastrocnemius.

If you've ever had a cramp in your gastrocnemius muscle (also known as a charley horse), you know how much pain this muscle can cause. To relieve a charley horse, quickly pull your toes toward you and hold for a few breaths, stretching and increasing circulation to the gastrocnemius (this is probably all the massage you'll be able to stand, but you can also grab hold of the gastrocnemius and pull it away from the bone).

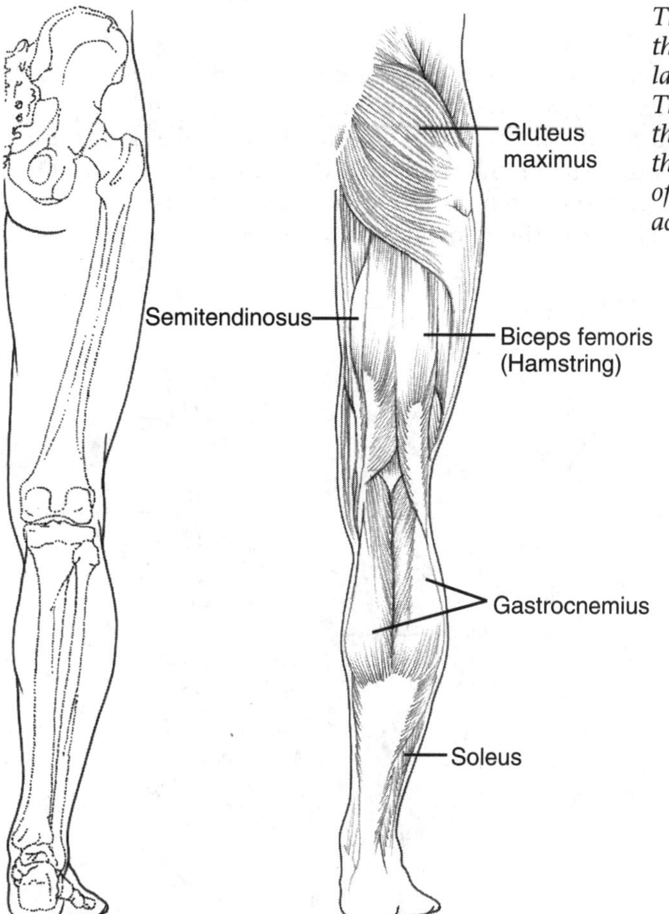

The gluteus muscles of the buttocks are multi-layered and run quite deep. The hamstring muscles of the back of the thigh and the gastrocnemius muscles of the calf are easily accessible to massage.

Hold on to Your Seat: Gluteus Maximus

Your *gluteus maximus* muscle is that great big muscle you sit on (see the previous figure). Yes, you know the one. This muscle is responsible for extending and rotating the thigh. You can feel it contracting when you walk uphill or after a few dozen leg lifts. This muscle holds a lot of tension, and because it is so large, it can be massaged quite vigorously. The gluteus maximus is easy to find. Lie on your stomach, and there it is, right between your hips and your upper thighs—you can't miss it!

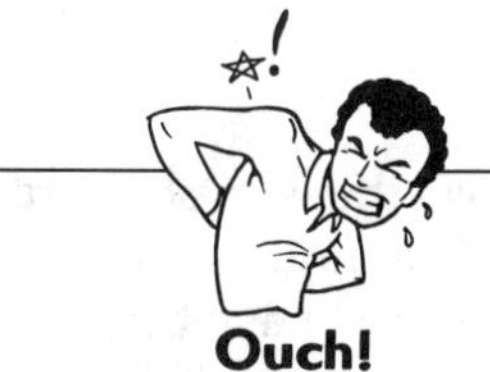

Ouch!

Never apply heat to a pulled or torn muscle. Heat will aggravate swelling. If you pull or tear a muscle, apply cold packs.

Let's Get Hip

Your hip muscles aren't as obvious as some of the others we've discussed. Deeper inside your body than, say, your quadriceps muscles, your hip muscles can nonetheless experience pain and strain. The two main hip muscles massage is concerned with are the *iliacus* and the *psoas*. The iliacus helps to flex the thigh, the hip, and the spine. It attaches to the hip bone and extends to the top of the thigh. The psoas muscle also flexes the thigh, the hip, and the spine. It runs from deep in the abdomen to the top of the thigh, along the spine.

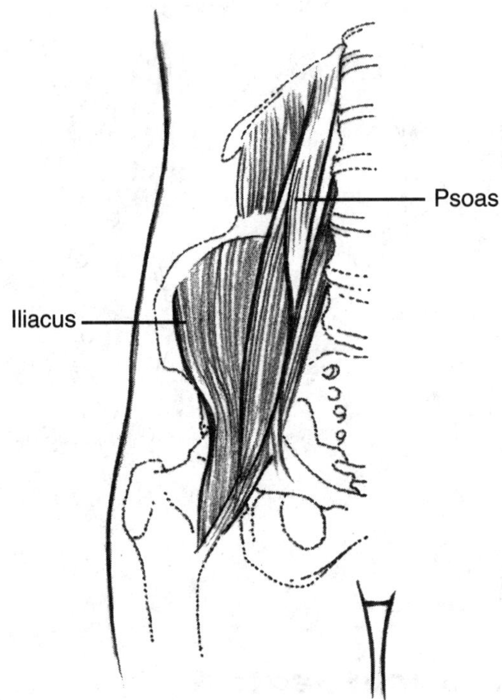

The psoas and iliacus muscles in front of the hip pictured here can have a significant impact on your posture. For example, if they're very tight, a forward-leaning posture can result.

Both these muscles are difficult to feel, but an experienced massage therapist should be able to find them with some deep tissue strokes. If you experience a lot of hip pain, you may have trigger points in the psoas muscle that a massage therapist could release.

Tummy Time!

Your stomach muscles may not feel the pain as often as some of your other muscles, but if you've ever decided to get back into shape with 100 sit-ups after months of life on the couch with a bag of chips, you know what it feels like to have sore tummy muscles! Massage can really loosen up and relax the muscles of the middle and lower abdominal area. Focus on the *rectus abdominis*, which are parallel, vertical muscles running from the upper chest to the pelvis, right in the middle of your torso; the *external obliques*, which are those muscles that wrap around the sides of your torso over your eight lower ribs (these are often sore after a session of side bends in aerobics class); and the *sartorius* muscles, which run diagonally across the thigh from the outer edge of the hip bone to the inner thigh just above the knee. The sartorius muscles are responsible for flexing and rotating the thigh and knee.

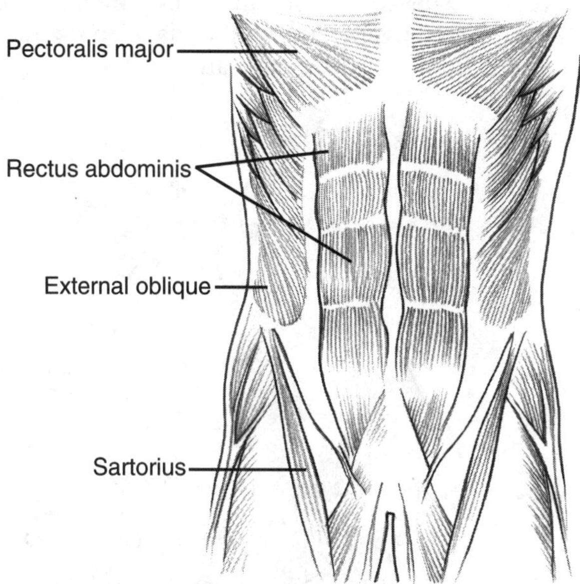

Notice the directions of the muscle fibers (lines). By becoming more familiar with the direction of the muscle fibers, you can give a more effective massage.

From the Waist Up

Now let's take a good look at your upper half, where the muscles may be smaller but are no less likely to need a good massage.

Open Your Chest and Breathe

Your upper torso is capable of many types of movement, from lifting your arms to twisting your body around to keeping those lungs moving productively. For massage, concentrate on the following muscles:

- The *deltoid* muscles cap your shoulders and consist of an outer, middle, and inner muscle. A shoulder rub targets these muscles.
- The *pectoralis major* extends from the center of your chest out to each armpit and helps you move your arms at the shoulder joint. This

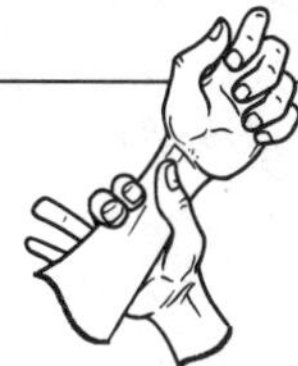

Your Finger on the Pulse

Stress can aggravate asthma attacks, during which bronchial muscles spasm, severely limiting air flow in and out of the lungs. Asthmatics can benefit from massage because it helps the entire body to relax and may lessen the severity of asthma symptoms. Percussion strokes (see Chapter 15, "Groovin' to the Massage Beat: Compression and Percussion") applied to the back can be beneficial for relieving chest congestion.

muscle gets pretty sore when you suddenly do a lot of weight lifting, moving heavy boxes, or swinging little kids around when you aren't used to it.

- The *serratus anterior* extends from the sides of your rib cage underneath your arm. If you decide to join your kids when they swing from the monkey bars, you may feel it the next day in these muscles.
- The *teres major* is a muscle that attaches to your shoulder blade in back and extends under your arm. People with larger chests tend to develop soreness in their teres major and can benefit from massage to this area.

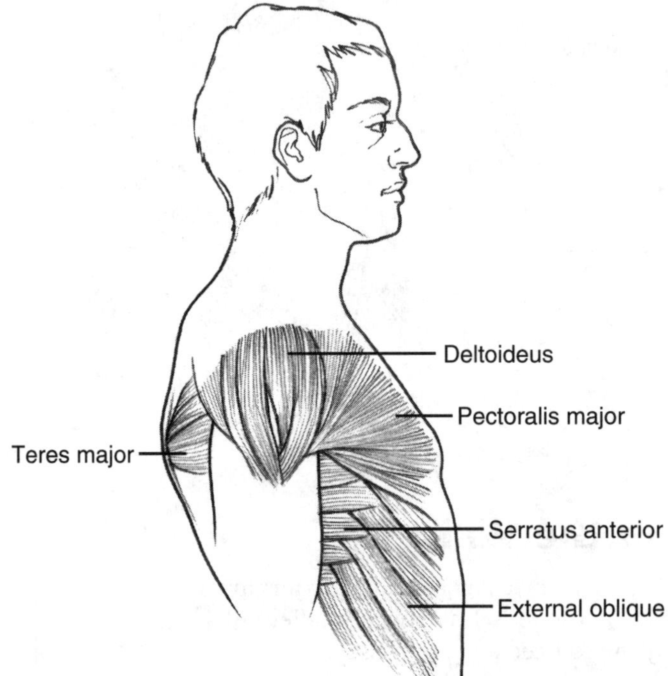

The muscles of the chest and shoulders help you with full arm movements. Supple muscles equal supple movements.

The Spine's Many Levels: From Neck to Back

Your poor spine takes plenty of abuse, too. After all, we weren't originally upright creatures. Suddenly (in evolutionary terms, anyway), our spines had to hold us up, support our heads, and handle a lot more gravity. Lots of muscles support the spine, and they can all feel the strain. Massage can easily reach many of these muscles, which is why backrubs feel so great.

For a back massage, concentrate on the following muscles:

- The *occipitalis* is located just above the ridge at the base of the skull.
- The *splenius* extends from the back of the neck on each side just below the skull diagonally toward the upper spine.

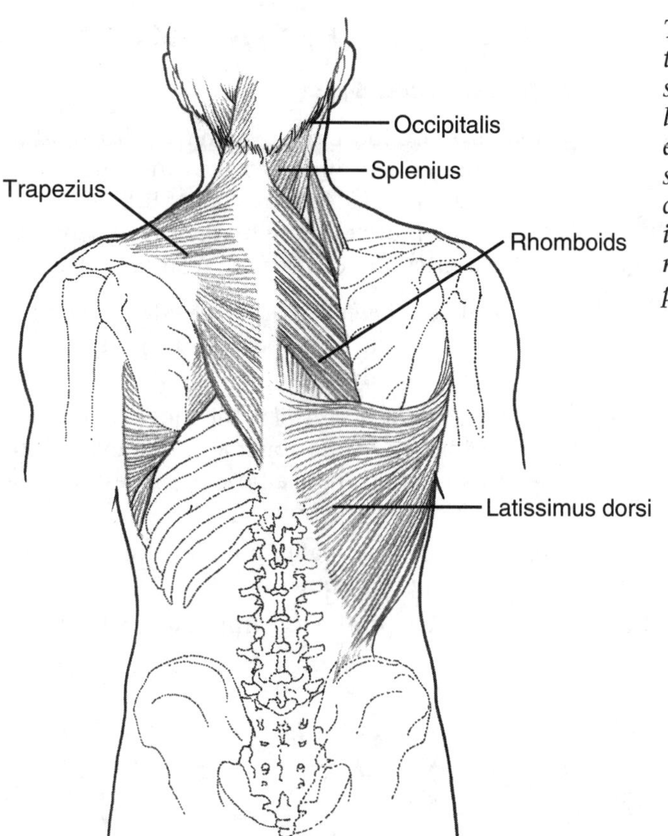

The spine separates the two sides of the back. The same complete and multi-layered set of muscles exists on each side of the spine. These muscles cushion the spine and internal organs and maintain our upright posture.

- The *trapezius* is a large, fan-shaped muscle that originates along a wide area from the base of the skull down a large portion of the spine and inserts at the shoulder. It's a big area of tension that can use lots of vigorous kneading.
- The *rhomboids* are located under the trapezius along the spine to the shoulder blade.
- The *latissimus dorsi* is another large, fan-shaped muscle; it attaches along the mid- to lower spine and extends up underneath the arm. There's lots of stress here, too, although the latissimus dorsi can't be massaged quite as vigorously as some back muscles because it encloses the rib cage.

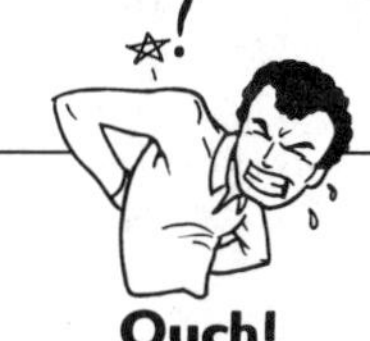

Ouch!

When giving a massage, never press directly on the spine. A professional massage therapist is trained to work on your spine in certain safe ways, but the novice should avoid direct pressure on the spine. Vertebrae can easily become misaligned, causing pain in the spine and in other areas of the body. Instead, concentrate on the muscles on either side of the spinal cord.

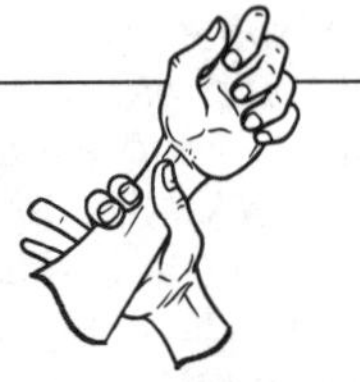

Your Finger on the Pulse

Frequent shoulder tension may be a sign that you aren't drinking enough pure, fresh water. Larger muscles collect more toxins, so help yourself relax by getting hydrated to help flush toxins out. Six to eight glasses of water per day is ideal.

The Weight of the World on Your Shoulders

Our arms do more than we may realize, and to give up control of them for a massage can be incredibly relaxing. The arms are made up of a lot of little muscles, but the following muscles more frequently experience strains and injuries and can benefit from massage:

- The *deltoids* are the triangular muscles that form the rounded shape of your shoulders, located in the shoulder girdle.
- The *biceps brachii* is the long, large muscle on the inside of your upper arm that extends from the shoulder to the elbow and is responsible for flexing the elbow.
- The *triceps* oppose the biceps and are the smaller muscles along the back of the upper arm responsible for extending the elbow.
- The *flexors* are the small, thin muscles in the forearm that flex the wrist and hand.

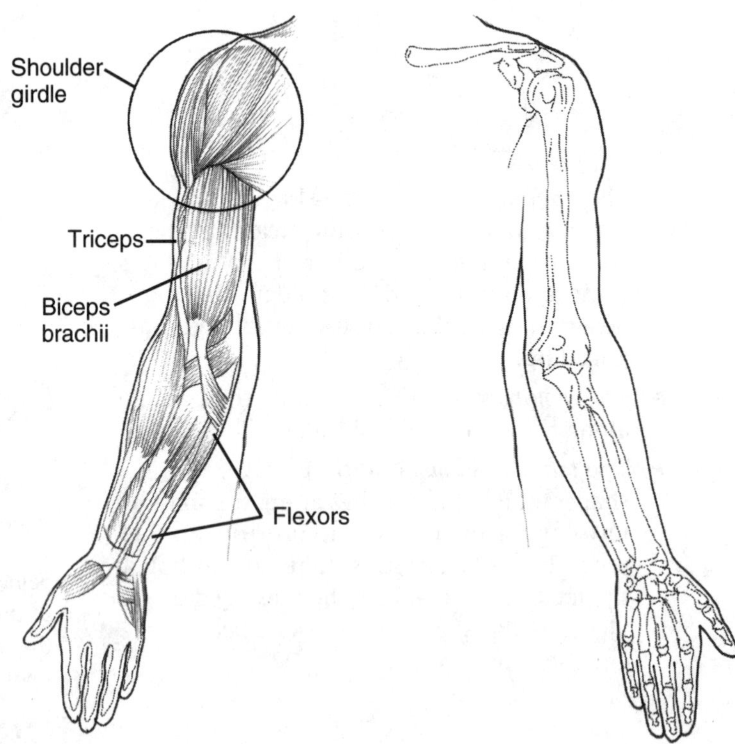

Overly tight shoulder muscles can have numerous side effects, such as decreased circulation and dexterity of hands and fingers, neck tension, and headaches. Time for a shoulder rub?

Geography of the Hand

Talk about little muscles—hands have lots of them, and they get a real workout if you work on the computer or do other fine-motor-coordination work such as sewing, electronic repair, or cooking. A hand massage can relax the whole body. The muscles to look for are the *flexors*, which begin in the lower arm (see the following figure) and extend through the palm towards each finger; and the *extensor* tendons of the fingers, which you can see when you look at the back of your hand and lift your fingers back. Range-of-motion exercises (see Chapter 17, "Goin' Round and Round: Increasing Range of Motion") as well as gentle compression feel good on the delicate hand, and helps to increase circulation.

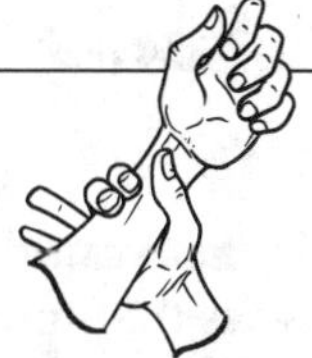

Your Finger on the Pulse

Have you seen those squeezable rubber-covered balls that are designed to relieve stress and are available in drug stores, discount stores, and novelty shops? They are also great for building hand strength. Pick one up for a couple of dollars and keep it on your desk. Squeeze and knead it whenever you get the chance.

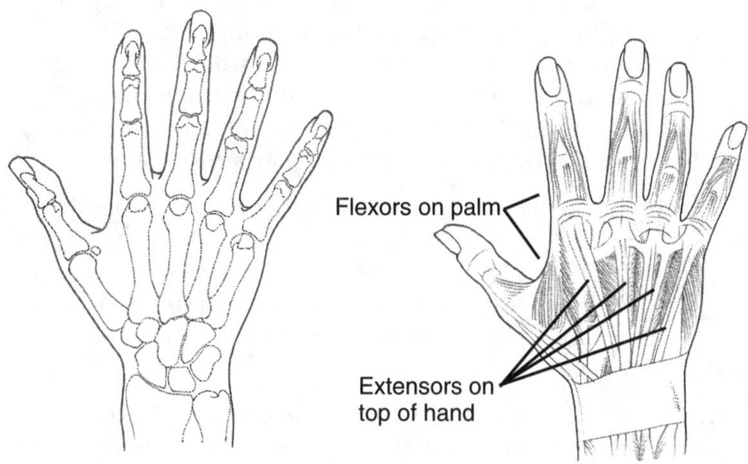

There are twenty-seven bones in the hand. Specific muscles support each movement of each bone joint. That gives a lot of room for tensions to take up lodging!

Such a Beautiful Face...and Scalp, Too!

We end our muscle tour with your beautiful face. If you didn't have muscles in your face, you wouldn't be able to make all those wonderful expressions that give you so much character. A face massage can be incredibly sensual and relaxing. Add a scalp massage, and your massage subject will be putty in your hands. For a face and scalp massage, concentrate on the jaw, the forehead, and the ridge in back at the base of the skull, all areas that hold a lot of tension. For more detail on how to give a good face massage, see Chapter 18, "Give Yourself a Hand: Self-Massage Techniques."

What Feels Right May Be Wrong: Homeostasis and Posture

Now that your tour is at an end, we hope you feel a little more enlightened about the muscles that move you. But how well do they do their job? Even the strongest and most able muscles can't hold you up straight if you don't use them the way they are meant to be used. In other words, unhealthy body habits can cause muscle stress, strain, and pain. You may be so used to that slump, that swayed hip, or that slouch that it feels comfortable. Little do you know what you are doing to your body!

Homeostasis is another word for a condition of balance or equilibrium. Your body's internal homeostasis changes constantly to meet your body's changing demands. Your heart and/or breathing slow or speed up, depending on your activity. Your temperature rises to fight infection, you sweat to cool your body, and your muscles grow or shrink depending on how often they are used. Even walking is simply falling forward, and then finding balance. The key is in how, or even if, we find balance!

When something throws off your homeostasis, your body gets out of balance, and illness or injury can result. Something as simple as crooked posture may be all it takes to send your health into a tailspin. How? Because incorrect posture uses your muscles unevenly, which can throw off all your internal workings. Rounder shoulders and a hunched-over back will contract your chest and compress your abdomen, putting strain on your breathing, digestion, and elimination functions, as well as putting undue stress on bones and ligaments.

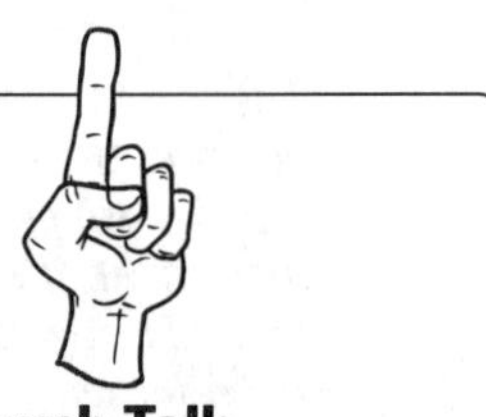

Touch Talk

Homeostasis is the tendency of a system (a body, a group, an ecosystem) to maintain an equilibrium or balanced state.

Ironically, however, your swayed posture may be what feels right to you. Do you remember being a teenager and having an adult tell you to sit up straight? If you tried, it was just plain uncomfortable, wasn't it? You were used to that rebellious teenager slump, and that's what felt right to your body.

Standing up straight, sitting tall, or walking correctly may make you feel like your homeostasis is all off. That's because habit is powerful and compelling. It can feel good to indulge in that swayed body posture, but it can also compromise your health.

Massage therapists are trained to examine your posture on your first visit to them. Are you standing and moving so that things are even on both sides of your body or is everything skewed to one side? Is one side held more tightly or does it move less freely? Are you standing tall and straight or are you all crunched down into yourself? Are you rotating one way or the other? A good massage therapist can make a personal assessment of what you need from a massage, beyond what you request, by looking at the way you stand and move. Then your massage can help your body to re-establish its true homeostasis, rather than what just feels right.

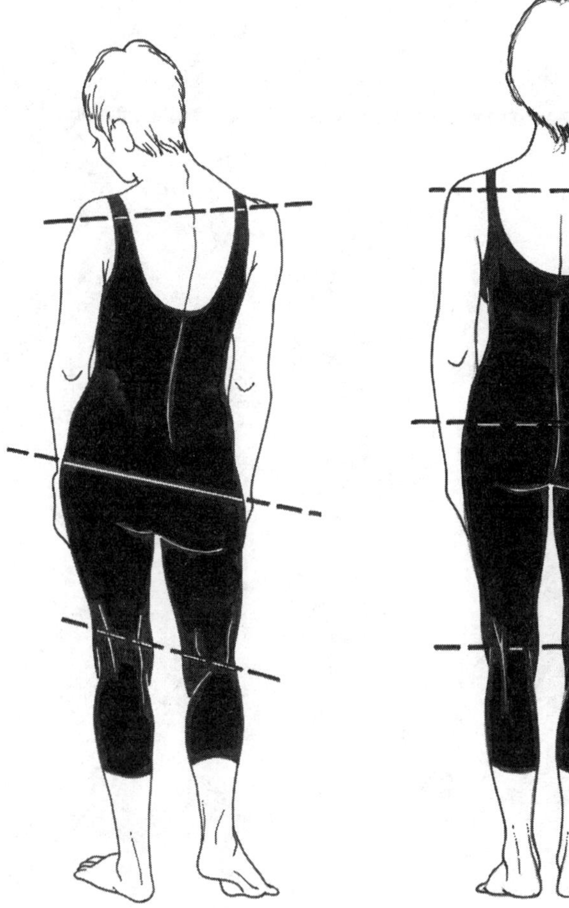

Incorrect posture throws your body alignment out of balance. You're not lined up! Imagine a string extending straight through your body and pulling up through the top of your head. As the string pulls up, feel your body move into a solid balance with your weight evenly distributed on both feet.

The Least You Need to Know

- ➤ Muscles are the primary movers of the body and the primary targets of massage.
- ➤ Muscles connect to the skeleton and to other internal structures via tendons and connective tissue.
- ➤ Each area of the body—feet, legs, buttocks, pelvis, stomach, abdomen, chest, spine, shoulders and arms, hands, face, and scalp—contains particular muscles that are more likely to suffer strain and most likely to benefit from massage.
- ➤ Good posture and the correction of unhealthy body habits through massage and movement re-education can help your body to maintain a state of balance.

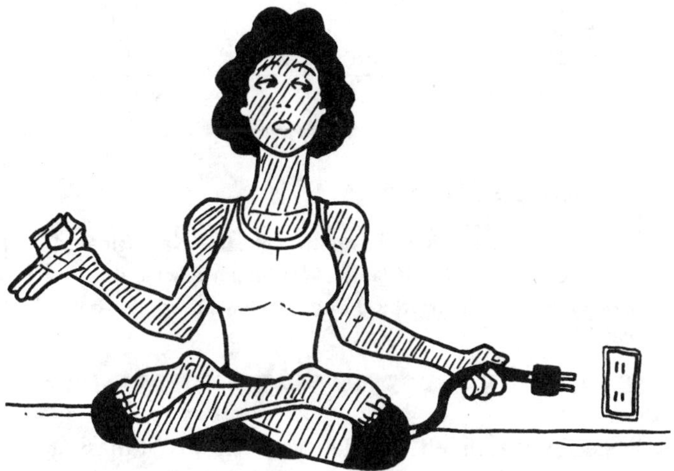

Chapter 7

Contact: Power Points

In This Chapter

- Understanding your body's life-force energy
- Learning where the energy is and how it flows through you
- Manipulating that energy via pressure points to keep it flowing freely
- Interpreting your body map for pain relief and better health
- Determining if you know your body or your mind better

Considering the broad and varied nature of bodywork, it wouldn't be fair to concentrate only on the Western conception of anatomy. Of course, almost everyone anywhere in the world knows that your heart is located approximately at point A, your lungs at point B, the abdominal muscles at point C, and so on. Anatomy is anatomy to some extent.

On the other hand, traditional Eastern medicine sees another sort of anatomy within and around the anatomy we Westerners have studied since that first titillating junior high anatomy lecture. Many Eastern traditions see the body as a sort of road map of pressure points and energy meridians, and it is this map that Eastern health care practitioners, including acupuncturists, acupressurists, and other bodyworkers, use to navigate the body toward health.

A Massage Minute

Many of the concepts around which Chinese medicine is based are thought to have originated with Huang-ti, the Yellow Emperor. The Yellow Emperor's Classic of Internal Medicine still influences the practice of Eastern medicine today. Huang-ti is thought to have lived between 2696 B.C. and 2598 B.C.

Westerners haven't ignored the Eastern wisdom, either. Plenty of schools of massage and bodywork have been built around the concept of pressure points and energy meridians, so to get the most out of massage, you should know just what and where these pressure points and energy flows are. Although numerous cultures and numerous traditions have slightly different energy focal points, we will give you an overview of some of the major Eastern-influenced energy concepts.

Your Body's Energy Systems and Hot Spots

Before you can truly understand the concept of energy flows and pressure points, you have to realize and accept that you can't see these pressure points or channels of energy on an X-ray or an MRI. According to many, however, they are as real as your pituitary gland or your big toe and can be felt, sensed, and manipulated for better health. In fact, several recent studies have demonstrated measurable electrical differences at pressure points, and some newly developed devices have even been developed to locate pressure points by measuring the differences in electrical conduction. Now that's what we call useful technology!

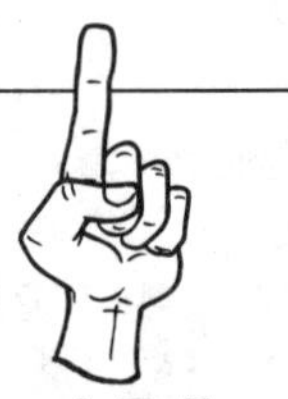

Touch Talk

Energy channels or **energy meridians** are specific channels that run through the body like rivers, through which life-force energy flows. Along these channels are **pressure points** where energy tends to pool or get blocked. Pressing or massaging these points can help to rejuvenate energy flows through the channels or meridians.

The Chinese Concept of Chi

Many people think of energy as that thing you often lack just when you need to finish a project or go to aerobics class. But Eastern medicine and many Western schools believe that energy, or life force, flows into, out of, around, and through the body. This energy or life force is known as *chi* (pronounced *chee*) or *qi* in China, *ki* in Japan, *prana* in India, *rlun* in Tibet, and *pneuma* in ancient Greece. Westerners tend to call it energy.

What is chi? A good question! You can probably find as many definitions as there are bodywork practitioners, but most would agree that chi is basically our energy essence. It is the force that animates us and gives us life. For centuries, Eastern cultures have expounded upon chi (or whatever they happen to call it) and its profound effects. Chi is everywhere; it's within us, in the environment, and throughout the whole universe.

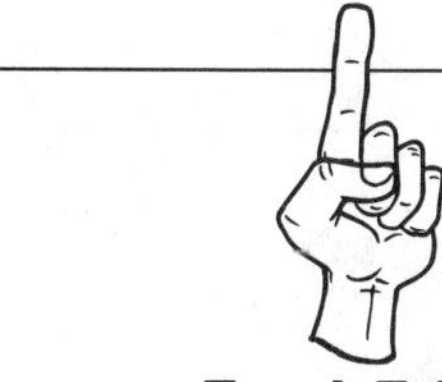

Touch Talk

The concept of **chi**, or life-force energy that flows through the body, isn't unique to the Chinese. In Japan, it is *ki*. In India, it is *prana*. In Tibet, it is *rlun*. In ancient Greece, it was *pneuma*. Westerners call it a number of things, all along the lines of "life-force energy." Many Westerns have also adopted the Eastern terms.

Once again, we Westerners eventually developed our own conception of energy, or chi. Albert Einstein himself "discovered" it with his theory of relativity. The concept that everything is energy, that even matter is made of energy (or potential energy), is quite similar to the ancient Eastern idea that everything is chi, and that even matter is frozen chi. Almost every culture has some version of this same idea—that we are, at our most basic level, pure energy, just like everything that exists. We are chi.

We don't, however, want to oversimplify the concept. Chi though we may be, that isn't all we are. Einstein would probably agree that, even if all matter is energy, matter is still different than energy when it is in its solid form. It has specific, measurable properties that energy doesn't have. The point is that chi isn't an easy concept to grasp, but grasping it isn't nearly as necessary as feeling it, allowing it to help you, and balancing it when it gets a little out of whack.

River of Life: Energy Channels

Learning how to sense or feel chi and knowing where it flows is the key to *pressure point bodywork*. When you are in perfect health, your chi flows unimpeded through specific channels that run like rivers through your body. These rivers of energy nourish your internal organs as well as your spirit and emotions, which are inextricably combined—a concept obvious to Eastern medicine but a little harder for Westerners to grasp. Free-flowing energy means all is well, physically and otherwise.

Sometimes, however, things go wrong, either physically, mentally, emotionally, or spiritually. Chi becomes blocked and energy doesn't flow freely somewhere along the line. Anything can block chi: too much heat or cold, too much aggravation or stress, too much moisture or dryness, or an injury. When chi is blocked, it's as if one of the rivers of energy in your body is dammed up and can't flow. This blockage in turn cuts off the energy supply from some areas and floods other areas. The result might be pain, tension, illness, swelling, depression, or just a feeling that something isn't right.

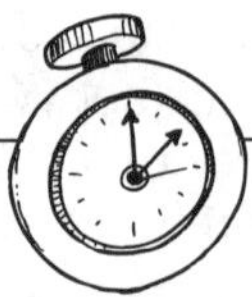

A Massage Minute

The concept of energy channels and pressure points is basic to Chinese medicine, but not to all Eastern systems of health. This system spread through Asia and is the foundation of the traditional medicine of the region, including Japan and Korea. However, the traditional medicine of India and Tibet, for example, has its own systems that differ markedly from the Chinese model. The meridian point model is known today in this country as Oriental medicine. However, all traditional science, including medicine, whether eastern or western, was originally based on a vitalistic or energetic view of the cosmos. Reductionistic science abolished this view from the European culture, eventually separating the concepts of "spirit" and "pheuma" (life essence or soul) from matter. Essentially, though, energy-based philosophies of health were once common to both Eastern and Western thought.

This blockage isn't like a blocked artery. The area won't suddenly become oxygen-starved and begin to lose function or suffer tissue death. Blocked energy isn't a matter of your foot falling asleep or your heart going into cardiac arrest—it manifests itself as an organic imbalance in your body-mind. Maybe coldness begins to overwhelm warmth, or your mental aspect begins to overwhelm your physical, or fatigue begins to overwhelm your waking state. Yet blocked chi can lead to physical dysfunction. According to traditional Chinese medical theory, if left untreated, chi blockage leads to lowered metabolic functioning and physiological pathology. One part of the body-mind can't be affected without all other parts being thrown out of balance.

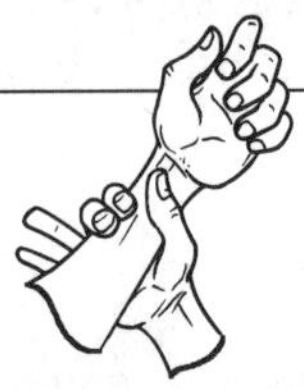

Your Finger on the Pulse

To charge your hands with chi before giving yourself or someone else a massage, place your palms together in front of you, then rub them vigorously, up and down. Every few seconds, clap your hands briskly. After about 30 seconds, shake your hands and wrists sharply towards the ground. Your hands should feel warm and energized.

When energy is blocked, it isn't a matter of finding precisely what is blocked and single-mindedly treating that isolated area. It's more a matter of working with the whole system to unblock and restore equilibrium. We're not saying blockages can't be precisely located; they can. But bodyworkers who practice this type of therapy treat specific areas by looking at the whole body-mind. Health problems and treatments are determined through a number of methods, including lifestyle questions, and therapy is administered by considering the entire energy network.

This way of dealing with health problems isn't always easy for Westerners to understand. We want a diagnosis, darn it! We can hardly call our mothers to say, "The results are in, Ma. I've got way too little chi in my left kneecap!" Nonetheless, this system works, and learning to adjust your thinking in this way can be enlightening. In addition, knowing where certain pressure points exist throughout the body and activating them is an important key to releasing specific blockages of chi, thereby releasing the river and allowing the body to better heal itself.

Under Pressure (Points)

Acupressure and shiatsu books are filled with diagrams of pressure points. Many bodywork systems are based on finding these points and stimulating them in some way: finger pressure, knuckle pressure, and a variety of other methods. A few of these pressure points have attained celebrity status. For example, have you heard that you're supposed to squeeze the flesh between your thumb and index finger when you have a headache? Thousands of pressure points have been charted by various methods, which differ according to the bodywork system you are using.

Are pressure points real? Good evidence exists that acupressure points can be located through electrical detection because these points have a lower electrical resistance than surrounding areas. Pressure points are located in the spaces between muscles and bones and can be felt, with practice, as very slight depressions, bumps, or areas of increased heat. Perhaps the best way to envision pressure points is to imagine that the river of your body contains offshoots here and there where the energy pools and rests while the main river continues to flow.

When the river of energy becomes dammed up somewhere, stimulation to these small pools of energy can be just the stimulus required to break the dam. Some pressure points may be flooded with excess energy, and stimulating them will equalize the imbalance. Other pressure points may be in drought, cut off and stagnant due to lack of energy flow from a block "upstream." Stimulation of these points might be likened to a little earthquake that shakes the ground loose and frees the dammed area, again equalizing the energy and restoring flow.

Massage can help relieve congestion in a muscle that can sometimes become a trigger point: a point that refers pain. Consistent massage or pressure over a trigger point, as seen in this drawing, can often break up congestion, dissolve trigger points, and release pain.

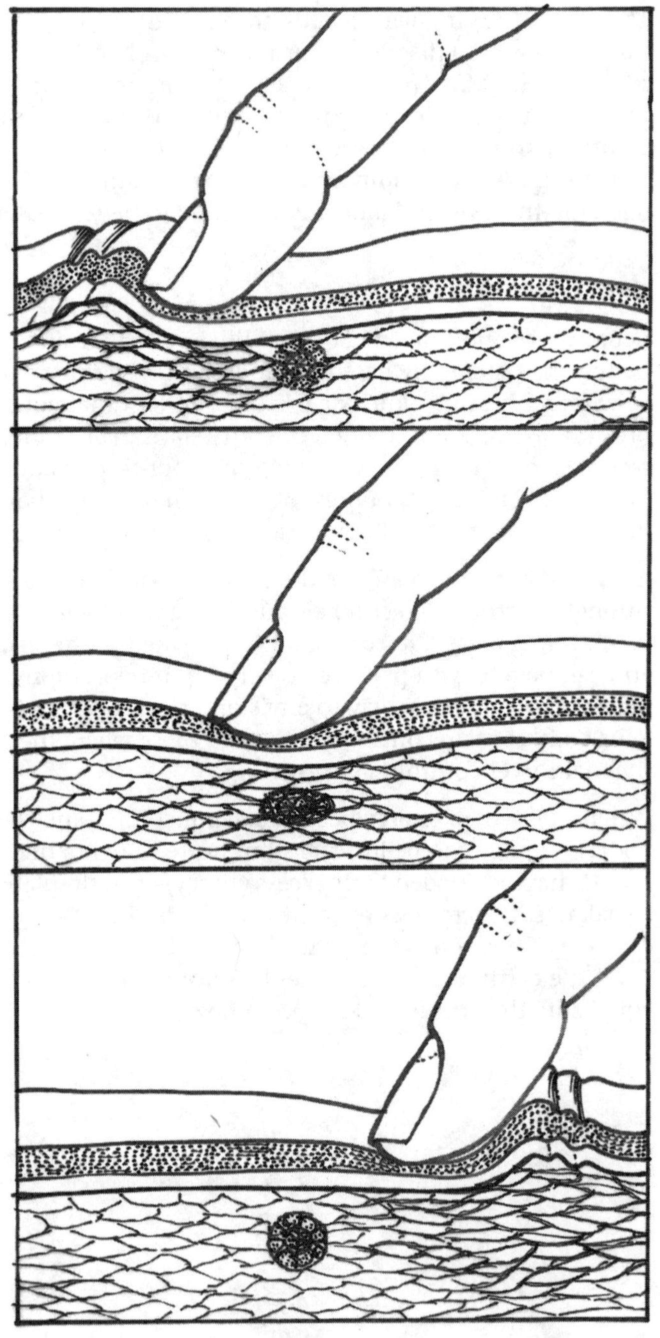

May the Life Force Be with You

Facilitating the free flow of chi may be the purpose of certain types of bodywork, but it can also be a concept you keep in mind as you go through life. When you experience pain or illness or an unpleasant state of mind, consider the possibility that your life force may be blocked somewhere in your body.

Even if the concepts of energy channels and pressure points are a little difficult for you to swallow—maybe you are incurably Western and perfectly happy that way—opening your mind to the possibilities of other ways of seeing can result in a wider sense of yourself and the world. You needn't make the word chi a part of your daily vocabulary if you don't want to, but it can't hurt to try a little acupressure or shiatsu on yourself now and then. You don't need to "believe" in chi to experiment with some of the less Western types of bodywork—all types of massage activate energy, and what you call that energy is really a matter of semantics. If you find that working with pressure points works for you and agrees with you, all the better! You'll have one more interesting view to add to your ever-expanding repertoire of self-awareness.

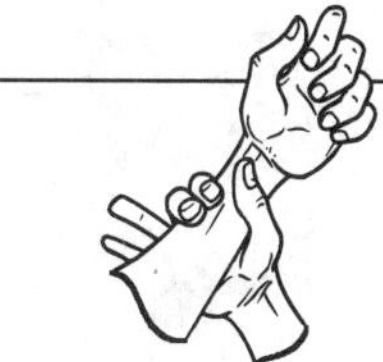

Your Finger on the Pulse

According to many massage therapists, the best way to find the exact location of a pressure point is to prod gently for a sunken or raised area, indicating that the spot is flooded or void of chi. The pressure point may not be in the area of pain but in the area corresponding to the afflicted area or system.

Do You Have References for that Pain?

Sometimes you know exactly where your pain is, and you want it to stop now! Maybe you've got a splitting headache or tennis elbow or a cramp in your calf muscle. Maybe you've got menstrual cramps or are suffering from a serious case of nausea. What can you do about it? Check your body map!

A Road Map to the Internal Organs

Bodywork therapies that deal with pressure points and energy channels have developed maps of the body showing exactly where energy meridians flow and pressure points exist. Although trained bodywork practitioners will be more experienced at finding your aggravated pressure points—in part because they know exactly where to look (or feel), and in part because they have developed a certain intuition for finding the aggravated areas—you can locate and manipulate your own pressure points with a little practice.

Each pressure point corresponds to certain organs or organ systems in the body. The points are usually not on the area of trouble, but they correspond to it because they are connected to it through an energy channel. Sometimes you can find these pressure points on your own. For example, an itch on your leg can sometimes be relieved by scratching somewhere else, such as your arm.

Ouch!

Suffering from lung congestion and an annoying cough that won't go away? Try massaging the hollows between each shoulder and collarbone for about 15 seconds on each side. Or try massaging the pads of your feet at the base of the second, third, and fourth toes and the grooves between the pads.

How do you find the right spot? Sometimes, you can just feel it. If you are experiencing pain or discomfort somewhere, spend some time reading your body map. Experiment with pressure in different areas that seem as though they might be the right place. Feel for small depressions or raised areas between muscles, bones, or joints that are more sensitive and warmer than surrounding tissue. If such intuitive prodding is a little too hocus-pocus for your logical sensibilities, consult a good pressure point map or try some do-it-yourself reflexology, acupressure, or shiatsu techniques described in a reliable book. (Like this one! See Chapters 11 and 12 for some techniques.) You'll be feeling better in no time.

Overcoming Energy Blocks and Obstacles

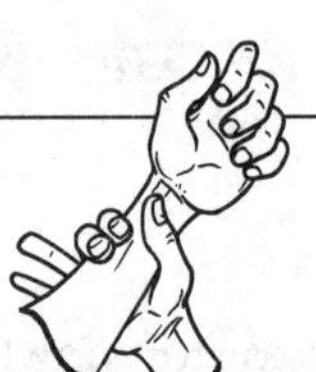

Your Finger on the Pulse

Does your overtaxed mind need a mental massage? Sit comfortably where you won't be disturbed for five minutes. Close your eyes and take deep, slow breaths. Imagine that each inhale fills your body with positive energy and each exhale empties your body of stress and negativity. Soon, you become light enough to float above where worldly cares can touch you. You are pure, clear energy.

As you're poking around for that exact spot on your foot that will relieve your earache, don't forget about the interrelationship between your body and your mind. Sometimes energy blocks can have emotional consequences rather than physical ones, or they can have consequences that are both emotional and physical, such as clinical depression or panic attacks.

Life is full of obstacles and challenges. You can accept the fact, or you can allow it to aggravate you to the point of sickness. According to Eastern medicine, the ability to deal with the aggravations of life is a sign of good physical health. Inability to deal with stress can be a sign of energy blocks, a cause of energy blocks, or both, perpetuating a vicious cycle. Just remember that blocked energy has physical, emotional, and spiritual manifestations and that life stress has physical, emotional, and spiritual consequences. As your body is relaxed through massage, remember to relax your mind correspondingly, or all that work will be for nothing.

You are probably reading this book because you are, more or less, on a journey of self-exploration. You want to feel better, and you want to understand your body and your mind a little better. You want to learn about yourself and how to be your best self. Overcoming energy blocks, whether you perceive these as chi blocked in your meridians or as a sort of symbolic emotional energy block, requires a whole body-mind approach. Step back from that magnifying mirror and look at the big picture. Your ultimate reward will be a better integration of your entire self.

Know Your Body, Know Your Mind

Knowing your body through bodywork means learning more about your mind. Which do you know better: your body or your mind? Chances are, you tend to favor one over the other, and if you do, you are faced with a great opportunity to further balance yourself.

Are you an athlete or a fitness buff who can't get through the day without a good workout? Or maybe you are an intellectual at heart and can go for days without getting your heart rate up because you're much more comfortable reading classic novels or your favorite news magazine. Maybe you have a physical disability that keeps you from certain activities, but you compensate by excelling in others. Would you rather spend time with your best friend jogging through the park, gossiping over coffee, joining your children on the playground, or analyzing the implications of the President's latest foreign policy announcements?

If you favor your body, that's great. Use your body knowledge as a pathway to your mind. If you favor the life of the mind, that's just as great. What does your mind tell you about the life of your body, and vice versa? Integrating body and mind, and letting each inform the other, doesn't mean that a beautiful body represents a deficient mind or a correspondingly beautiful mind. Along the same lines, a body with physical challenges doesn't imply a superior intellect or a correspondingly disabled mind. The state of your body and the state of your mind are simply highly individual clues for you to decipher as you travel toward self-discovery. The connection is by no means simple and is highly personal.

When you get right down to it, we are all energy. In essence, we are neither our bodies nor our minds. These are superficial hints as to who we are. And just who are we? Not anything that fits entirely under any label: not wholly strong, weak, smart, stupid, beautiful, ugly, athlete, teacher, laborer, scholar. The one label that might apply to all of us is "student." We are each students in a learning process about ourselves and our own intricate body-mind connections.

How do you begin to discover yourself and the way your body and mind interact? Ask yourself some searching questions:

- How would you say you are physically different than others?
- What do those differences mean to you?

- How can you reframe your physical challenges as positive learning or growth experiences?
- What are some of your physical attributes, and how can each be a roadway to growth?
- Do you typically think first or act first?
- What would happen if you tried it the opposite way?
- How do you think better body care would enhance your mental state?
- How do you think better attention to your mental health and processes would enhance your physical state?

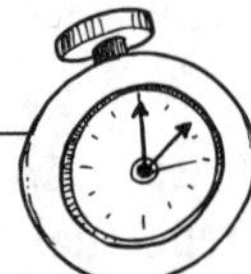

A Massage Minute

Heart disease has been linked to both physical inactivity and to a cynical or negative attitude, another example of how the body and the mind both influence health.

Pathways to Freedom

Whoever you are, you can work toward balance, integration, and self-actualization. This work will involve the whole you, not just your favorite part. Keeping this in mind (or in body) will help you to get the most benefit from bodywork and from mindwork, too. Getting a massage is one step along a path you can choose to follow—or, more accurately, a path you can choose to blaze because it is your own personal path. The ultimate you waits at the end of the road, and the journey is lifelong and as worthwhile as you choose to make it. (And you thought you were just going to learn about how to give a good backrub!)

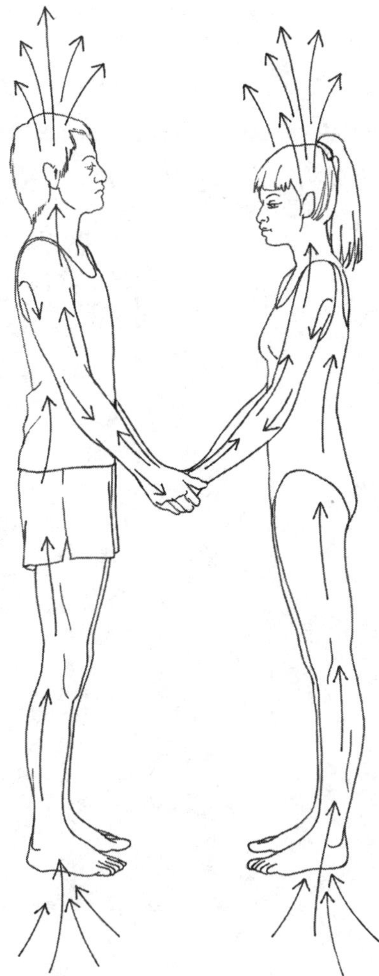

Massage opens energy pathways so the life force can flow easily through our bodies, producing an optimal state of health.

The Least You Need to Know

- According to Eastern notions of health, the body is a complex network of energy channels and pressure points through which the life force energy, also called chi, constantly flows.
- The life force can become blocked within the energy meridians, and the activation of pressure points throughout the body can help to unblock it.
- Your outsides are a road map to your insides, and your insides are a road map to your outsides.

Chapter 8

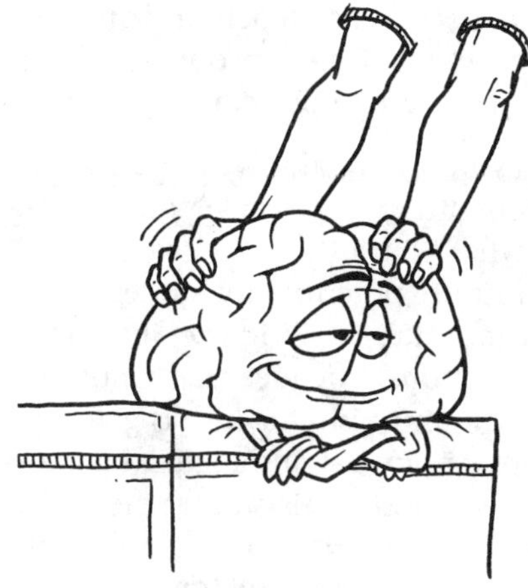

Putting Your Mind to It

In This Chapter

- Can massage make you smarter?
- Listening in on the body-brain conversation
- Why your emotions and intellect are inseparable allies

You know (at least by now) that massage can have great physical benefits and psychological benefits, such as relieving stress and anxiety. But massage has more of a mental component than the mere alleviation of negative conditions such as stress. Massage can make your brain work better.

Massage Makes You Smarter

"Get smart" could be the catch-phrase of modern society. Certain drugs, herbs, and other remedies that promise increased brain activity and cognitive enhancement abound. Self-help books about intelligence—what it is, how much of it you've got, and how to get more—are flying off the bookshelves. When a television news show airs a special about something that makes you smarter, it seems everyone is watching.

Who wouldn't want to be smarter? But not everyone wants to pop three handfuls of herbal supplements each day, and few have the time for radical changes in behavior. Can massage help? You bet! In many ways, massage can make you smarter than you are right now. No, it can't change your potential intelligence, but it can help you to get closer to fulfilling the potential you have. You've probably heard about how little of our brain power humans use—1 percent, 5 percent, or 10 percent, depending on the source. Whether such a thing can be measured is one issue, but most people won't deny that we've all got the potential to be smarter than we are in our daily lives.

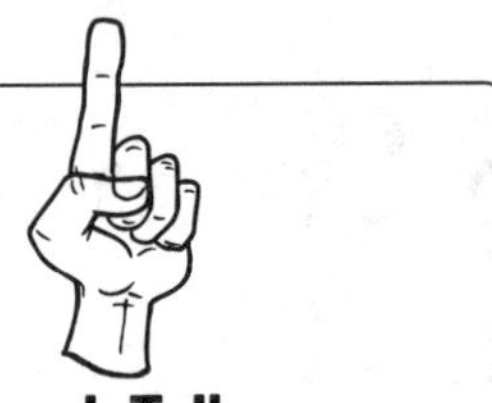

Touch Talk

I.Q., or Intelligence Quotient, is a number that signifies a person's mental development. It is obtained by multiplying the person's mental age (determined by a test) by 100 and then dividing the result by chronological age.

But let's start with an assumption, and we hope you will agree: Intelligence is more than your grade point average or your SAT scores or what your fifth grade teacher determined to be your future potential for success. Intelligence includes the ability to recognize, manage, and properly express emotions. The idea that emotions are an important component to intelligence is gaining increasing support as psychologists and medical doctors alike recognize that life success consists of far more than pure intellectual ability. Just because you score 150 on an I.Q. test doesn't mean you'll have the intelligence to succeed in the professional world, have satisfying personal relationships, or be able to maintain a deep sense of well-being and happiness.

With this expanded definition of intelligence, it may be easier to understand how massage can have a profound effect. Massage and other forms of bodywork operate on the brain and body in multiple ways that potentially enhance intelligence. *Somatics* is a type of bodywork that teaches mindfulness in movement, which links the body and mind to increase the effectiveness of both. Other activities, such as meditation and breathwork, which can be used in conjunction with massage, increase physical and mental awareness to enhance brain function and overall intelligence.

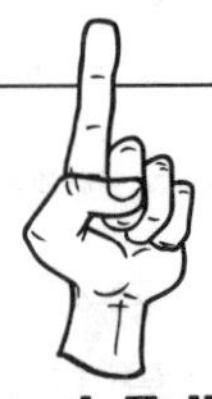

Touch Talk

Somatics is a broad term that can be applied to many types of bodywork in which the student is actively taught techniques for increased self-awareness and self-mastery—to move, feel, and exist with consciousness and forethought. The word *somatic* means "of or relating to the body."

On the physical level, massage has several potent effects on brain function. First and most obvious is enhanced circulation. Better circulation to the brain means that more nutrients, such as oxygen and glucose, will be delivered to the brain so that it can run more efficiently. Also, the elimination of toxins will be enhanced, keeping waste products from accumulating and inhibiting brain function.

To expand the definition of intelligence even further, researchers, especially those involved in holistic health research, are finding evidence that consciousness, emotion, and memory extend beyond the nervous system into the soft tissues of the body. Reports abound of intense emotions or repressed memories being released as certain areas of the body are massaged, especially when the massage is working on deep tissue, such as with certain intense Swedish massage strokes, myotherapy, or Rolfing (see Chapter 11 for a more detailed discussion of deep tissue massage).

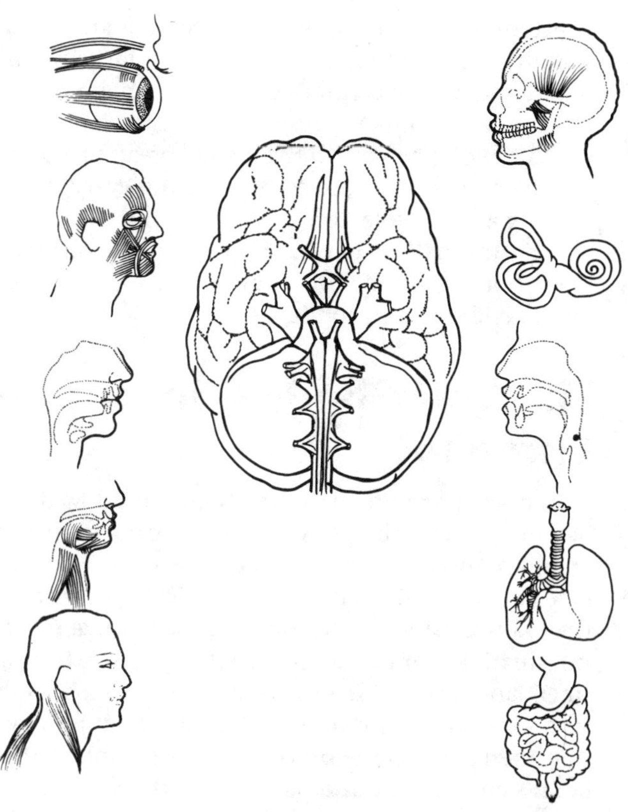

From the muscles to the sensory organs, such as the eyes or the inner ear, to internal organs and body systems, such as the lungs or the digestive system, the brain communicates directly with every part of the human body. Massage keeps the dialogue open, free, and healthy!

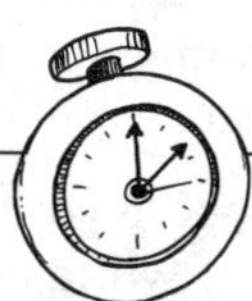

A Massage Minute

People don't all learn in the same way. Because bodywork involves re-education, knowing your learning style can help you to get the most from your bodywork experience. According to one theory, *concrete perceivers* learn by actual experience. *Abstract perceivers* learn by observing and then analyzing what they observe. *Active processors* understand by using learned information in a practical way, and *reflective processors* understand by reflecting on learned information.

Every cell has a *cytoskeletal structure*, and every cytoskeleton is connected to its external environment. Connective tissue, which is woven throughout the entire body in and around organs, muscles, and bones, may serve as a sort of primitive circuit board,

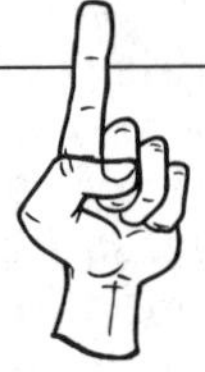

Touch Talk

Cytoskeletal structure is sometimes referred to as the cell's individual nervous system. Connected on a molecular level to the body's entire tissue matrix, the cytoskeletal structure gives the cell its shape. Some researchers believe the cytoskeleton is a storehouse for cellular memory, which can then be communicated to the rest of the body through the tissue matrix.

registering vibrations of every movement and storing that information in a method certainly far more rudimentary than the central nervous system, but quite possibly with similar consequence. Because massage works directly on connective tissue, breaking apart *adhesions* between muscles and keeping everything moving and flexible, it may promote the release of stored information, encouraging our conscious awareness of our emotional lives, and in turn, increasing our intelligent reactions to life.

The Brain-Body Conversation: Listen In!

How does the brain talk to the body, and how does the body talk back? The physical processes are immensely complex and beyond the scope of this book, but we'll give you a simplified overview. To do anything at all, the brain needs information, and the brain gets that information from your senses: what you see, hear, feel, smell, and taste. When the brain receives sensory input, it processes the information, deciding what to do with it. It then delivers the processed information to the brain's emotional center (also called the *limbic system*), which makes a judgment call based largely on both instinctual responses and stored past experiences. The emotional center then prompts the body to act appropriately.

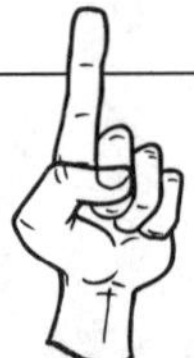

Touch Talk

Adhesions are abnormal connections between tissues, such as muscles stuck together with connective tissue, that are caused by injury, stress, or misuse. Massage can break apart adhesions to restore normal function to muscles and connective tissue.

Suppose you're walking down the street, and you see a huge white dog standing in your path. Your eyes send the signal of what you've seen to your brain. Your brain registers "big white dog in my path," and then sends this signal to your limbic system. If your past experience with dogs has always been pleasant, your emotional response will be far different than if you were attacked by a big white dog when you were a small child.

In either case, your limbic system will most likely temper your reactions with an instinctual response that a big white dog could be potentially dangerous. (This is, of course, a necessarily oversimplified description of a complex process.) Then, depending on who you are and what your past experiences with dogs were like, your limbic system may tell your body to turn around and run, to proceed with caution, to walk confidently around the dog, or to approach the dog in a friendly manner, hoping it will let you pat it on the head.

What does all this have to do with being smart? Our very consciousness of existence is due purely to our sensory input and our brain's interpretation of it. A multitude of different factors in every individual can influence the reactions in the brain, and those reactions determine what is variously interpreted as intelligence (or a lack of it!). In other words, not everyone's brain works in the same way. Even beyond differences in past memories stored in our brains, people have minutely different and individual brain structures, brain chemistries, and bodies. Add to that a lifetime of physical and emotional experiences stored in both brains and soft tissue, and you've got a whole world full of individuals who will perceive and react to life in their own unique ways.

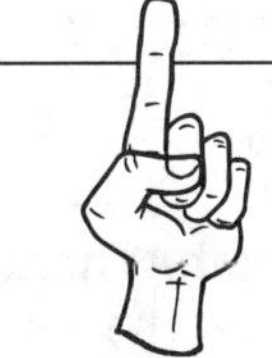

Touch Talk

The limbic system is the brain's emotional center. A more primitive area of the brain (present in evolution long before higher brain functions evolved), the limbic system reacts to sensory signals and cues the body to act without analysis or interpretation.

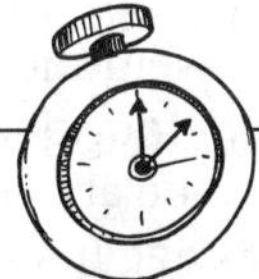

A Massage Minute

Proof that massage may improve brain power and function: Some experts suggest that gentle massage can be great therapy for Alzheimer's patients. Massage therapists report that, even though Alzheimer's patients may not retain the memory of a massage or the massage therapist even immediately afterwards, some patients seem less agitated, more receptive, and more communicative during and after massage.

On the other hand, there are more and less successful ways to act and react when living in a complex society. You could say that people who learn from experiences are more intelligent than people who make the same mistakes over and over again. You could say someone who is able to integrate his or her rational and emotional sides is more intelligent than someone who denies one side in favor of the other. You could also say that awareness of one's physical, emotional, mental, and spiritual state constitutes intelligence. Most people would agree with these definitions of intelligence before they would say intelligence equals being good at calculus or having a large vocabulary. Because massage works on the whole body, increasing overall awareness, enhancing sensory function, releasing repressed memory, calming the emotional mind, and clearing the rational mind, massage certainly has the potential to make you smarter.

Emotions in Motion

The part of the brain that deals with emotions (the limbic system) is more primitive and has existed far longer than the part of the brain that deals with rational, logical thought. When confronted with an extreme circumstance such as danger, our senses channel the data to our rational center so it can interpret an appropriate response, and then inform our emotional centers so they can produce a feeling, such as fear or anger. This feeling can then prompt a physical response, such as fighting or fleeing.

More recent discoveries have revealed a circuit that travels directly from the senses to the limbic system. While our higher brain is processing information logically, our limbic system receives just enough information to react almost instantaneously to an emergency. Before we have even registered that the noise behind us is a car, we may leap out of the way. Before we even realize what we smell is smoke, we may already be headed to the baby's room. Rational thought isn't always involved when action is warranted. Sometimes we act on an instinctive level of intelligence, where mind and body are even more closely linked.

Our emotions often govern us, whether good or bad, and intelligent control over our emotions is an important step to overall intelligence. Note that control over emotions does not mean denial of emotions—emotional denial can have disastrous effects on the mind and on the body. Part of emotional control is emotional acknowledgment. You have to know what you feel to be able to understand and control what you feel. Emotional awareness is where massage fits in.

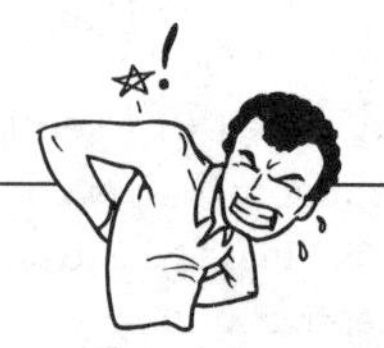

Ouch!

Instinctive emotional reactions can save lives, but they can also be inaccurate because they aren't processed through the rational brain. For example, if someone has a gun, he or she may shoot at a strange noise in a dark house before realizing it is someone harmless—a family member, a friend, or a pet. Instincts are important for our survival, but they can't always be trusted.

Our emotions aren't stuck into some isolated little pocket deep into our brains, even if a particular area of our brains controls emotional responses. Everything that happens to us is imprinted upon our bodies. Your individual posture, stance, and habits of movement are all products of your experience, and much of that experience is emotional. You might have a slight limp from a skiing accident or a scar from an elementary school jungle gym fall, but you might also store your job stress in your neck muscles, your failed relationships in your lower back, and your low self-image in your slumped shoulders. On a more positive note, your optimistic attitude might be revealed by the spring in your step, your happy marriage by your easy posture, your inner contentment by your serene facial expression. It's all there in your body. You are a living, breathing, moving photo album of your past experience.

But the photograph album isn't fixed. You can slide the pictures you don't like out of their pockets and replace them with newer ones, and massage can help. As massage works on the body, it can release the negative emotions stored there. No, it can't erase negative experiences. Those will always be a part of your past, but it can help your body to focus on and embrace the positive experiences, both those in the past and those to come. After all, no photo album can hold pictures of every moment of your entire life. You have to pick and choose which moments to display. Much of this work you must do on your own, though massage, and many other forms of bodywork, can make your job a little easier by adjusting your body so that it becomes a template far more suitable to positive emotions.

Gesture and Movement: Mindfulness in Action

Your body at rest can reveal much about you, but so can your body in motion. Movement can do more than reveal your emotional condition. The way you move can influence the way you feel and the way you think—and vice versa. Even more significantly, you can learn how to move mindfully and with a consciousness that can change your inner life.

Many types of bodywork, which fall under the general category of somatics, teach students how to move mindfully, truly fusing body and mind. Bodywork that deals with gesture and movement involves a personal exploration. As opposed to passively receiving massage, the student of somatics actively learns how to perceive and how to pay attention to specific movements again.

If you get the chance, watch a child at play. Children delight in the movements of their own bodies. They truly experience movement, and it is part of their consciousness. Most of us lose this consciousness as we grow older, however. Movement becomes habit and a part of the subconscious. Most of us live in our minds, not in our bodies, as adults. Our bodies perform the necessary tasks for living. They are a means to an end. They are no longer an end in themselves.

Somatics reminds us what it feels like to move mindfully. Somatics teaches

- How to move based only on internal impulses, not external rules or demands
- The mind to make a conscious decision to move before any movement takes place
- Movement that reflects or releases the psychological state

Your Finger on the Pulse

Try this exercise for increasing your self-awareness through movement: Stand in the middle of a room. Close your eyes. Feel where your body exists in space: your feet, your legs, your hips, your stomach and back, your chest, your arms and hands, your neck, and your head. Notice everything, but don't move until you feel an inner impulse to move. Then, notice how the movement feels.

Many early practitioners of somatics in Europe worked in close contact with Sigmund Freud, believing that the internal perception of the body was directly linked with the psychological state.

Internal perception of the body by the mind is indeed what somatics is all about, no matter the specifics of the technique. Somatics teaches active self-awareness and conscious self-regulation and adjustment in response to that self-awareness. It is a dynamic process in which body and mind are indistinguishable.

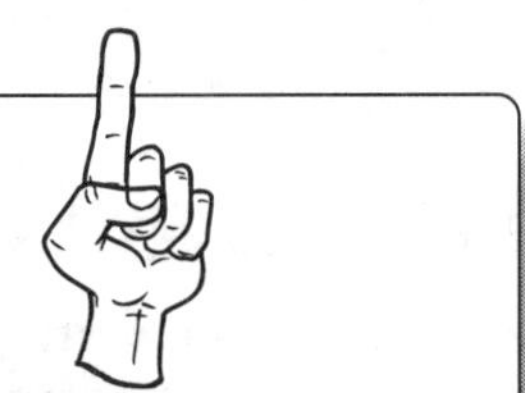

Touch Talk

Creative visualization is a technique for attaining what you desire, such as material possessions, spiritual goals, or certain life situations, by regularly visualizing yourself already in possession of what you desire. The theory goes that because everything is essentially energy, thoughts (energy) can influence matter (energy), and creating a mental template of what you want will affect the physical reality.

You can begin to become more self-aware by making an effort to notice yourself more often. Every so often throughout the course of the day, notice how you feel. Be specific. Where do you feel tension? Where do you feel relaxed? How are you standing or sitting or walking or talking or gesturing? What's on your mind? In other words, notice yourself from the inside out.

Learning to move with consciousness can bring increased awareness to every aspect of your life. Too many of us barrel through our days with barely a thought to the journey because we are so intent on getting to work, getting home, getting the house clean, getting that project finished, getting to sleep, waking up, and getting to work again. Mindfulness through somatic bodywork reminds us who we are by continually asking the question "Who are you?" through the medium of gesture and movement.

Meditation and Massage

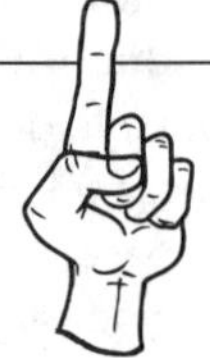

Touch Talk

The **Lotus position** is a seated yoga pose in which the legs are crossed and each ankle is placed on top of the opposite thigh. Often used for meditation, this position is said to resemble the beauty and symmetry of the lotus flower.

Another less physically active way to ask yourself who you are is to practice meditation. Although not bodywork (meditation is more mindwork), meditation is a wonderful way to prepare your mind for a massage and also to retain the benefits and relaxed sensation of a massage after it is over.

Meditation means different things to different people, whether it's a particular technique taught in a school, class, or seminar; *creative visualization;* or simply meditating in your own way. Your personal meditation could involve anything from sitting quietly in the *Lotus position* for an hour each evening to relaxing and focusing your mind when you walk from the parking lot to the office each morning. The purpose of all meditation is the same: to clear your head of the flotsam and jetsam of daily living. Clearing out this stuff makes you better able to focus on your massage or whatever life experience you want to experience fully.

Let Your Breathing Do the Thinking

What is the one thing that binds us, physically, to our universe? It is part of the universe, we take it into ourselves, transform it, and then release it. You guessed it: breath. Breath is energy and life. If you stop breathing for more than a few minutes, you will die. Deep breathing helps you to thrive. According to yogic philosophy, breath is pure energy and can nourish the body even better than food and replenish the body more effectively than sleep. Knowing how to breathe means knowing how to thrive. Deep breathing feeds your body, your brain, and your spirit.

But breathing isn't bodywork—or is it? You can certainly learn deep breathing techniques in the same way you can learn movement techniques. You can also incorporate deep breathing before, during, and after your massage experience. When receiving a massage, people often let out an unexpected and surprisingly deep sigh. This sigh is a sign that the body is truly breathing, oxygen is moving, and toxins are being eliminated. When you are breathing deeply during a massage, the point of the exhalation is a great time for the massage therapist to go a little deeper into the soft tissue. Massage therapists may also synchronize the rhythm of the massage to the massagee's pattern of breathing. Deep breathing can also help you to hold onto the relaxed state after a massage is over.

Mastering control over the breath is an important step toward self-awareness. In conjunction with massage, it can be the key to a new level of intelligence that involves a deep body-mind awareness and the integration of your rational, emotional, and instinctual minds.

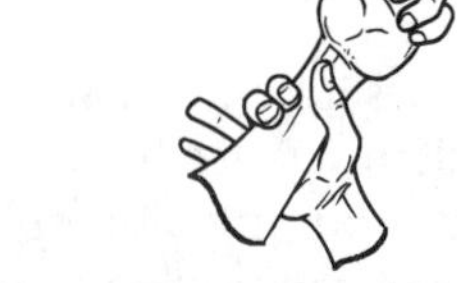

Your Finger on the Pulse

Try this breathing exercise in preparation for massage, during massage, or in conjunction with the massage strokes. Take your right hand and place it on top of your left shoulder. Inhale deeply. As you exhale, slowly slide your hand down your shoulder, all the way down your arm to your fingertips. Feel the tensions release out of your whole arm.

Be a Know-It-All

What does it mean to know it all? Certainly, no one person can be aware of every existing fact, and no one can have every possible experience. On the other hand, because we exist in our own minds and everything we see, do, know, and understand comes from our own brains (a highly subjective point of view at best), maybe we can know it all. Considering that each person's only possible perspective is a necessarily personal one, knowing it all is really nothing more than knowing yourself completely, and that doesn't sound like such an intimidating goal.

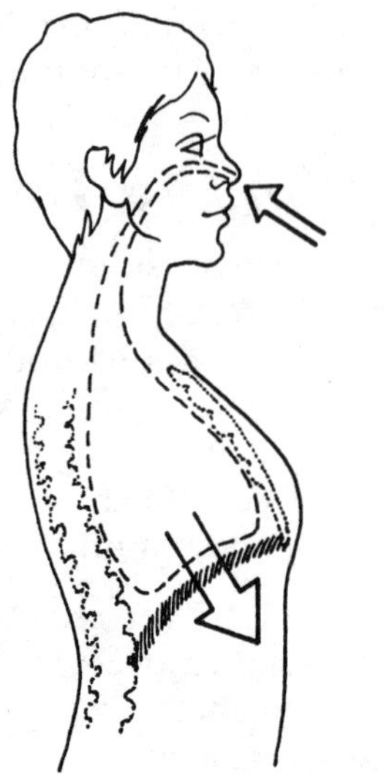

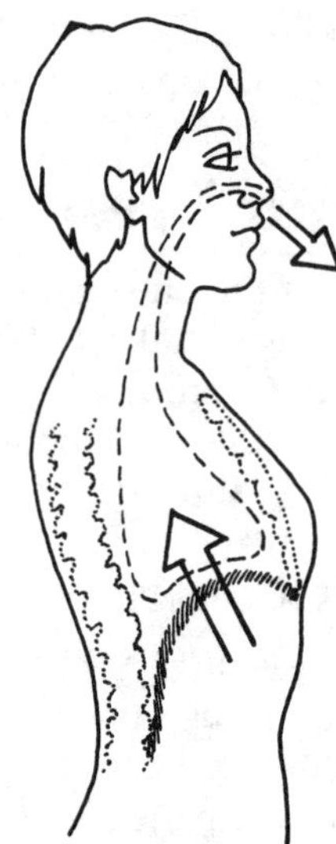

The diaphragm muscles move downward during inhalation and upward during exhalation. Take a few deep breaths and feel the rhythm of the diaphragm as it moves.

Or does it? You are by no means a simple organism. Your brain alone contains depths modern science has only begun to plumb. Add to that the rest of your complicated body, your ineffable spirit, your elaborate personality, and the minutiae of your experience from conception to this very moment, and knowing yourself may not seem so simple after all. Yet what could be a more interesting area of study? Working to know your body and optimize your mind are goals worthy of your time. Let bodywork become a part of your life, and know thyself.

The Least You Need to Know

- Massage not only enhances brain function but increases emotional self-awareness and other intelligence-enhancing traits.
- Your brain and body talk back and forth so you can react best in any situation.
- Somatics is bodywork that teaches increased self-awareness and self-mastery through movement.
- Meditation and deep breathing enhance both massage and body-mind intelligence.
- To know thyself is to know all!

Part 3
Massage Basics

This section gets down to the business of getting, or giving, a massage, whether at home or from a massage therapist. We'll advise you on how to set up a personal massage space at home; we'll help you create a mood, decide what to wear (or not to wear), and offer some tips on massage products and equipment. We'll teach you how to build up your hand strength and establish a massage rhythm, and we'll give you a little more encouragement on the importance of touch.

For those of you who would like to try a professional massage (and we highly recommend it!), we'll advise you on how to find the right massage therapist for you, where to find qualified therapists, and even whether your insurance might cover the treatment (it very well might).

Next, the big question: What kind of massage should you get? We'll brief you on many of the most popular techniques out there, including Swedish massage, Esalan, structural integration, Rolfing, trigger point therapy, hydrotherapy, sports massage, manual lymph drainage, craniosacral therapy, applied kinesiology, and reflexology. We'll talk about some of the more esoteric techniques, such as polarity therapy, orthobionomy, Reiki, the Alexander technique, yoga, qigong, Trager, Aston-Patterning, and Feldenkrais. Finally, we'll explore the Oriental techniques, including acupressure, acupuncture, shiatsu, and Jin Shin Do. Then all you'll have to do is choose. (Oh, and we'll give you a quiz to help you do that, too!)

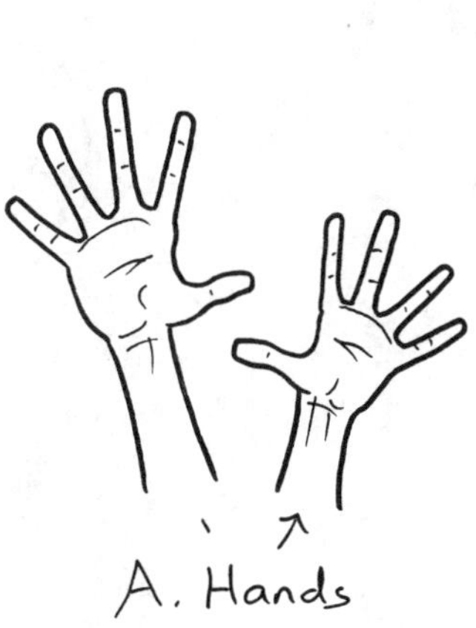

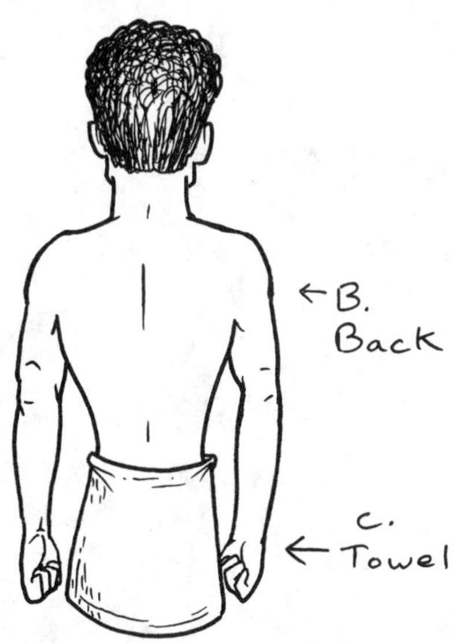

Chapter 9

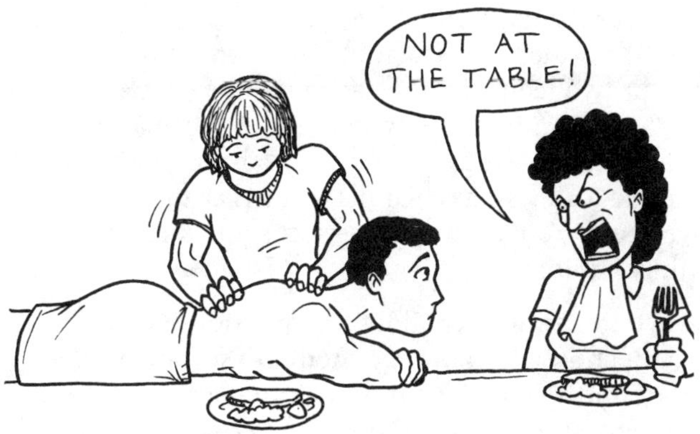

Getting, or Giving, a Massage at Home

In This Chapter

- How to create the ultimate massage area in your home
- How to determine the best time for a massage
- A few tricks for helping those tired hands last a little longer

Now that you've learned so much about the body and the wonderful benefits of massage, you're probably eager to get started. But before you skip right off to Appendix C to try some massage routines for yourself, we suggest you read a little bit further. In this chapter, we'll tell you how to get good and ready for the ultimate home massage because, although massage can be done anywhere (while watching television, while waiting for dinner to cook, while sitting at your desk), it's always much nicer if you can create the ultimate massage environment in order to keep all your senses attuned to the experience.

As long as you're thinking about home massage, don't forget your options: Massage can be learned and effectively practiced through books like this one. You can also supplement your "book learnin'" with a variety of audiotapes and videotapes that show and tell how to perform various types of massages, from infant massage to simple Swedish massage techniques to do-it-yourself shiatsu. (See the back of this book to order Joan Budilovsky's massage audiotapes and videotapes: *The Art of Massage Made Simple*; *Foot Massage: Body, Mind, and Sole*; and *Swedish Massage 101*.)

Setting Up Your Massage Area

If you plan to make massage a part of your regular home life (and we suggest you do!), you'll want to have an area specifically set aside for massage. No, you don't need to force your two teenagers to share a room so you can have a "massage room." Any massage area can also be used for other purposes, but creating a great place in your home for massages will make it easier to perform or receive them. You'll have the perfect spot all ready for you, fully equipped.

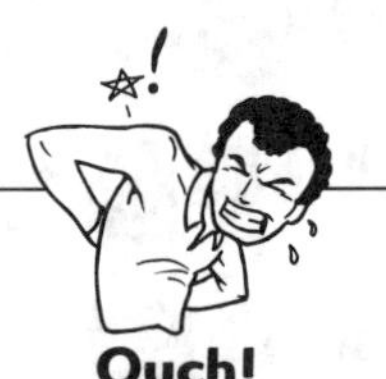

Ouch!

Lots of people give home massages on a bed, but beds are too soft to provide the proper resistance necessary for a good massage and may be too low for the person giving the massage to maintain the best position. A floor with a cushy carpet or some blankets can work if the massager uses pillows to cushion his or her knees while working.

Unless you have an incredibly tranquil household, the room you choose for massage shouldn't be one in the center of traffic. You'll want to maintain a serene atmosphere, so a back bedroom, study, or any other room where you can close the door and shut out the outside world is ideal. The room should be clean and inviting; good ventilation is also important—if you can open the window on a beautiful day, all the better, unless the massage recipient finds an open window distracting due to noise or temperature. The room should be big enough for the recipient to lie or sit comfortably and should give the massager plenty of room to maneuver.

If you've got the space, keep your massage room supplied with the following equipment:

- Small and large pillows and/or bolsters
- A few clean sheets
- A light but warm blanket
- Clothing hangers and somewhere to hang them
- A comfortable robe
- A clock
- A box of tissues and a wastebasket
- A live plant for extra oxygen

A well-supplied massage area will allow you to get or give the perfect massage at a moment's notice.

Assuming the Position

If you aren't a massage therapist, you probably won't want to invest in an expensive professional massage table, even though they do provide the ultimate surface for a great massage. Massage tables allow the person massaged to lie face down without craning his or her neck to either side, and are often adjustable to different positions and heights.

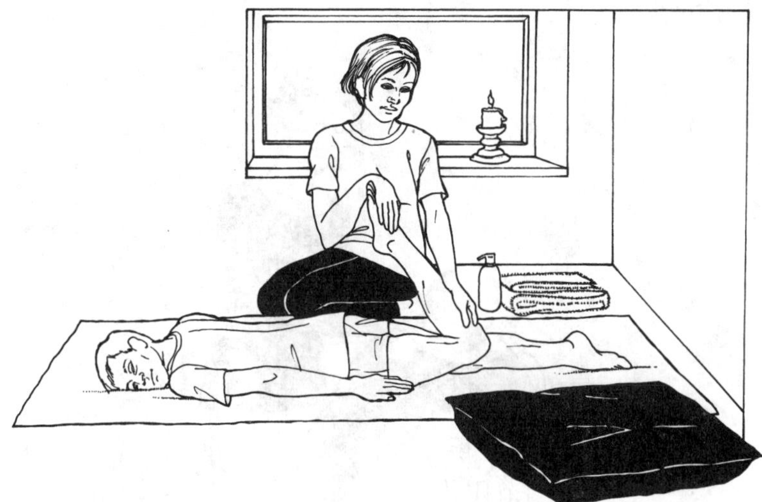

If you don't have a massage table, you can use the floor! Keep a large pillow handy. If you're the one giving the massage, you may want a pillow to cushion and protect your knees from the hard floor. Or try placing a large pillow between the back of your thighs and your calves. When you sit back, it will take some strain off of your bent knees.

In the absence of a professional massage table, and if your knees (or the rest of you) just aren't up to giving a massage on the floor, you'll need to consider what furniture to provide in your massage area.

Will you want your massage recipient to be seated or lying down? When most people imagine a massage, they envision receiving it while lying down, and this is the best position for a complete, full-body massage. If you choose to go this route, you'll need a home massage table, but that doesn't mean you have to buy one. Most people have something in their homes that will suffice (even if it's the dining room table).

Whatever table you choose, it should be sturdy and stable. You don't want a table that rocks back and forth or creaks with every massage stroke. The ideal massage table height should be level with the outer wrist bone of the person giving the massage, when he or she stands next to the table with arms hanging down. Massage tables should be about 29 inches wide and 76 inches long (shorter is fine if your massage recipients can fit fully onto the table without any body parts hanging over the edge) to allow easiest access to the massage recipient. (A very tall person's feet may hang over the edge of the table, which may become uncomfortable. Lots of pillows can alleviate some of the discomfort.) Your massage table must also be padded, either with a couple of inches of foam, a few folded sleeping bags or quilts, or whatever other padding will be comfortable but relatively firm. (Bed mattresses are too soft, but the right size exercise mat might be perfect.) Make sure the padding cushions the table edges and corners.

Chairs are great places for quick massages, especially those that concentrate on the back, neck, and arms. Some massage therapists make their living visiting people's offices and offering massages during breaks or lunch hours, right there in the office chair. Seated massage is also good for older people or anyone who might be more comfortable seated than lying down.

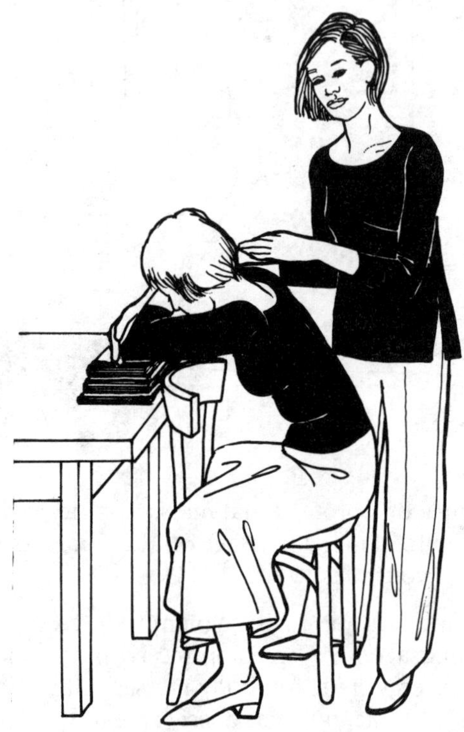

You can use a stack of books to adjust the chair's height when giving a seated massage at the office. If it's easy to find one, look for a pillow to use as a cushion over the books and chair back. If you can't find a pillow, go as is!

If you plan to give a massage to someone who is seated, the best chair is one with no arms and a comfortable, padded back. The massage recipient can sit backwards in the chair with his or her arms and head resting on the padded back. This position offers comfort to the recipient and full access to the back and arms. Some padded office chairs are ideal for chair massages and are height-adjustable. A stool scooted up to a desk or table, on which the receiver can rest his or her arms and head, is another option.

Massage Aids

If you want to get a little more fancy, you can also purchase a variety of massage aids that can benefit both the massage recipient and giver. Massage aids can add a different dimension to massage by utilizing the benefits of different temperatures or types of stimulation and also by making the giver's job a little less strenuous.

The types of massage aids most available for use in the home are hot and cold packs, heating pads, and vibrators. You can use hot and cold packs on injured areas, but exercise caution. Heat dilates blood vessels and increases circulation to an area, and cold can stimulate an area if applied briefly or numb and reduce circulation to an area if applied for longer periods. The wrong treatment could have an injurious effect. A cold pack over the eyes for a tension headache or a heat pack or heating pad over the abdomen for menstrual cramps are two good examples of ways you can use heat and cold during a massage to make the experience more pleasant.

Vibrators are another good way to increase your massage repertoire. We're not talking about those kind of vibrators they sell in the back of certain brown-paper-wrapped magazines, but the kind specifically meant for use in therapeutic massage. You can use vibration to loosen tight muscles, increase circulation, or generally impart a feeling of relaxation. Some vibrators strap to the hand; others are held with one or two hands and moved over the back, arms, and legs. Vibrators may move back and forth or in a circular or thumping motion. Light application of the vibrator on muscle tissue tends to be relaxing; using firmer pressure tends to be stimulating. Don't overuse vibration equipment, though, or it could numb the area.

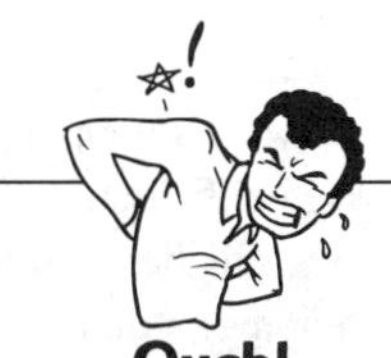

Ouch!

During a massage, you may want to experiment by applying hot or cold treatments to the recipient. Never apply heat or cold packs or heating pads to an injury without prior approval from your physician. Applying heat to an area that's swelling, such as a sprained ankle, would increase circulation to the area and make things worse. Applying the wrong type of treatment can aggravate injuries and prolong healing.

Choosing the Right Time

When would you like a massage? Any time you can get one? Good answer! However, some times are better than others, and the rules differ from person to person.

Massage for Wherever You Are

The best way to determine when you would benefit most from a massage is to look at your day. When are you the most stressed? First thing in the morning, when you're rushing around to get everyone, including yourself, to wherever they need to be?

Mid-day, when your morning workload has overwhelmed you? Late afternoon, when you hit that dreaded energy slump and can't function for one more minute? Or in the evenings after work, when you collapse, your head buzzing with everything you didn't accomplish?

A Massage Minute

Everyone's temperature fluctuates slightly during the day, usually between about 96 and 100 degrees Fahrenheit. This fluctuation is directly related to your energy level: When your temperature is higher, you feel more energetic. When your temperature drops (as it usually does near bedtime), you'll feel much lower on energy and ready for a snooze. Your energy level during massage can directly affect your massage experience and the way a massage works on your body.

Your time of peak stress is a good time for a relaxing massage, whether it's a chair massage on your lunch hour or a full-body massage from your partner at the end of a long day. On the other hand, those times when you're relaxed and feeling great can be ideal for massage. Your mind will be fully able to take in the experience without straying to your excessive obligations or worrying that you should be getting something done. Your body will already be relaxed, so massage can move beyond relaxing you to working on improving your circulation and body functions on a deeper level. Although the difference between how you feel before and after a relaxed massage might not be as dramatic as after a massage given when every muscle is clenched, regular massages when you're already relaxed may have an even more pronounced benefit on your health.

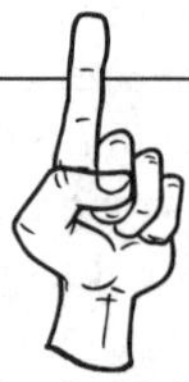

Touch Talk

Circadian rhythms are your internal rhythms of temperature, hormone levels, and energy. Circadian rhythms vary among individuals (especially between morning people and night owls), but most people tend to have high energy in late morning and late afternoon, an energy slump an hour or two after lunchtime (siesta time), and the need for a long period of sleep beginning a few hours before midnight.

Circadian Rhythm: The Rhythm of Life

Another way to look at your day when scheduling massage is to examine your *circadian rhythms*. These internal rhythms affect your temperature, energy levels, and even hormone levels throughout the day. If you are a morning person who functions best before noon and has a horrible time accomplishing anything in the evening, you might find that late afternoons or evenings are good times for an energizing massage (though not too close to bedtime). If you're a night owl and find it torture to get up before 10 or 11 a.m., a morning massage might help you to get through the day.

On the other hand, just as receiving a massage when you're feeling relaxed can be extremely beneficial, so can receiving a massage when you're at your energy peak. Morning massages for morning people or evening massages for night owls can feel incredible and further enhance those feel-good, high-energy periods of your day.

Setting the Mood

Now that you have the time and the place, you need to set the mood. Creating the right ambiance can make massage even more pleasurable and relaxing. It can help to release your mind and engage all your senses in the massage experience. Give your massage experience visual appeal by keeping your massage area clean and aesthetically pleasing. The massage itself and the comfort of your massage table or chair will appeal to your sense of touch. And don't forget the powerful influences of hearing and smell.

Enya, Anyone? Or Mostly Mozart?

Music can add a whole new dimension to your massage experience. Maybe you love the spiritual quality of New Age music. Maybe classical is your ultimate favorite. Maybe soft jazz will relax you every time. You can even purchase CDs and tapes that feature the sounds of nature, such as running water, wind in the trees, rain, or ocean waves. Equip your massage area with a tape or CD player, and you'll soon find yourself transported by the combination of relaxing touch and sound that takes you away from it all or, better yet, brings you back to yourself.

Getting "Scents"ual: Candles and Incense

Using scented candles, incense, and other forms of aromatherapy can add yet another dimension to your "scents"ual experience. Scented candles add visual beauty as well as a pleasing aroma to a massage area. Incense can perfume a room beautifully, although the massage recipient (and also the giver) shouldn't directly inhale the smoke—keep it in the background.

Although everyone reacts to aromas differently, the following scents tend to invoke the following reactions (some people are sensitive to oils, so test a drop or two on a small patch of skin before applying over a large area):

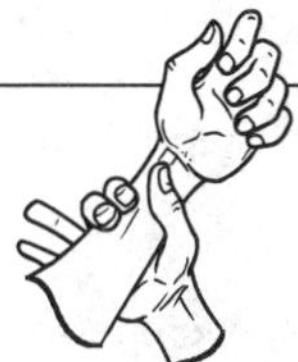

Your Finger on the Pulse

Like the idea of a musical massage, but not sure what music to try? Consider new age, classical, soft jazz, earth sounds, ocean sounds, chanting, or anything else that helps your mind to relax. Avoid music that engages your mind with busy lyrics or a hopping rhythm. The key is to keep it simple and soft.

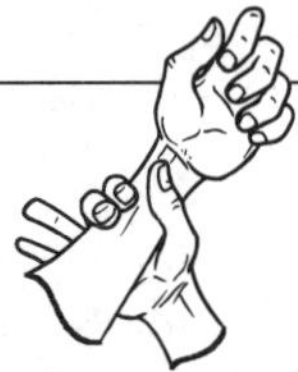

Your Finger on the Pulse

Ayur-Veda, an ancient Indian system of health, recommends a sesame oil self-massage each morning to relax and balance the body. Warm a quarter cup of sesame oil (not too hot!), undress, stand in the shower or bath, dip your hands in the warm oil, and massage your body from scalp to feet, firmly stroking muscles and gently massaging joints. Then, shower in warm water.

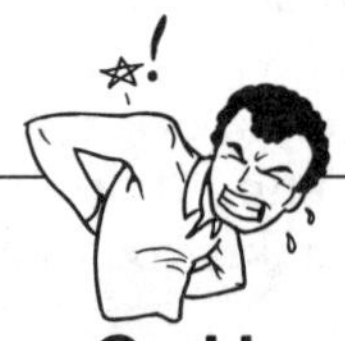

Ouch!

When receiving a massage, your body isn't in motion and may tend to feel cold, especially in your extremities (feet and hands), more so than if you were moving around the house. Always keep a supply of light, soft blankets handy for warmth. Warm muscles respond much better to massage than cold muscles, and cold can make you feel more tense, too.

- Chamomile is soothing.
- Cinnamon is warming.
- Eucalyptus is invigorating.
- Geranium is balancing.
- Lavender is restorative and healing.
- Lemon is reviving.
- Pepper is strengthening.
- Sandalwood is grounding.
- Tea Tree is cooling.

Other aroma options include aroma diffusers or essential oils warmed in warming rings that can be placed over light bulbs. Another popular option is to use essential oils or other scented preparations as massage oils.

Everyone reacts differently to different aromas, however, so make sure any scented oil you use is pleasant to both giver and receiver. You may be crazy for the scent of vanilla, but the person you're massaging may not share your enthusiasm. Experiment with different scents and the sensations they invoke: relaxation, serenity, energy, joy. For a more detailed discussion of aromatherapy and massage, see Chapter 19.

To Dress or to Undress, that Is the Question

Should you disrobe when getting a massage? Your answer to that question probably depends on a few factors, such as who's giving you a massage, how long you want the massage to last, and whether you expect company (or kids) to come bursting into the room at any moment. A massage is best performed on bare skin, so if the situation warrants it, disrobing is probably the best option. Professional massage therapists typically drape the body with a sheet and undrape only the area they're working on at the moment. This technique allows for less stress due to modesty, and the important temperature factor (it can get pretty cold lying there in your skivvies!).

If the person giving you a massage is your partner or close relative and you feel perfectly comfortable around them when in your birthday suit, great! You might still want a cover to keep your muscles toasty, but you'll feel more relaxed about whatever part is uncovered. If, on the other hand, you aren't quite comfortable being totally naked, no problem. Almost any type of massage can be performed over light clothing, especially if arms, legs, and neck are exposed. If you only have a few minutes for a quick relaxation massage, anyway, you won't have the time for the whole undressing-massage-dressing routine.

How Much Is Enough?

How long would you like your massage to last? You might answer that question with a question: "How long have you got?" Many massage recipients have groaned despondently when they sense their shoulder or head or foot massage is coming to an end: "Tell me you're not done yet!"

A professional massage usually lasts about an hour, but a home massage can last anywhere from a few precious minutes to an hour or more—if the massage giver's hand muscles can last that long! How long the giver of a massage can last without muscle fatigue, especially if he or she isn't a professional massage therapist, depends on a few factors, including the intensity of touch, basic hand strength, and the use of lotions and oils.

Light, Moderate, or Firm to the Touch

A gentle, feathery massage is easier to sustain over long periods than a firm, deep tissue massage. If you prefer to receive a vigorous massage with lots of muscle behind it, you probably shouldn't expect your partner to be able to keep it up for an hour. A light touch can be sustained much longer. When you're giving the massage, probably the best technique, especially while you're building up your massage muscles, is to alternate deep and light strokes.

If you aren't used to giving a massage, you might not last long at all. Some people have very little hand strength, and anything beyond a light stroke results in muscle cramps or fatigue after just a few minutes. You needn't be ashamed of your weakling hands, however. Take action with these easy steps to building hand strength.

(1) Put palm out and down.
(2) Pull gently back with your other hand.
(3) Hold for three breaths.
(4) Repeat these steps with palm up and palm in. Do both hands.

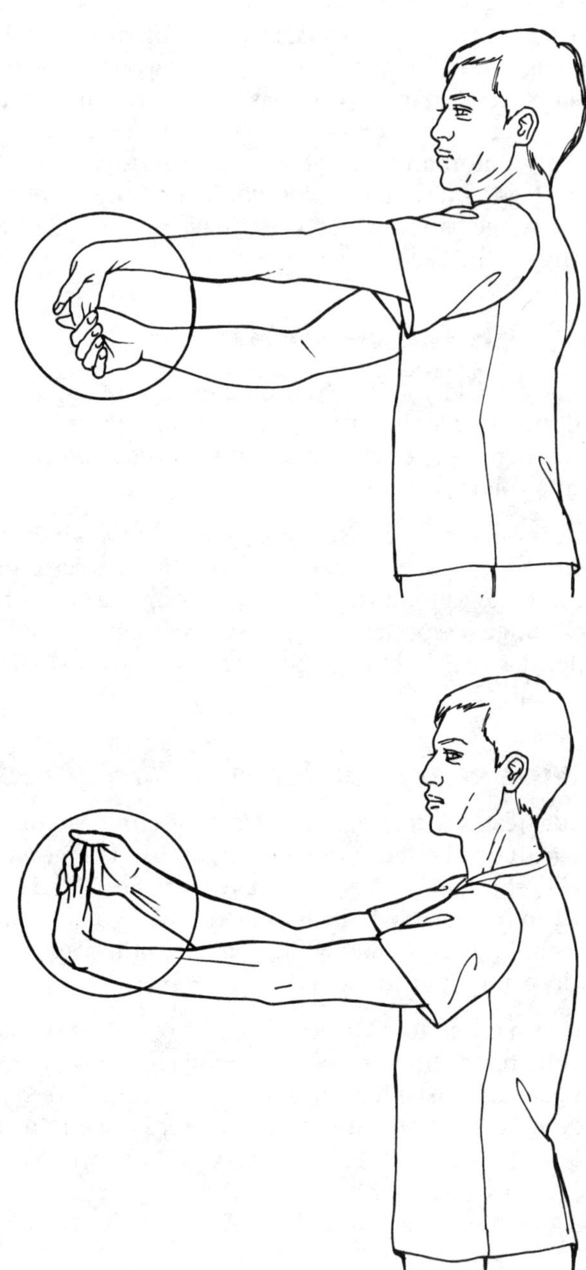

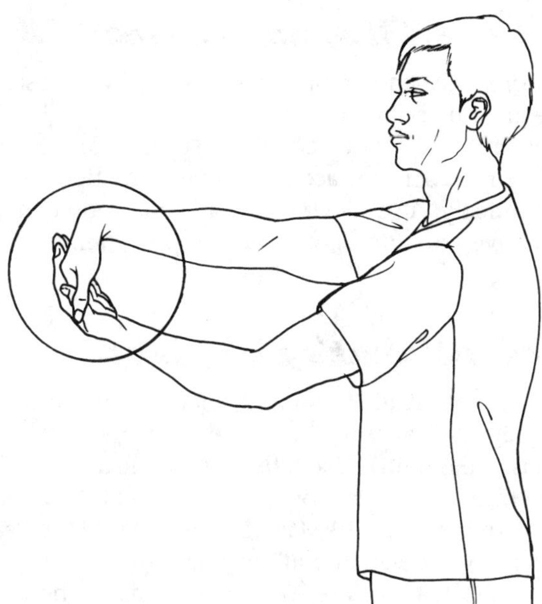

Another way to offer an extended massage is to keep in touch, literally. If you need to rest your hands for a bit, keep them on the skin of the person you're massaging. Remember earlier in this book when we talked about how giving a massage can be as beneficial as receiving one? Part of this benefit has to do with the energy that flows between giver and receiver through touch. Keeping in constant touch with the person you're massaging will help to keep your energy replenished.

Establishing a Rhythm

Random stroking here and there can lead to boredom on the part of the massage giver, which often causes the massage to be cut short. Having a plan for a massage and finding a rhythm are good ways to know how much is ahead of you as a massage giver and where you're going. When you've mastered the various massage strokes in Part 4, check out Appendix C for some massage routines (although massage never has to be routine!), and then find the pace that works for you and for your receiver. Massaging to relaxing music can help you establish a rhythm, too. Finding your rhythm is where massage becomes an art form. It's like learning to play music: Basic scales on the piano can be boring to learn and practice, but once you've got them mastered, you can create a masterpiece!

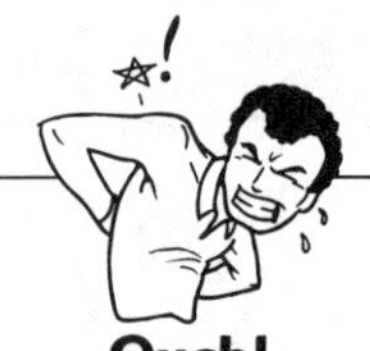

Ouch!

In general, avoid mineral oil as a massage oil because it clogs pores. Stick with vegetable, fruit, and nut oils, which smell nice and react well with most skin types.

Lotions, Oils, and Cremes, Oh My!

Lotions, oils, and cremes can make massage easier on the giver by reducing the friction of skin on skin. Not all lubricants are created equal, however. Some produce a silky or slippery surface; others become sticky or soak in too quickly. Also remember that some people may have sensitive skin and may request or prefer an unscented product.

A Finish that's Just Right

When that dreaded moment, that moment when the massage is at an end, does at last arrive, how do you end gently and gradually? Ending a massage is a little like telling someone a piece of news. The way you tell it will largely determine their reaction. You don't want to stop the massage abruptly and announce sharply, "That's it! Massage over. See ya!" Instead, gradually slow your rhythm, lighten your touch, and allow your strokes to impart the gentle message that the massage is coming to a close. You might consider holding the massagee's feet for a moment or so, for grounding. Last of all, quietly thank the person who has put enough trust in you to receive a massage.

Last but not least, don't forget that after you've given someone a massage, you've forged one more bond. No matter how long-term or intimate your relationship with someone, every massage bonds you yet again. Don't take these bonds lightly—they're the bonds that sustain you and help your life to thrive. Never forget the importance of touch, and your life will be fuller, greater, healthier, and more loving.

The Least You Need to Know

- You'll be more likely to give (and receive) massages if you have a properly equipped massage area set up in your home with just the right ambiance.
- Older people and people who may be uncomfortable lying down can benefit from receiving a massage in a seated position.
- Every individual has internal body rhythms that can determine the best time for a massage.
- Giving a massage can be physically tiring, but there are ways to increase your endurance, such as alternating between firmer and lighter touches, using lotions or oil, building hand strength, having a plan, and taking advantage of the flow of energy from the person you are massaging.

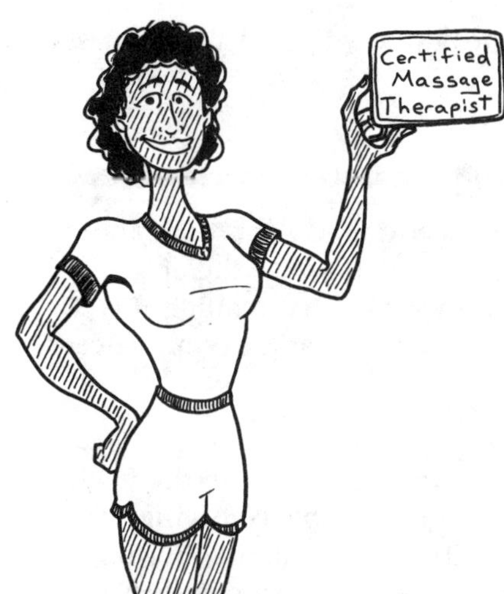

Chapter 10

Getting a Massage from a Massage Therapist

In This Chapter

- How to choose the right massage therapist
- Where to get your massage
- Will your insurance cover your massage?
- What happens during a typical professional massage session

Sure, you're willing to participate in home massages whenever you can, but maybe you're also pretty excited about the prospect of getting a real professional massage from someone with extensive training. You won't regret it! That is, you won't regret it if you choose your massage therapist with a little care. Know your massage goals (remember listing your personal massage goals in Chapter 4?), and then find a therapist who's qualified and, just as importantly, whom you feel you can relate to.

What Makes a Massage Therapist?

Just what is a massage therapist, exactly? Well, that depends where you live. Different states, counties, and even cities have different (or sometimes nonexistent) licensing, certification, or registration requirements for massage therapists. The educational requirements for these licenses vary dramatically, too.

If you live in a state where massage is completely unregulated, you'll want to be even more careful about whom you choose. On the other hand, sometimes the very best massage therapist for you won't have any kind of formal certification at all. Enthusiastic recommendations by people you trust are often the best way to find a great massage therapist.

Playing by the Rules

The first step is to understand the differences between licensing, certification, and other forms of professional credibility. Does your area require massage therapists to be licensed or state-certified? Practicing without a license in a state that requires it is illegal. Call your state licensing agency to find out if massage therapists require licensing in your state.

Certification, on the other hand, isn't legally required to practice massage, but it can be a good indication of adequate training, competence, and knowledge in the field (depending on the certifying organization). One of the most reliable certifying organizations is the National Certification Board for Therapeutic Massage and Bodywork (NCBTMB). The NCBTMB requires certain qualifications for certification and also administers an exam. Those who pass can put the initials *NCTMB* (nationally certified in therapeutic massage and bodywork) after their names for professional use. A massage therapist who is NCTMB-certified has proven that he or she has the skill and knowledge to practice the massage therapy profession.

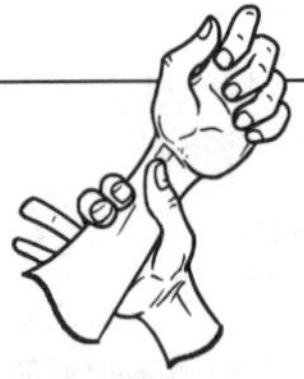

Your Finger on the Pulse

When interviewing massage therapists, ask where they were trained, whether they are licensed (if required) and nationally certified, how they were trained, whether they belong to any professional associations, and what massage techniques they specialize in. Also ask them to describe their personal philosophy on massage and bodywork.

The NCBTMB is accredited by the National Commission for Certifying Agencies to assure high standards in the national certification process. If your massage therapist is certified by some other organization (other certification credentials include Licensed Massage Therapist (LMT) or Certified Massage Therapist (CMT)), you might want to check their requirements, which may or may not uphold rigorous standards for certification. Many are good indications of competency; others aren't.

Membership in a professional association is another indication that your massage therapist takes his or her profession seriously. The two most well-known professional associations are the American Massage Therapy Association (AMTA) and the Associated Bodywork & Massage Professionals (ABMP), but there are many others, such as the American Oriental Bodywork Therapy Association (AOBTA), the International Massage Association (IMA), and other associations geared toward specific bodywork practices. Some professional associations do more for (and require more from) their members. Some may provide liability insurance and some basic information. Others have stringent educational prerequisites and continuing education requirements and require adherence to an established code of ethics to secure and maintain membership.

Many massage schools and programs are accredited, which means they follow certain requirements established by accreditation agencies or associations. Accreditation is just one more quality control measure, assuring consumers (and massage-therapists-in-training) that the program meets certain standards. For example, the Commission on Massage Therapy Accreditation (COMTA) offers massage schools accreditation if they adhere to a wide variety of quality control measures, such as extensive self-evaluation, an approved curriculum, and periodic site inspections. On the other hand, a very small percentage of massage schools are accredited. Many more are "AMTA-approved." Even so, some great schools have no COMTA or AMTA association at all.

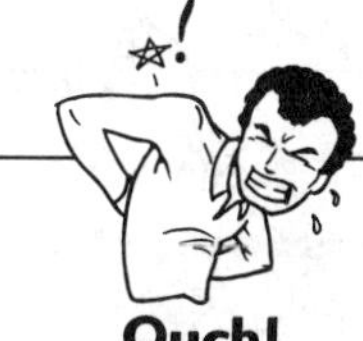

Ouch!

If you prefer a particular gender for a massage therapist because you think your massage experience will be erotic or in any way sexual, you are under a false impression. Although a professional massage is most definitely a sensual experience, it is not about sex.

When searching for a massage therapist, keep in mind that the most qualified, certified, educated massage therapist in the world still might not make you, personally, feel as comfortable as you do in the hands of the elderly German woman down the street who mastered bodywork in Europe before the war and never received a single piece of paper that proves it. Go with what feels right for you.

Male, Female: Who Are You Comfortable With?

Some people couldn't imagine receiving a massage from a massage therapist of the same sex or of the opposite sex. The preference is wholly personal. Whatever your reasons, even if you can't quite explain them or even if you know they aren't quite logical, you need to feel comfortable while receiving your massage. If you can't relax, it doesn't matter why. Some people simply feel more comfortable with one or the other gender. You don't have to explain yourself.

Where to Go to Get Your Massage

Maybe you know just the type of massage therapist you'd like and just what you want to get out of massage, but you aren't sure where to look. These days, massage therapists seem to be popping up everywhere, working out of fitness clubs, visiting you at the office, even conducting business in malls and airports! The following sections detail some of the other places you can seek and find a massage therapist.

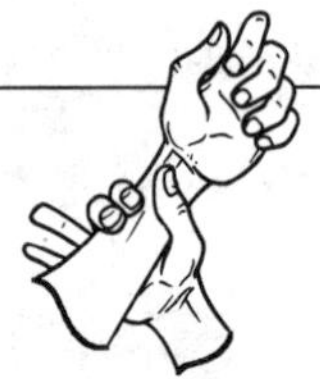

Your Finger on the Pulse

Big cities are replete with bodyworkers, but smaller cities and especially small towns or rural areas may offer an extremely limited choice, if any. If you can't find a good massage therapist near you, don't despair. Learn some basic techniques on your own. Or consider training as a massage therapist—you'll probably end up with more business than you can handle!

The Home Business Massage

Many massage therapists are in business for themselves, and do the bulk of their business from their homes. Getting a massage at the home of a massage therapist can be a comfortable, informal experience that is more pleasant to many than the public setting of a health club or clinic. Massage therapists who work from their homes are professionals, but may also be your best bet if you want to form a bodyworker/client relationship with someone that is unintimidating and relaxed. Some home-based massage therapists will occasionally travel to a client's home.

Don't Come to Us, We'll Come to You

The easiest place to get a massage is in your own home, and lots of massage therapists are happy to oblige. Because massage is a relatively portable business, many independent massage therapists will come to your home, set up their massage tables, give you a great massage, and then leave. This option is great for people who are too busy to get to one more place of business in the course of the day, who are homebound for health reasons, or who can't ever seem to get out of the house because of family obligations, a home business, lack of transportation, or whatever. Of course, the disadvantage to a home massage is that you're stuck in the middle of all your habitual distractions. Setting up a massage area at home can help to counteract this effect.

The Gym (Yes, the Gym!)

If you belong to a gym or fitness center, chances are, they employ a massage therapist (or a whole bevy of bodyworkers). Depending on the gym, massage may or may not be included in the price of membership, but having massage available at the place you go to work out is convenient and makes for good timing—post-workout massages are great for keeping muscles functioning at their peak. Be sure to inquire about your gym's requirements for hiring massage therapists. The gym should be aware of and follow all required regulations for your area.

The Spa, Resort, or Retreat

If you've got vacation time coming up, or if you just need a break, consider a day, a weekend, or (what luxury!) a couple of weeks or more at a spa, resort, or retreat. These health- and/or indulgence-oriented spots are the new vacations-of-choice for many, and the options abound. From outdoorsy dude-ranch settings to the poshest of posh salons, many spas, resorts, and retreats offer massage as part of their get-away package. Pricey? Usually. But oh, so worth it!

The Office: Is Your Employer in Touch?

Massage at work? What next—complementary chocolate cake with your coffee? Actually, more and more employers are seeing the very real benefits of allowing on-site chair massage at the office. According to a Touch Research Institute study, office workers who received 15-minute chair massages every day for a week performed significantly better on math tests and showed lowered signs of job stress compared to a control group. If massage can translate to a more efficient staff with higher morale, what employer wouldn't see the light? It's a win-win situation.

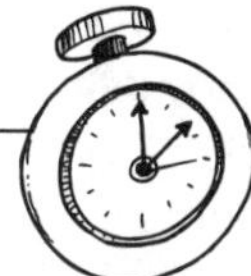

A Massage Minute

Office massages needn't be all about your back, shoulders, and neck. What about those poor hands, banging away at the computer keyboard all day long? According to the Touch Research Institute, massage helps to stretch tendons and relieve the pain of *carpal tunnel syndrome*, a debilitating condition originating in the wrist and caused by repetitive hand movement.

Clinics: What the Doctor Ordered

Because massage is becoming increasingly accepted as a legitimate therapy in the medical mainstream, many physicians have begun to prescribe massage for certain conditions, and in many cases, physicians leave the treatment details up to the massage therapist's expertise. Massage clinics may seem more medical in atmosphere than other massage environments, which some people prefer. They are almost certain to maintain stringent standards for their massage therapists, even in the absence of local regulations. Best of all, when you receive a physician-prescribed massage at a massage clinic, chances are your insurance will cover the cost if the referring doctor deems the massage a medical necessity (ask your doctor if this is a possibility). More insurance companies are becoming enlightened to the benefits of such coverage.

Are You Covered? Insurance and Massage

Why on earth would a big insurance company want to pay for your massage? As massage gains more publicity as a legitimate treatment for certain medical problems from broken bones to degenerative disease, more insurance companies are jumping on the "covered" bandwagon. With people seeking alternative therapies with increasing fervor, insurance companies are realizing that the way to win customers is to give them (at least to a profitable extent) exactly what they want.

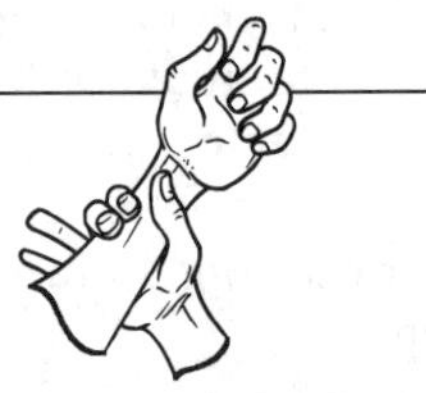

Your Finger on the Pulse

If you are lucky enough to live in a city that has a massage school, you may be able to receive a massage from students for a nominal fee. Many massage schools maintain clinics where massage therapy students can meet their requirements for a given number of massage hours. Call your local massage school for clinic hours, cost, and other details.

But how can covering massage be profitable? For an insurance company, paying for massage therapy is cheaper than paying for physical therapy, something most insurance companies already cover when a doctor prescribes it. If massage therapy can achieve the same (or even better) results, reason the insurance companies, then medical bills will be lower. That means less out-of-pocket expense for the insurance companies and great benefits for you.

If your doctor recommends massage for you but your insurance company doesn't cover massage, write a letter to its corporate headquarters explaining that such coverage is cost-effective. Cite some of the statistics listed throughout this book. While you're at it, write a letter to your state representatives encouraging legislation that will offer incentives to insurance companies to cover massage therapy and other proven alternative therapies.

Your First Session

You think you've found the perfect massage therapist, the perfect setting, and you're ready to go. Nervous? You don't have to be, but if you are, it isn't surprising. It's easy to feel a little vulnerable, especially the first few times you receive a professional massage, so we'll give you a peek into the process. After all, isn't most of what we fear the unexpected? Because we can't cover the typical process involved in every type of bodywork, we'll just give you an idea of how the typical Swedish massage session works, because Swedish massage is the most common type of massage practiced in the United States.

When you first meet with your massage therapist, you'll probably be asked a series of questions and/or be asked to fill out a health questionnaire. Your massage therapist will need to know any health problems you might have (be completely honest—your massage experience will be the better for it) and also will want to talk to you about your massage goals. Are you seeking relief for lower back pain in particular, or do you want to reduce overall stress in general?

Next, your massage therapist will leave the room or give you some sort of privacy to undress. You should only undress to the extent you feel comfortable. (Many people undress down to their underwear.) You'll lie on a padded massage table, and to assure modesty and warmth, you'll be covered with a towel and also a sheet.

Your massage therapist may put on music and will probably use some sort of massage oil. She or he should also ask you to speak up if anything at all makes you uncomfortable or inhibits your ability to relax: the music, the scent of the massage oil, or any aspect of the massage itself, including strokes that are too soft or too hard. Your massage therapist will typically uncover only the body part being worked on, and then re-cover it before moving on to the next part. (In the case of towel draping or diaper draping, only the breasts and genitals are kept covered.) The normal sequence involves hands and arms, legs and feet, chest and abdomen, then (after the client turns face-down) the backs of the legs and the back.

Swedish massage is a technique that can be learned, but every massage therapist is different (and so is every massagee!), so your massage will be unique, influenced by your massage therapist's individual style and the ways in which he or she is tailoring the massage to your needs. Sessions typically last for about an hour, but they can be as short as 30 minutes or as long as 90 minutes.

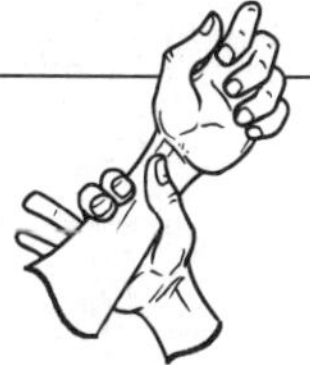

Your Finger on the Pulse

To get the most out of your professional massage, take a few preparatory measures. Don't eat anything within an hour or two of your massage. Spend a few moments in quiet meditation just before your massage. Most importantly, be open-minded to the experience. Try not to pre-judge what it will be like or how you will feel.

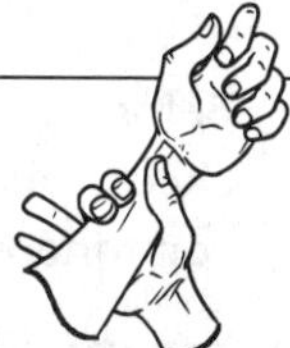

Your Finger on the Pulse

Post-massage, remember to drink lots of water to flush out toxins, move slowly for awhile to savor the relaxed feeling in your body, and carry that relaxed feeling throughout your day, recollecting it whenever you feel stress.

After the massage is over, your massage therapist will probably allow you to rest for a few moments in private to revel in that relaxed feeling. You'll then get up, get dressed (showers or towels are often available to remove oil), and go on with your life, but how much nicer the rest of your day will be!

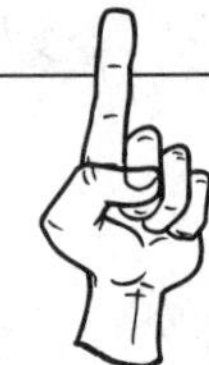

Touch Talk

Chiropractors treat disease and other medical problems by manipulation of the musculoskeletal system. **Osteopaths** typically combine traditional medical treatment with structural manipulations and a holistic perspective.

Massage and Chiropracty

Although you could also receive a massage in a doctor's, obstetrician's, or dentist's office, chances are greater that a massage therapist is somewhere on the premises if you visit a chiropractor. Massage therapy and chiropractic care are frequently practiced in conjunction. *Chiropractors* (doctors who treat disease and other medical problems by manipulation of the musculoskeletal system) and *osteopaths* (doctors who combine medical treatment with structural manipulations and a holistic perspective) view health care much in the way a massage therapist does. Because osteopaths are technically considered physicians, they can prescribe medication on a limited basis. Both osteopaths and chiropractors can order X-rays and other medical tests, and both are likely to be covered by insurance.

The Least You Need to Know

- Before choosing a massage therapist, check your area's licensing requirements, check your therapist's credentials, and establish a rapport to make sure you feel comfortable.
- You can find massage therapists in all kinds of places these days, from the gym to the mall to your office.
- Your insurance might cover your physician-prescribed massage.
- A massage therapist can be a part of your holistic health care team.

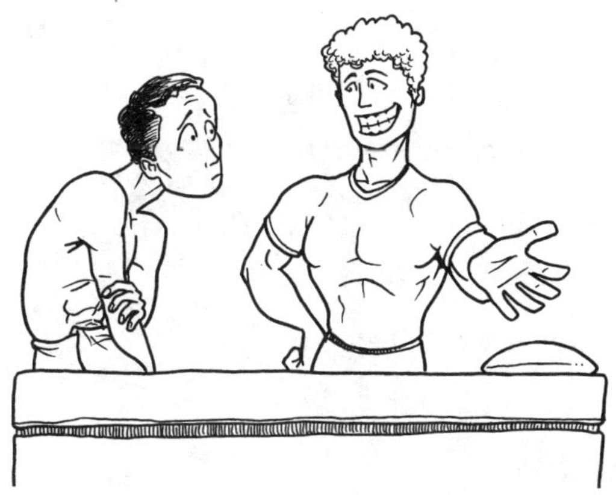

Chapter 11

Welcome to the World of Massage

In This Chapter

- What kind of massage is best for you?
- Relaxing massage therapies
- Deep tissue massage therapies
- Targeted massage therapy
- How to choose and find the appropriate bodyworker

Now that you're primed and prepped, let's get specific. We've been mentioning a lot of types of massage, and you may be wondering how they all differ. Knowing the differences can help you tailor your massage experience. Even small towns may have several pages in the phone book devoted to different types of massage and bodywork, so whom do you call? That depends on what you want.

Get Quizzical: What Kind of Massage Do You Need?

The type of massage you need depends on several factors, including your individual massage goals, your particular health problems and physical strengths, the way you typically use your body, and your philosophy of healing. Take this quiz to determine your primary massage needs:

1. At the end of the day, I am typically:
   - A. Energized.
   - B. Dead tired.
   - C. Emotionally depressed.
   - D. Suffering from some isolated pain, such as a headache, lower back ache, or wrist pain.

2. If I could change one thing about my health, it would be:
   - A. To become more stress-resistant.
   - B. To be more physically active.
   - C. To improve my mental health.
   - D. To get rid of a specific, chronic problem, such as arthritis, migraines, or a weak back.

3. My greatest hope for my massage experience is that it will:
   - A. Help me to relax.
   - B. Increase my physical performance.
   - C. Brighten my mood.
   - D. Alleviate a specific condition.

If two or three of your answers were A, you're seeking a massage for the purpose of relaxation and stress reduction. If two or three answers were B, you're looking for an adjunct to your active lifestyle. If two or three answers were C, you're seeking emotional release and mood enhancement from massage. If two or three answers were D, you're hoping massage will help with a specific problem. If all your answers were different, you expect a lot from your massage—and you can get all that you desire.

Massage can do all of the above, and Swedish massage alone can address all four goals, so Swedish massage is almost always a great choice. Other types of massage, however (including the many variations on Swedish massage), may address your specific problem equally well, and you may prefer certain types over others. Read on to get the low-down on the individual benefits of some of the more popular forms of massage therapy. (Chapter 12 covers even more types of bodywork, but it focuses on some of the less well-known types of bodywork and on the Oriental techniques, which are quickly gaining in popularity.)

Relaxation

You know you need to relax. You wish you could relax. Your body is telling you on a daily basis that you have to relax. But actually relaxing is a different story. For many, relaxation seems virtually impossible, and the desire for at least short-term relief from stress is probably the number-one reason why most people initially seek out massage.

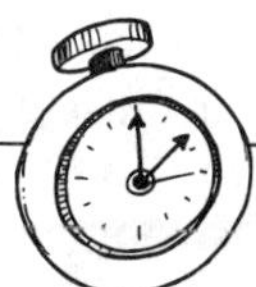

A Massage Minute

Many studies have demonstrated the effect of attitude towards stress on the immune system. Everyone experiences stress, but not everyone handles it in the same way. People with a feeling of control over stressful situations are less likely to get sick and tend to recover from illness more quickly. People who feel overwhelmed or helpless about their situations are less resistant to disease and often take far longer to recover. In other words, negative reactions to stress apparently repress immune function. The response to stress, not the presence of stress, is what matters.

If you suffer from the ill-effects of stress: tense muscles, inability to concentrate, insomnia, headaches, irritability, depression, forgetfulness, and minor aches and pains, to name a few, you're certainly not alone. Stress could be considered an epidemic in this country, and although a few of us thrive on it (especially in low dosages), many of us frequently find ourselves limping along under its prodigious weight, barely able to make it to the ends of our long and hectic days.

Which type of massage is great for lifting the weight of stress from tightly knotted shoulders and teaching us, slowly but surely, how it feels to be truly relaxed? Swedish massage is probably the number one choice for relaxation. After a good Swedish massage, you'll wonder how you could have gone on for so long without letting yourself feel this good.

Swedish Strokes for Soothing Folks

Swedish massage, the most popular form of massage in the West and the primary technique taught by most massage schools, is a malleable art, but it has some definite consistencies among practitioners, including specific strokes (see Part 4 for more detailed discussions of massage strokes). Swedish massage can be soft, gentle, firm, deep, energizing, relaxing—or all of the above! Different massage therapists tend towards different techniques, but you can also explain your massage goals to your massage therapist to be assured of obtaining the desired effect.

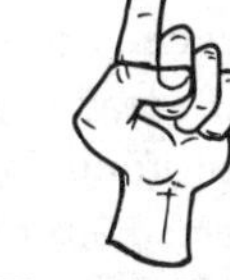

Touch Talk

Swedish massage is a popular form of massage based on a system developed by Per Henrik Ling (1776–1839) of Sweden. Ling developed a system of movements called Medical Gymnastics based on the then-fledgling science of physiology. The Ling System was also called Swedish Movements or the Movement Cure and spread through Europe, and then the United States. In the United States, the technique was known as The Swedish Movement Cure and eventually evolved into what we now call Swedish massage.

You might think light, gentle strokes would be the most relaxing, and they certainly are, but other strokes can relax your muscles, too. In general, light movements are most effective over bony areas of the body where tissue is thin, such as the face, the hands, and the knees, but deeper, stronger strokes are more effective for areas of the body with lots of muscle or thicker tissue covering, such as the shoulders, thighs, and buttocks. In other words, a general Swedish massage in which all strokes are used and varying pressure is applied can make for an ultimately relaxing experience.

Esalan: A One-Way Ticket to Shangri-La

Esalan is a variation of Swedish massage developed at the Esalan Institute in Big Sur, California. The essence of Esalan is sensuality. At the Esalan Institute, massages are given outside in the California sun on a cliff overlooking the ocean. The crash of the waves, the gentle whisper of the wind, and the warm embrace of the sun are integral to the Esalan experience. When practiced elsewhere in the absence of such dramatic scenery and ideal weather conditions, music often plays a significant part of the experience.

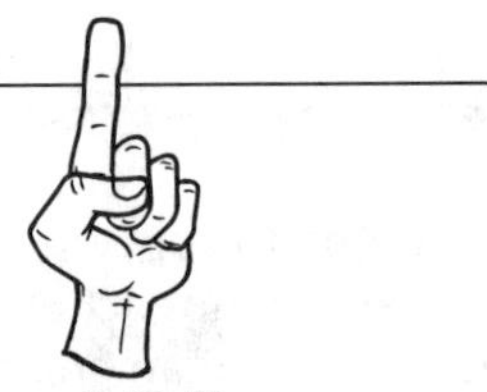

Touch Talk

Esalan is a combination of Swedish massage and sensory awareness techniques that includes passive joint movements and deep tissue work in a nurturing and, ideally, an aesthetically pleasing environment. The technique is named after the Esalan Institute in Big Sur, California, where Esalan massages are given outside on a cliff overlooking the ocean.

Although the basis of the massage itself is Swedish, strokes tend to be longer and more fluid, connecting the whole body. One stroke may extend from toe to crown, as opposed to concentrating on one body part at a time, as in a traditional Swedish massage. A classic Esalan massage is also less encumbered when it comes to clothing. Typically, both massager and massagee are completely undraped (yes, we mean buck naked!). Still, an Esalan massage isn't sexual. It is purely, wholly, intensely sensual. According to Esalan practitioners, this form of massage is highly individual, but the goal is profound relaxation and release. For those who can't make it to Big Sur, Esalan is practiced elsewhere, sometimes in a modified form and with some degree of draping. For those who embrace its theory and are uninhibited by its practice, Esalan can be a heavenly and even deeply spiritual experience.

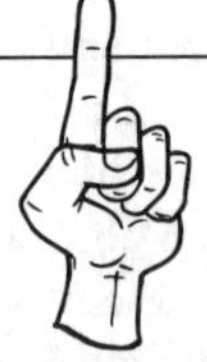

Touch Talk

Deep tissue massage is a general term referring to several variations of Swedish massage that concentrate on freeing the body's connective tissue through intense physical manipulation.

Let's Get Deep: Deep Tissue Massage

Deep tissue massage is a lot like what it sounds like—massage that gets right into the heart of the muscles and connective tissue. There are no soft, feathery, superficial strokes in this type of massage, but you won't come out bruised and battered, either. Because of their anatomy training, massage therapists know just where to access the deeper levels of tissue and how to loosen up contracted muscles, break apart adhesions, and generally get things moving where they've gotten a little stuck.

But deep tissue massage works on more than the physical level. It releases emotions and traumas from where they have been repressed and stored within your body. An intense session can leave you feeling drained—but drained of negativity, pent-up frustrations, and painful memories you hadn't previously been able to release. Depending on the way Swedish massage is practiced, it can certainly manipulate the deeper tissues of the body and is, essentially, deep tissue massage. However, other forms of deep tissue massage have evolved over time.

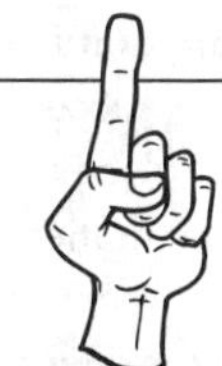

Touch Talk

Structural integration is a general term (originally it referred to what is now known as "Rolfing") for a type of massage that works to integrate the body's structure by reorganizing it through physical manipulation of the body's muscles and connective tissue so it can exist in better harmony with gravity.

Structural Integration

The purpose of *structural integration* is to move the body, which invariably slips, slides, and unconsciously forces itself into a crooked mess, back around its central axis. This process is accomplished by manipulating muscles and connective tissue at the deepest level over a series of sessions, after which many clients report a marked feeling of physical and psychological balance.

Rockin' and Rollin' Rolfers

Many people associate *Rolfing* with pain, and many are afraid to try it for that reason. Rolfing needn't be painful, however. It addresses the body at its deepest structural level, coaxing it into balance. People who have been Rolfed frequently report intense emotional release during or after a Rolfing session, and many admit that at times, it can get a little uncomfortable. But loyal followers wouldn't trade the experience because the short-lived pain is both bearable and well worth the result. A type of structural integration, Rolfing manipulates deep muscles and connective tissue until they are realigned and the body itself is changed in appearance through better posture, alignment with the pull of gravity, and the glow that comes from the serene sense of contentment often evident in the wake of a Rolfing session.

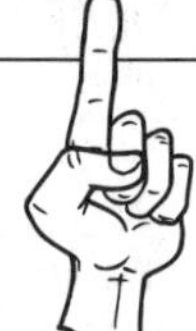

Touch Talk

Rolfing, or the Rolfing Method of Structural Integration, is a form of structural integration developed by Ida P. Rolf, Ph.D. Its purpose is to restructure the body in response to gravity through deep tissue manipulation and to correct misalignments caused by bad habit and trauma.

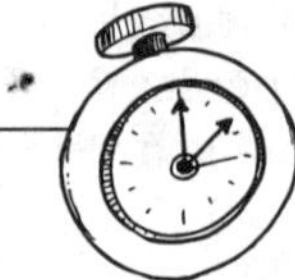

A Massage Minute

Dr. Ida P. Rolf (1896–1979), who developed the Rolfing Method of Structural Integration, had a profound effect on many later schools of deep tissue bodywork. She began her work after being successfully treated for a kick from a horse by an osteopath, who put a broken rib back into place and restored her breathing. Eventually combining her thorough studies of osteopathy, yoga, homeopathy, and many other forms of bodywork, Dr. Rolf developed a system in which soft tissue can be readjusted and manipulated into balance, allowing the body to better utilize its vast energy stores for physical and psychological healing. She once said, "I don't know why it works, I only know that it works."

My Oh My: Myotherapy and Other Trigger Point Therapies

When you abuse your muscles through years of misuse or from a single incident such as a car accident or athletic mishap, they don't take it lightly. They actively protect themselves, often by tying themselves in tight little knots to prevent future abuse. Back in the 1800s, medical practitioners noticed a phenomenon in muscles: a small, hard spot that was painful to the touch, but that seemed to relieve pain when pressed and held. Treating these hard spots, or trigger points as they are now called, is the heart of trigger point therapy.

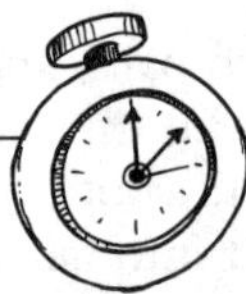

A Massage Minute

Bonnie Prudden (born in 1914) began to wonder about pain when her own arthritic hips produced pain in parts of her body that weren't clearly linked to the hip joints. After she awoke with a stiff neck on a climbing expedition, a doctor friend exerted extreme pressure on a painful spot in her neck, and her stiffness dissolved instantly. Bonnie Prudden then began a journey of discovery, during which she worked with a number of doctors who referred patients to her. She experimented with trigger points with tremendous success, relieving the patients' pain. Eventually, she founded the Institute for Physical Fitness and Myotherapy in Stockbridge, Massachusetts. She has since become the most known and influential name in the field of myotherapy.

Ideally, trigger point work can trick the muscle into letting go by interrupting the reflex involved in maintaining chronic tension. The greatest value of this is the client's awareness of where chronic tension is and the experience of letting it go. What was habitual has the potential of becoming a matter of choice. *Myotherapy* is one of the better known schools of trigger point therapy, made famous by Bonnie Prudden.

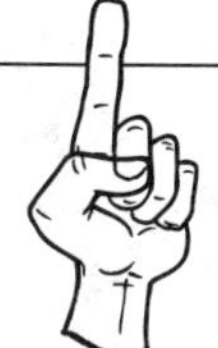

Touch Talk

Myotherapy is a type of trigger point therapy made popular by Bonnie Prudden. Trigger point therapy is a term referring to several types of therapy in which trigger points, or sensitive areas in tight muscles that cause pain in various parts of the body, are pressed firmly until the tension releases.

Myotherapists have an intimate knowledge of anatomy and common trigger points. They also know that trigger point locations vary among individuals, and they are trained to seek them out. Myotherapists apply deep pressure with their fingers, knuckles, or elbows to the trigger point for approximately seven seconds; pain relief is often immediate and permanent, although sometimes several sessions are required.

Myotherapists will often instruct family members or the client on how to continue to treat a problem at home. Myotherapy and other trigger point therapies are most effective for jaw, neck, back, hip, sciatic, and shoulder pain.

Targeted Massage

An all-over massage can be just the ticket, but sometimes you need some specific help. Whether that help comes in the healing power of water, the therapeutic power of sports massage, or the targeted healing of reflexology, massage has an answer.

The Wonderful World of Hydrotherapy

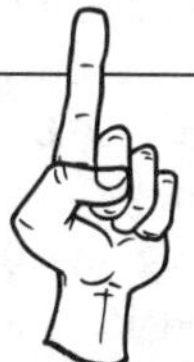

Touch Talk

Hydrotherapy, or water therapy, uses the healing power of water in conjunction with massage or movement or simply for soaking, streaming, spraying, or otherwise applying water, in its various forms and temperatures, to the body.

Humans, like the earth, are largely made up of water, so it's no wonder humans have always been fascinated by the sea. After all, for nine months after conception, when we are in the amniotic fluid in the womb, we are aquatic creatures. Maybe that's why *hydrotherapy*, which is the use of water for therapeutic purposes, feels so good.

Hydrotherapy comes in many forms, including but not limited to baths (mineral baths, salt baths, shallow hip baths, steam baths, and foot baths), showers, saunas, ice packs, heat packs, hot tubs, even natural hot or cold springs. Methods of application might include differing types of showers, shower heads, hoses, and sprayers; herbal wraps (sheets soaked in "teas" made from herbs steeped in water, then wrapped around the body); and seaweed and mud wraps, in which the body is soaked or wrapped in these substances.

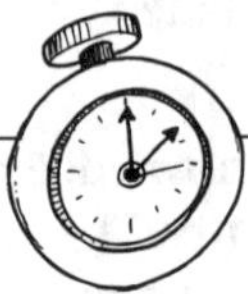

A Massage Minute

Heat's effects on blood: It thins blood, reduces the amount pumped to the heart, raises body temperature, increases inflammation, and dilates blood vessels.

Cold's effects on blood: It thickens blood, increases the amount pumped to the heart, lowers body temperature, reduces inflammation, and constricts blood vessels.

Because the skin is permeable and filled with a fine network of blood vessels, it is highly susceptible to the application of heat and cold, an important part of hydrotherapy. Applying cold packs to the skin constricts the smaller blood vessels but increases blood flow to deeper tissues, lowers temperature, slows breathing, contracts muscles, slows healing, stems bleeding, dulls pain, slows fluid accumulation, and reduces inflammation and swelling. The application of heat dilates small blood vessels, draws blood to the skin surface, thins blood, raises temperature, increases breathing rate, relaxes muscles, increases the rate of healing, encourages swelling, eases muscle pain, encourages drainage from injured areas, reduces congestion and pressure, speeds digestion, and induces a relaxed state.

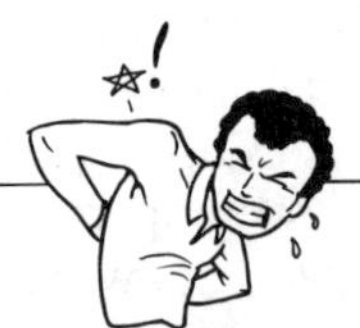

Ouch!

You can apply heat almost as long as is comfortable, although soaks in hot water should usually be limited to 15 or 20 minutes. Cold applications should be limited to 10 to 15 minutes on and 10 to 15 minutes off. Cold or hot packs should be removed immediately if you experience any signs of discomfort, irritation, pain, numbness, tingling, shivering, if the skin turns bluish, or if body temperature goes above or below normal.

To make your own cold pack, mix equal parts alcohol and water and pour into a heavy-duty freezer bag. Freeze it, and you've got a "slushie" to put on injured areas such as sprains or pulled muscles (but put a thin towel between your skin and the bag to protect your skin). To make your own moist heat pack, fill a heavy sock with raw rice, close it securely, and cook it on high in the microwave for one minute (put a thin towel between your skin and the sock to protect your skin from any overcooked rice).

The skin is a delicate sense organ, and hydrotherapy can be an excellent therapy for the entire system. Some forward-thinking bodyworkers even practice bodywork in the water, such as water yoga and watsu (shiatsu in the water).

Watsu was invented in 1980 by a poet and shiatsu master named Harold Dull. Shiatsu's stretching and pressure point techniques are practiced in warm water, where a client's muscles can truly relax and where a therapist can manipulate, stretch, and work on the body in ways that would be virtually impossible without the increased buoyancy and decreased weight water imparts. Watsu can be extremely effective for the physically disabled, who can find relief from their normally limited movement, and watsu often seems to work therapeutic magic on the emotionally disabled, as well. Many who have experienced watsu claim they quickly enter a transcendent state.

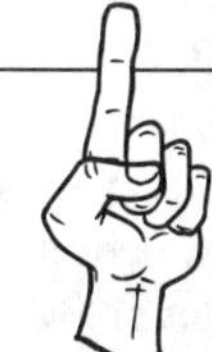

Touch Talk

Sports massage is a variation of Swedish massage specifically tailored for the athlete. Sports massage lessens the chance for injury, decreases recovery time, and optimizes performance.

Water yoga involves the practice of modified yoga poses in the water, assisted by a qualified yoga teacher. Water yoga's advantages are similar to watsu's: the body is able to move in ways it cannot on dry land, and practicing yoga in the water is relaxing and therapeutic.

Be on the Winning Team: Sports Massage

If you're an athlete, whether by profession or just for fun, you know that your body is your tool. For peak performance, your body has to be in peak condition. Unfortunately, the harder you work and the more you push yourself, the more likely you'll be to experience injury, which can sideline you when you'd much rather be back out there in the game.

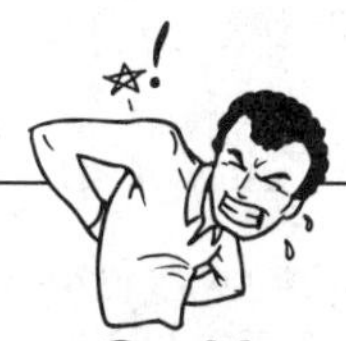

Ouch!

If you can't get a massage before a workout, make sure you take the time to warm up properly. Five to ten minutes of aerobic activity to warm muscles, followed by basic stretching exercises, will prime your muscles for competition and decrease the likelihood of injury. Warm down after your workout, too, to help flush toxins out of muscles and reduce muscle soreness.

Enter *sports massage*. Another variation of Swedish massage, sports massage is tailor-made for the athlete. When administered before an athletic performance, sports massage can loosen and activate muscles, flushing them with nutrients and thereby increasing performance and minimizing the chance of injury. After a workout, sports massage can speed healing of injured tissue and reduce recovery time and the muscle pain that almost inevitably accompanies a limit-pushing performance.

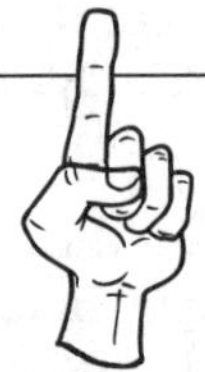

Touch Talk

Manual lymph drainage was developed by Dr. Emil Vodder and wife Estrid in the 1930s in Europe. This technique facilitates the lymphatic system's processes by massaging the body with slow, light strokes. Widely practiced in Europe, where it is often used to alleviate post-surgical pain and swelling, manual lymph drainage is more recently becoming popular in the United States.

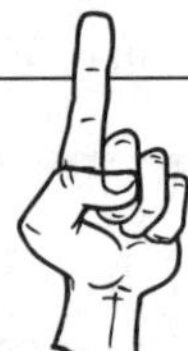

Touch Talk

Craniosacral therapy involves gentle pressure and manipulation of the craniosacral system, which are the bones and soft tissues of the skull, face, vertebrae, and sacrum (the bones at the base of the spine). This technique balances the flow of cerebrospinal fluid, which is thought to balance the entire body. The name for the therapy was coined by Dr. John Upledger, an osteopath.

Sports massage focuses on facilitating fluid movement throughout the body and lengthening muscles, as well as breaking apart adhesions that may have formed from injuries. The two main strokes sports massage utilizes are compression and percussion. A sports massage therapist may also use trigger point therapy to keep muscles released, flexible, and pain-free.

Manual Lymph Drainage

You probably don't thinkmuch about your lymphatic system, but you would certainly feel it if it stopped working! Waste products would accumulate in your body, you'd feel tired and run down, and your immune system would eventually fail. *Lymph massage*, or *manual lymph drainage*, is a system of massage related to Swedish massage that requires a detailed knowledge of the lymphatic system because it specifically focuses on encouraging the flow of lymph throughout the body. Massage strokes involve compression movements to help pump lymph through the body and focus on areas where lymph tissues are most concentrated (usually in muscle tissue) and in areas of concentrated lymph glands. Lymph massage helps the body to eliminate toxins more efficiently, encourages a balance in internal chemistry, and normalizes organ and immune system function. (See the section "The Circulatory System" in Chapter 5 for an illustration of the lymph system.)

Get Heady with Craniosacral Therapy

Your brain doesn't just rattle around in a dry skull—it floats in cerebrospinal fluid. This fluid isn't just limited to the inside of your skull, however. It extends all the way down your spine to your sacrum. Your skull itself, once a soft enclosure of plates only loosely attached at birth to permit a more flexible passage through the birth canal, has since fused into solid bone. According to craniosacral therapists, however, the plates of the skull, joined by joints, expand and contract with the movement of cerebrospinal fluid, and this movement is essential for proper body functioning.

Sometimes, the skull bones can become minutely misaligned, hindering the natural movement of the skull plates. Such misalignment can even be a result of a baby's journey through the birth canal if the skull doesn't readjust into the proper shape. Cerebrospinal fluid movement can be hindered, and any of the mechanisms along the spinal cord could be adversely affected. In *craniosacral therapy*, the skull bones are readjusted and aligned to facilitate movement and to enhance the circulation of cerebrospinal fluid. The result can be pain relief, especially when head or jaw pain is the problem.

Get Testy with Your Muscles: Applied Kinesiology

Applied kinesiology is a complex process of testing muscles to determine muscle weaknesses, which are directly related to the various systems of the body. Particular muscle weakness could indicate anything from diabetes to allergies. Treatment involves three aspects: chemical, structural, and mental. Treatment plans typically include different massage therapies; nutrition, vitamin, and mineral counseling; and behavioral modification. Applied kinesiology's muscle testing and lifestyle modification prescriptions aren't for the novice.

Touch for Health is a simplified, user-friendly version of applied kinesiology. Dr. John Thie, a colleague of applied kinesiology's founder, Dr. George Goodheart, made the concepts behind applied kinesiology available to the masses by writing a book called *Touch for Health* that describes a wide range of muscle tests anyone can do, plus appropriate treatments.

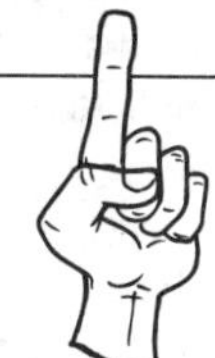

Touch Talk

Applied kinesiology is a technique that first tests muscles for strength and range of motion, analyzes posture and lifestyle, and then prescribes an appropriate treatment program, which may include particular massage techniques, acupressure work, craniosacral work, a specific diet, vitamin and herb use, and exercises meant to mobilize joints.

Playing Footsy: Reflexology

He's got the whole world in his foot? Well, maybe not the whole world, but according to *reflexology*, you've got a map of your whole body on the bottom of your foot, on your hand, and on your ear, too. The theory of reflexology holds that the body is divided into 10 vertical zones, and each zone reaches from head to foot. Firm pressure on the appropriate area of your foot, hand, or ear, where each zone connects, can stimulate and stir areas of stress or blockage to promote healing and

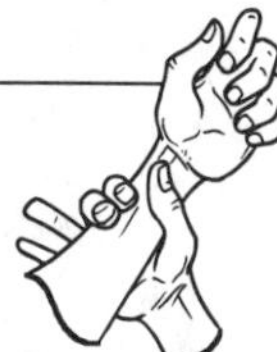

Your Finger on the Pulse

Here's an example of reflexology in action: To stimulate brain function and clearer thinking, squeeze the tip of your thumb with your opposite thumb and index finger, then pinch all around the tip, making seven slow circles around the tip, never completely releasing pressure. Repeat on the other thumb.

relaxation. Reflexologists don't claim that their method cures. Instead, like many other forms of bodywork, reflexology signals the body to heal itself.

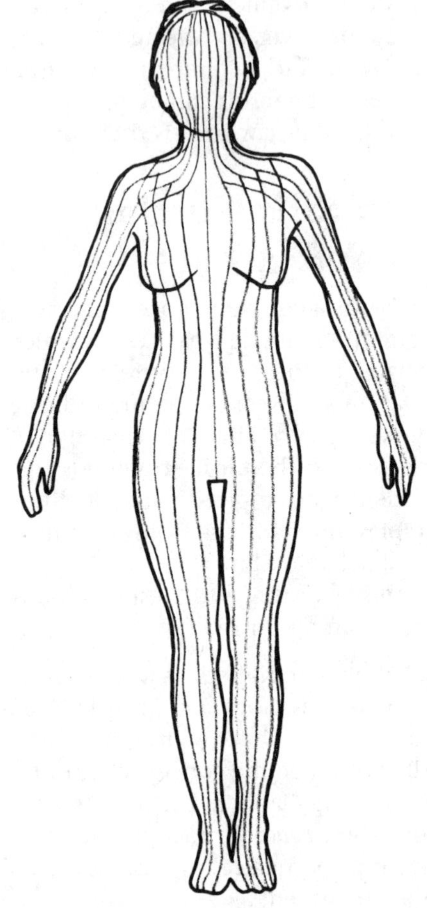

Zones from head to toe correlate with points in the hands, feet, and ears. The organs and systems of the body run within particular zone lines.

Another great thing about reflexology is that it lends itself to self-treatment. It's easy to massage your own feet, and with a little study and a good foot map in front of you, you may be able to relieve some of your own stress and minor pain, such as a headache, a sore shoulder, or a stiff neck, by taking your feet into your own hands.

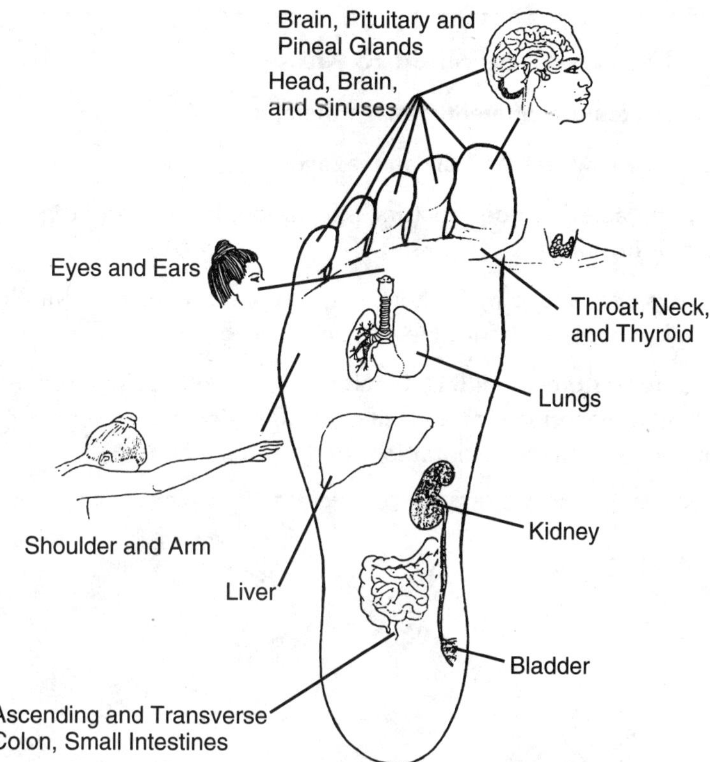

Here are some of the important reflexology areas on the bottom of your right foot. Note that the stomach and heart are on the bottom of your left foot.

Eenie, Meenie, Meiney, Mo...

Now that you know some of your many choices, how do you pick which one to try? Some systems naturally appeal to people more than others, and if you feel particularly drawn to a certain kind of bodywork after what you've just read, look around for a good, reputable practitioner. Keep in mind that alternative health practitioners aren't always listed in the yellow pages, so you might have to do some hunting. Ask around in your local natural or health food store, health club, chiropractor's or other alternative health care practitioner's office, or even an alternative bookstore. Ask friends and friends of friends. Or surf the Internet for professional organizations.

The Least You Need to Know

- Different massage needs require different massage therapies.
- Relaxing therapies include Swedish and Esalan massage.
- Deep tissue massage therapies include structural integration, Rolfing, and trigger point therapies such as myotherapy.
- Targeted massage therapies include hydrotherapy, sports massage, manual lymph drainage, craniosacral therapy, Touch for Health, and reflexology.
- Ask around at health food stores, health clubs, chiropractors' offices, or alternative bookstores to find a practitioner of a specific massage therapy that interests you. Or call a professional massage organization for a referral.

Chapter 12

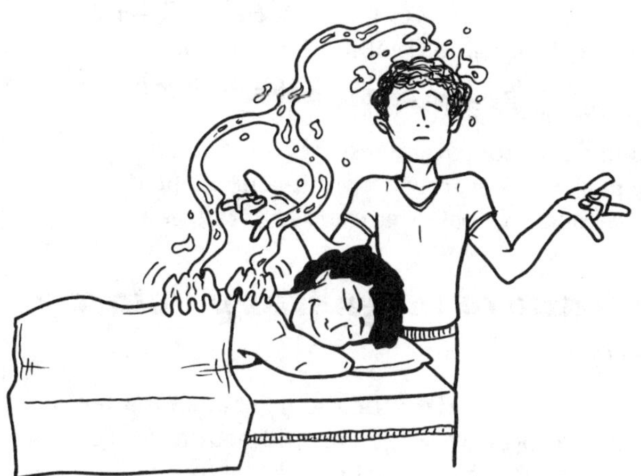

More Kinds of Massage

In This Chapter

- Bodywork and energy balancing
- Bodywork and movement
- Integrating your body and your mind
- Oriental bodywork techniques

Although Swedish massage is the most popular type of massage in the United States, it's by no means the only type. In fact, so many types of bodywork exist that we couldn't begin to brief you on all of them. Choosing which ones to mention was tough, and if we've left out your favorite type, we apologize. We've tried, however, to give you a good sampling of most of the more prominent or well-known methods.

That's not to say that a method we haven't mentioned doesn't have value. This book is a starting point, and if a certain type of bodywork interests you, you can go further in your research (see Appendix B, "Let Your Fingers Do the Walking: Suggested Reading," for other sources of information). This chapter covers energy therapies, somatic methods, and Oriental techniques.

Energy Therapy

According to the theory behind *energy therapy*, your body is surrounded and permeated by a vibrant energy field—the universal life force called chi, prana, or energy (see

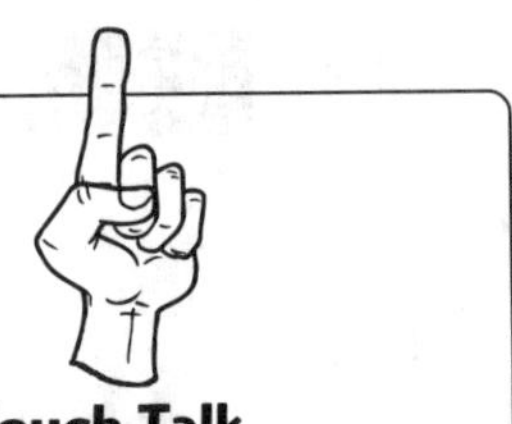

Touch Talk

Energy therapy is a type of bodywork that manipulates, unblocks, and balances the body's energy field.

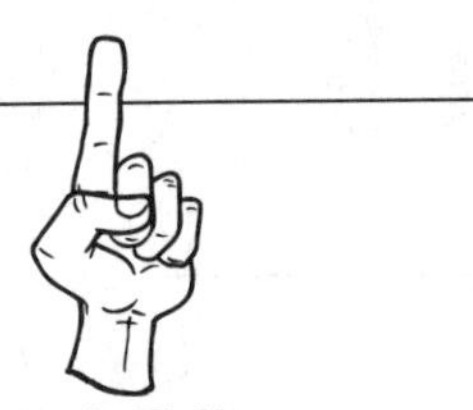

Touch Talk

Polarity therapy was founded by Dr. Randolph Stone (1890–1981), who emigrated to Chicago from Austria in the early 1900s. A doctor of chiropracty, osteopathy, and naturopathy who traveled widely and was well-versed in Oriental and East Indian theories of healing, Dr. Stone based his technique on a combination of osteopathy, acupuncture, and Ayur-Veda to balance the body's energies.

Chapter 7, "Contact: Power Points"). Humans—and all other physical forms, for that matter—are manifestations of this energy, and it flows through us as it flows through the universe. When this energy becomes blocked or unbalanced, the result is disease. Energy therapy goes straight to work on the energy field, putting it back into balance in order to restore health.

Your Natural Magnetism: Polarity Therapy

Polarity therapy is based on the theory that all matter is polarized with positive, negative, and neutral energy fields. According to polarity therapy, the human body is polarized in this way: the head is positively charged, the legs and feet are negatively charged, and the trunk is neutral, although to some extent the entire body is an ever-shifting mosaic of energy fields. Keeping the human body's energy fields balanced and flowing is the goal of polarity therapy.

How do you balance energy? That depends largely on the individual and on the practitioner, but most polarity therapists use a combination of pressure point work, gentle body massage and manipulations, diet advice (because food imparts energy to the body—a vegetarian diet is usually recommended), counseling to emphasize a positive frame of mind, and energy-balancing exercises you can do at home. Largely based on the theories of Ayur-Veda, polarity therapy encourages the individual to take charge of his or her own care. Polarity therapists use two-handed contacts to facilitate energy movement between the client and the therapist.

Go with the Flow: Orthobionomy

Translated as "correct application of life principles," *Orthobionomy* is a system of bodywork invented by a British osteopath, Dr. Arthur Lincoln Pauls. Orthobionomy combines the martial arts principle of following the body's natural energy flows with the techniques of massage therapy and osteopathy.

For example, when a muscle is injured, the body tends to curl around it. When people feel pain, they tend to lean in toward it. When people feel emotional distress, they may physically withdraw. In an orthobionomy session, the practitioner moves the body and/or energy fields into the blockage, even exaggerating the body's natural response. Generally, this gentle, supportive, almost cradling action helps release the blockage. By nurturing the body in these supportive ways, the practitioner helps the body to open and blossom.

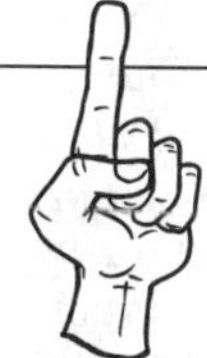

Touch Talk

Ayur-Veda is considered the oldest (over five thousand years old) system of scientifically based health care. Literally translated as "science of life," Ayur-Veda combines diet, exercise, meditation, and a regular routine into a philosophical system of energy balancing. Ayur-Veda has recently enjoyed a surge of popularity in the West because of the writings of Deepak Chopra, M.D.

Cha-Cha-Chakras: Reiki

Like polarity therapy, *Reiki* (pronounced *ray-kee*) works with energy. Rather than working with pressure points and moving the body, the Reiki practitioner places his or her hands on the receiver at certain specific points corresponding with the *chakras*, or energy centers, and the endocrine glands. (One theory has it that the chakras shuttle energy to the endocrine glands, which affect many aspects of our bodies and minds.) The touch is held for a long time, usually three to five minutes. According to the theory of Reiki, chakras are energy entrance points, so placing one's hands over these areas draws the universal life force into the body.

Reiki retains an aura of mystery because practitioners generally don't reveal their secrets. Supposedly, everyone is theoretically able to channel universal energy, but most of us have become blocked. To practice Reiki, you have to go through a series of initiations with Reiki masters to overcome what's blocking you. After this special training, the Reiki practitioner is able to channel energy directly into the bodies of others, not by using his or her own energy, but by channeling the universe's energy.

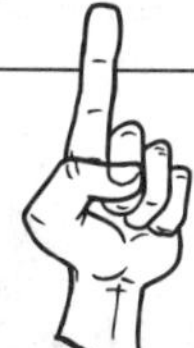

Touch Talk

Orthobionomy is a bodywork technique developed by Arthur Lincoln Pauls. *Ortho* means "to correct or straighten," and *bionomy* means "study of life processes." According to Dr. Pauls, orthobionomy restores the body's natural understanding of itself by safely and slowly moving the body in the direction of its habitual holding patterns that are blocking energy and/or causing pain.

The Western anatomical model of the human body's musculoskeletal and nervous systems (left) is complemented by the seven energy centers, called chakras (right), which store and release the body's life force.

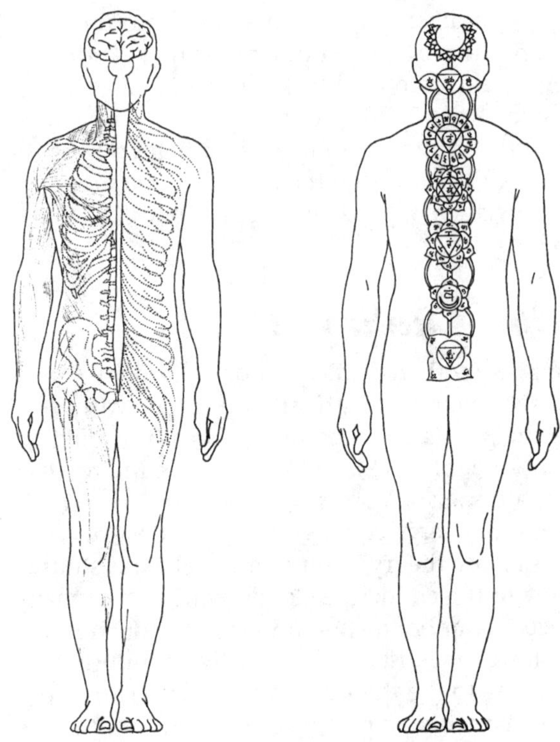

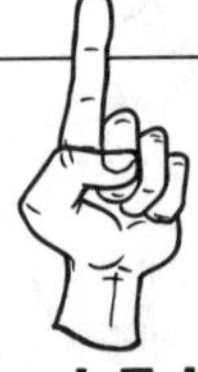

Touch Talk

Chakras are centers of psycho-spiritual energy in the body. The seven primary chakras are located at the base of the spine (Saturn), on the spine behind the pelvic area (Jupiter), behind the stomach area (Mars), behind the heart (Venus), in the throat (Mercury), in the middle of the brow (Sun), and at the crown of the skull (Thousand-Petalled Lotus). There are also many subtler chakras.

Teach Your Body Well: Somatic and Psychophysical Therapies

Moving, thinking, touching, feeling, holding, releasing—we do these activities all the time, often combining two or more simultaneously. But how often do we notice what we do? The purpose of *somatic* and *psychophysical therapies* is to teach you how you're using (or misusing) your body and mind, and then direct you toward a more productive and conscious existence. All of these therapies are based around the goal of complete integration of the body and mind, but each takes a slightly different approach.

Alexander the Great: The Alexander Technique

F.M. Alexander (1869–1955) was an actor who lost one of his most valuable assets: his voice. Encouraged by doctors to "save" his voice by not speaking, he would regain it periodically, only to lose it again. Frustrated by a lack of real help from doctors, Alexander began to study his body and the way he used his voice. He soon discovered that he and many of the rest of us regularly misuse our bodies, crunching down instead of expanding, tensing instead of relaxing, and tightening into strange and crooked knots and positions in preparation for movement. The result, over time, is that the body stops working as well. We lose our voices, we stutter, and we experience chronic pain.

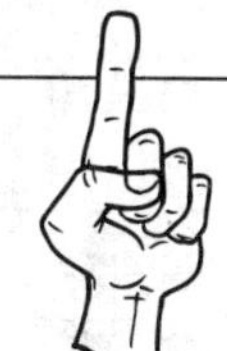

Touch Talk

Psychophysical therapies are types of bodywork that work with both the body and the mind in terms of how they affect each other, such as how an emotional trauma can cause physical distress to the body. Releasing repressed emotions, for example, can correct physical dysfunction.

Many people think the Alexander technique is about posture, and it is, but it's also more than that. It's about using your body in a way that doesn't inhibit functioning, and that means learning to lengthen and expand rather than shorten and contract. This takes some practice and lots of mindfulness.

The Alexander technique can be applied to any movement. You can practice mindfulness and adjustment before you speak, perform, lie down, begin typing, go jogging, or do anything at all. This technique will increase your awareness of the processes that precede and accompany movement.

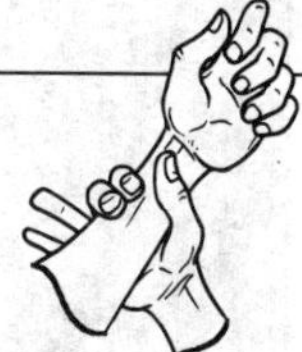

Your Finger on the Pulse

Notice how you are sitting right now. Stand up. How did you stand up? Most people curl in then push up. The Alexander Technique teaches you to work with your body flow. For example, imagine your head floating up and leading your body effortlessly after it into a standing position. *Voilà*—an Alexander technique!

Yoga: The Internal Massage

Yoga may not look like massage on the outside, but it's most definitely massage on the inside. On the outside, many yoga movements look like they're imitating things: the tree, the lightning bolt, the mountain, the bridge, the plow, and the lotus, to name a very few. True, capturing the energy essence of these models is part of yoga. But yoga movements are also specifically designed to open certain chakras, compress or release certain internal organs, mobilize energy, and, in general, do all the things massage can do.

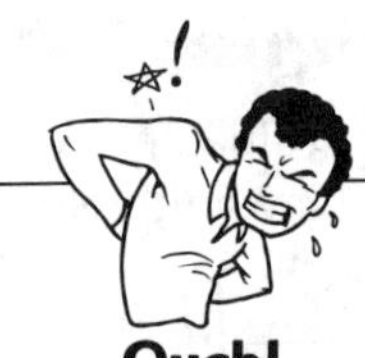

Ouch!

Yoga is great for relaxation, fitness, and internal massage, but some yoga poses are very advanced. Trying the hardest poses before you're ready could result in serious injury. Best to progress at a gradual pace, ideally under the guidance of a knowledgeable instructor.

For example, the photo below shows Joan in a yoga position called the bow. This pose is meant to imitate the bow of an archer held taught. Because an archer's bow that's ready to be released is a potent storehouse of potential energy, the bow pose is a high-energy pose that decreases laziness and feelings of malaise.

Now, look at the drawing on the next page; it shows a rocking bow. As you rock in the bow pose, the ground massages your abdomen. Your spine is stretched in a direction opposite from what it's accustomed to, so it becomes more flexible and supple. Your back muscles store energy that's released when the position is released, invoking a completely relaxed feeling. (For more on yoga poses and their internal massage-like effects, check out our companion volume *The Complete Idiot's Guide to Yoga*.)

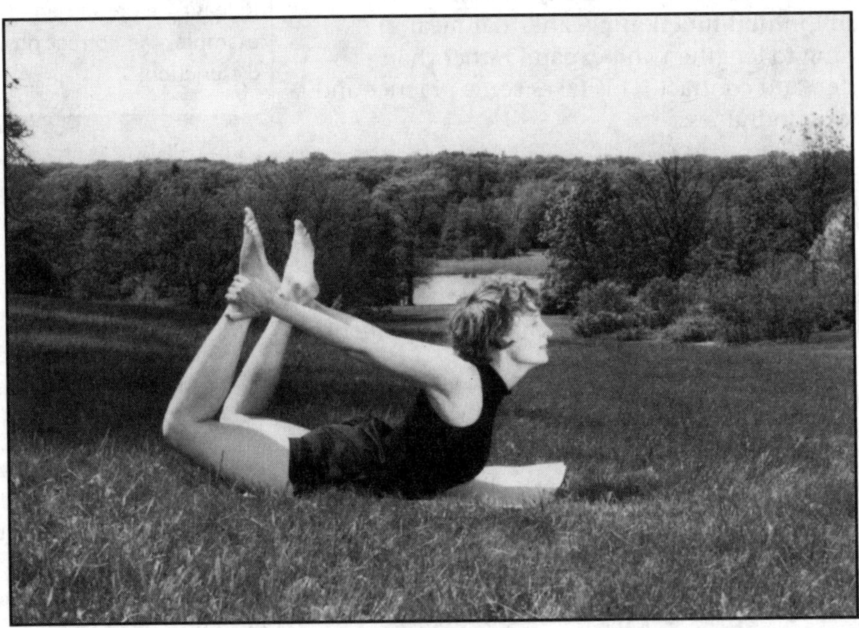

Joan performs yoga's bow pose. (Photograph by Saeid Lahouti)

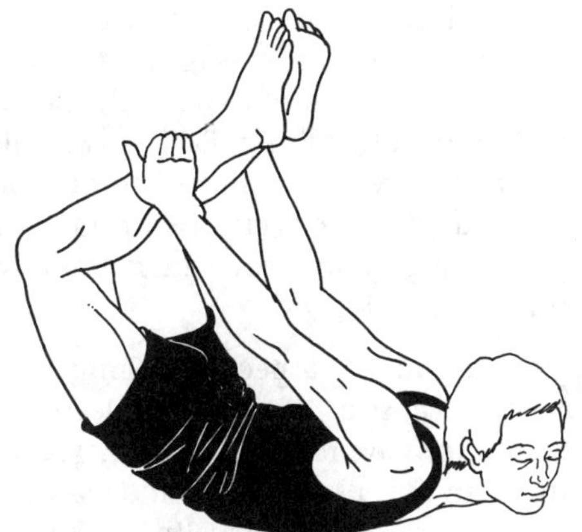

Rocking bow massages the internal organs of the torso and the abdominal muscles.

Groovin' in the Movin': Aston-Patterning

Like so many other bodyworkers, Judith Aston studied with Ida Rolf (see Chapter 11, "Welcome to the World of Massage"). Because she was a dance teacher and movement instructor, however, Aston transformed the Rolfing technique into her own dynamic version of movement re-education and fitness training. *Aston-Patterning* builds body strength and endurance, improves balance, and helps each person to find his or her own natural body positioning and movements. The result is more graceful movement, better physical health, and pain relief. Aston didn't believe each person was meant to be perfectly straight. Instead, her program is tailored to each body.

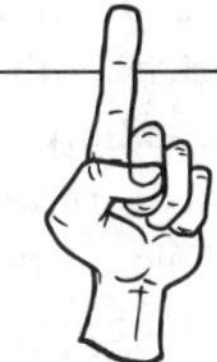

Touch Talk

Aston-Patterning was founded by Judith Aston and involves movement re-education that combines the techniques of Dr. Ida Rolf with patterns of movement. It has grown to include fitness training and ergonomics.

Massage, Movement, and Mind: Hellerwork

Joseph Heller, the creator of *Hellerwork*, also studied with Ida Rolf and was the first president of the Rolf Institute. (He's a former aerospace engineer and is no relation to Joseph Heller the novelist.) He later studied with Judith Aston, founder of Aston-Patterning. He took the concepts he learned from these two masters—massage from Rolf and movement from Aston—and added a third component: mind. Hellerwork, then, is a system that equally combines attention to these three M's: massage, movement, and mind.

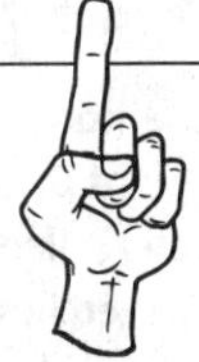

Touch Talk

Hellerwork was founded by a former aerospace engineer and student of Ida Rolf, Joseph Heller. Hellerwork combines movement re-education, massage, and dialogue between client and massage therapist.

A Hellerwork treatment consists of 11 90-minute sessions, each focusing on a different area of the body (its physical and mental aspects). The massage portion of each session consists of deep connective tissue massage in an attempt to align the body with the force of gravity, à la Rolfing. Each session also involves instruction in movement, and all along, you'll experience lots and lots of conversation, from what to expect at the beginning to how you can carry on with what you've learned at the end.

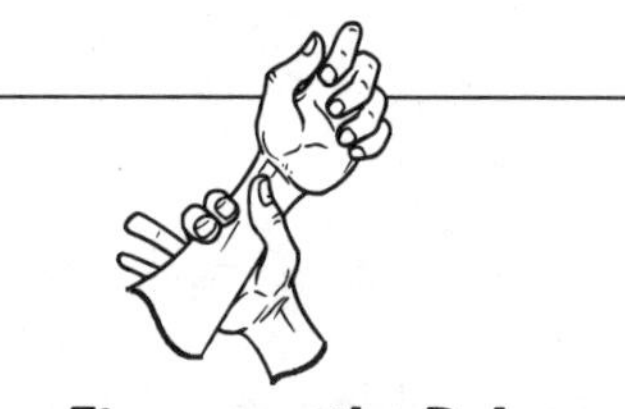

Your Finger on the Pulse

Bodywork that involves movement re-education is popular with actors, dancers, and other performers whose bodies are their tools, but even if your paycheck doesn't depend on your body condition, don't forget that your primary profession is life, and to get the most out of life, you need a body that moves well and feels great.

Dialogue (the "mind" aspect) is an important part of Hellerwork because as the body is released and corrected, emotions are released. Talking about them helps to bring them out, purge them, and clarify them. The result is an energized, freed feeling that can be permanent if you continue to utilize Hellerwork techniques after the treatment ends.

Mind and Muscle: Trager

If you like a nice, peaceful, quiet massage with no verbal communication between you and that person turning your muscles to little pockets of peacefulness, the *Trager method* might take some getting used to. Trager work, also known as *psychophysical integration*, isn't anything like a traditional Swedish massage. Instead, the Trager bodyworker gives you constant feedback on what your body is telling him or her. The movements are pleasurable and playful, consisting of shaking, vibrating, and soft kneading, to remind your body what it feels like to feel good.

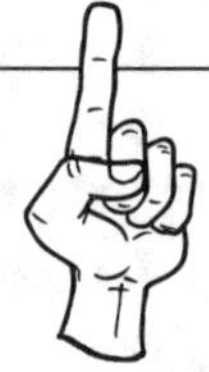

Touch Talk

The **Trager method** was founded by Milton Trager, M.D. It combines painless touch (called **psychophysical integration**), exercises the client performs, and mental/movement exercises (called **Mentastics**) to release blockages in the body as an approach to healing.

Beyond that, a Trager practitioner will attempt to communicate to your subconscious through talk and through the touch communication with your body so your subconscious can then talk your muscles and the rest of your body back into a state of ultimate health. You'll also be taught a set of do-it-yourself movement/mind exercises called Mentastics (mental gymnastics). According to Milton Trager, M.D., who invented the Trager method, pain, blockages, and all physical problems begin in the mind. His goal was to uncover the soul of the individual, freeing the mind and, therefore, healing the body.

Moving to a New You: Feldenkrais

Just as we only use a small part of our brain power, we also use only a small number of movements compared to the possibilities inherent in our bodies. Moshe Feldenkrais, D.Sc. (1904–1984), believed that as young children, we learned how to move in set patterns, and our minds and bodies stick to those patterns, missing out on most of the possible movements our bodies can make. The *Feldenkrais method* re-educates the body and mind by exposing the student to movements beyond those in his or her comfortable repertoire. The Feldenkrais method consists of two parts: one-on-one functional integration lessons and Awareness through Movement classes.

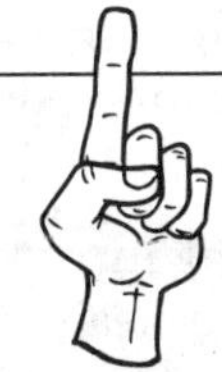

Touch Talk

The **Feldenkrais method** was founded by Moshe Feldenkrais, D.Sc., an Israeli physicist from Russia who developed a system of movement re-education meant to optimize human function by raising a client's awareness about limiting movement patterns and habits.

Bodywork from the Orient

We've already talked a lot about the different ways Eastern and Western culture view the treatment of disease and health itself. We've talked about energy meridians and chi, the life force that flows through everyone's body and that's accessible in certain areas of the body called pressure points. This section gets a little more specific and tells you about some of the techniques that access and manipulate chi for pain relief, health maintenance, and superior life performance.

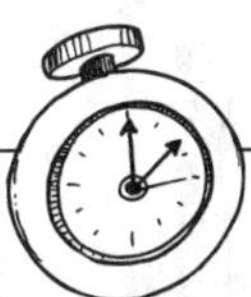

A Massage Minute

According to the National Institutes of Health Office of Alternative Medicine, there are approximately 6,500 acupuncturist practitioners in the United States, and the American Oriental Body Work Therapy Association has approximately 1,600 members.

Cultivating Your Energy: Qigong

Qigong, or *chikung*, as it is also known, is the art of cultivating and enriching your life force for better physical, mental, and spiritual health. Widely practiced in China, qigong comes in several forms, including Confuciust, Taoist, and Buddhist. All of these forms incorporate form (the body), energy, and mind to promote longevity and healing.

Qigong incorporates posture, movement, self-massage, breathwork, and meditation for self-healing. The effects of qigong are best achieved when the student learns from an experienced teacher and then practices with devotion. Thought to originate from the ancient Taoists, qigong is also sometimes practiced in conjunction with the martial arts.

Qigong body movements can open the qigong system of energy flow you see in the drawing.

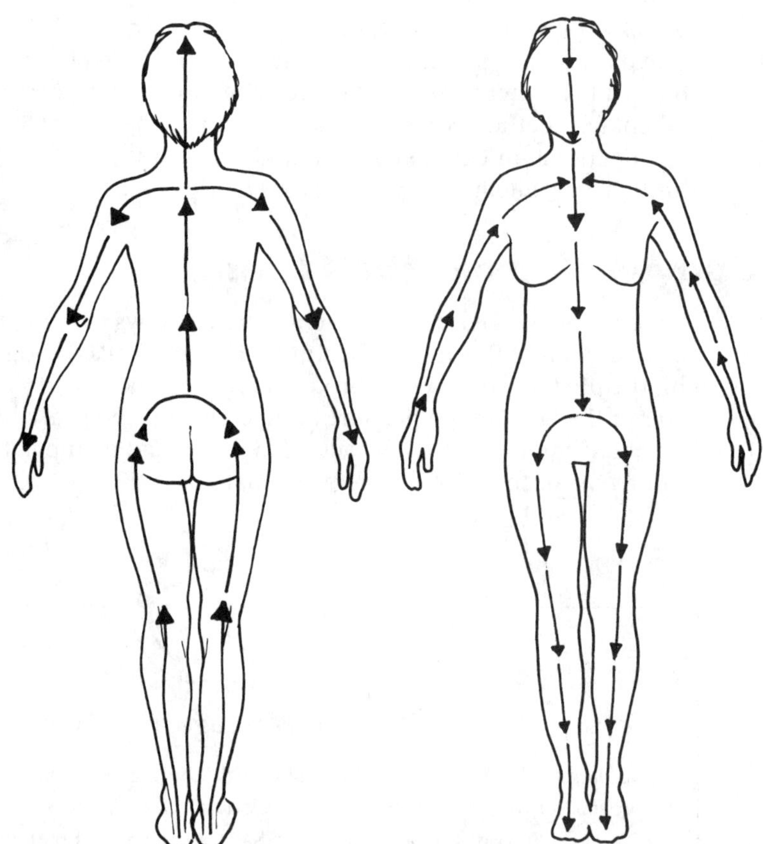

Under (Acu)Pressure

You've probably heard of *acupuncture*, that method of healing in which hair-thin needles are inserted into pressure points to relieve pain and heal disease. Once regarded as on-the-fringe, acupuncture is now a common method of treatment in the United States, and many insurance companies now cover acupuncture treatments.

Different doctors and scientists have various theories on why it works, but there's little doubt that acupuncture, an ancient Chinese medical technique, does work.

Acupressure also originated in China and combines pressure and massage to treat the same areas delineated by acupuncture theory. Like many other forms of Chinese medicine, acupressure techniques moved from China to Korea to Japan, where they were embraced and developed.

Many people prefer acupressure over acupuncture. Acupressure is less invasive than acupuncture because acupressure involves applying pressure to areas of blocked or stagnant chi with fingers, thumbs, elbows, or even electrical currents instead of needles. It's something you can do to yourself if you know how. Like many other forms of bodywork, acupressure has evolved into many different schools and methods.

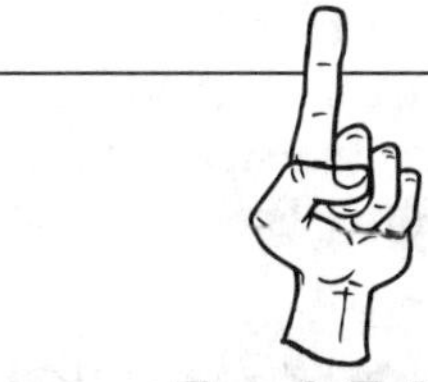

Touch Talk

Acupuncture, a method of healing in which needles are inserted into certain areas of the body to free or reactivate stagnant chi, was developed centuries ago in China. Originally, needles were made from bone and stone. Later, they were made from steel. Some historians believe an original purpose for acupuncture was to lance infections.

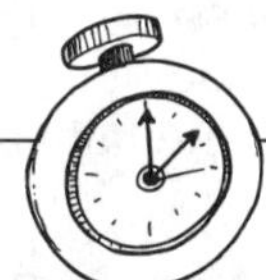

A Massage Minute

Moxibustion, a technique similar to acupuncture and acupressure, was developed in ancient China in areas where the climate was cold. Rather than using needles or pressure to activate chi on pressure points, moxibustion involves burning small, cone-shaped bundles of herbs directly on the skin over pressure points to activate the areas with heat. Still commonly practiced in China today, moxibustion is much less popular in the West. Moxibustion should only be performed by a practitioner with formal training in Chinese medicine.

Kudos to Tsubos! Shiatsu

Although many people usethe terms *shiatsu* and *acupressure* interchangeably, acupressure is a more encompassing term that includes shiatsu. Shiatsu is a particular method of acupressure developed and refined in Japan that combines pressure, usually exerted with the thumbs and fingers, with long massage strokes over energy meridians. According to some shiatsu practitioners, stroking and massaging the meridians is just as important, if not more important, than activating the pressure points (or *tsubos*, as they are called in Japan). Although you can find books on "self-shiatsu," according to many, shiatsu can be administered only by a practitioner, whereas acupressure can be self-administered.

Meet Your Acupoints: Jin Shin Do

Jin Shin Do, translated as "The Way of the Compassionate Spirit" or "Body-Spirit Way" is another school of acupressure developed in the late 1970s by Iona Marasaa Teeguarden. Jin Shin Do combines ancient Oriental techniques (Japanese acupressure, Chinese acupuncture theory, Taoist theory, and yogic breathwork) with certain Western theories of psychotherapy and body-mind management. This technique appeals to many Westerners because of this East/West synthesis.

Jin Shin Do is different than traditional acupressure in two ways. One way, as we've said, is that it utilizes Western psychotherapy by combining acupressure treatments with specific psychological techniques. Two, it bases its acupoints on 8 energy channels in the body that work in conjunction with the traditional 12 energy meridians. These eight channels are called the *strange flows*, and Jin Shin Do helps to open these channels to keep the life force moving more freely and in a more balanced manner.

According to Teeguarden, the body is a metaphor for the psyche, and we can feel our emotional and spiritual lives in our bodies if we only learn how. In Jin Shin Do, acupoints are direct lines to your body-mind, and activating them will help to keep you in better touch with yourself—literally and figuratively.

A Massage Minute

Wilhelm Reich (1897–1957) was a psychiatrist whose work was based on the idea that the body and mind are inextricably linked. He believed that disease is a direct result of psychological trauma, which becomes trapped in the body in a process called *armoring*. Reich believed that the body could be segmented into areas that hold individual emotional experiences. Jin Shin Do acupressure is based in part on Reich's theories of the segmented, armored body.

Choosing a Massage that's Right for You

Choosing the right kind of bodywork depends largely on what appeals to you, what you want to work on in your personal development, and what your physical, emotional, and spiritual beliefs happen to be. If you're attracted by the Oriental techniques, visit an acupressurist or a practitioner of shiatsu. If you are a dancer or an actor, try one of the movement therapies. Maybe you like the idea of balancing your energy, or trying yoga, or combining psychotherapy with bodywork. Talk to different practitioners and, if possible, their clients. Do a little research, then start experimenting. Most of all, have fun, and enjoy how much better you feel!

The Least You Need to Know

- Some types of bodywork deal with the manipulation and treatment of the body's energy field. These types of bodywork are considered energy therapy.
- Some forms of bodywork, known collectively as somatic and psychophysical therapies, deal with movement re-education and the combination of psychotherapy techniques and body-use patterns.
- Oriental techniques focus on energy flows and pressure points.
- Your mind and your body are not separate. Healing means making the connection between your body and your mind; it means opening up your life to your body-mind connection.

Part 4
Different Strokes for Different Folks

This "how-to" part consists of chapters or sections on each of the main strokes commonly used in Swedish and other types of massage. First, we'll introduce you to the long, flowing strokes of effleurage. Then, we'll explain how to knead the body into submission with petrissage. We'll teach you how to administer compression and percussion strokes to loosen up and energize the body; then we'll explain the details of friction and vibration strokes. After that, we'll show you some range-of-motion techniques, which are great for reminding the body what it can do, as opposed to what it always tends to do. After this part, you'll be ready to give a proficient and wonderful massage. (But don't stop reading yet—there's more to come!)

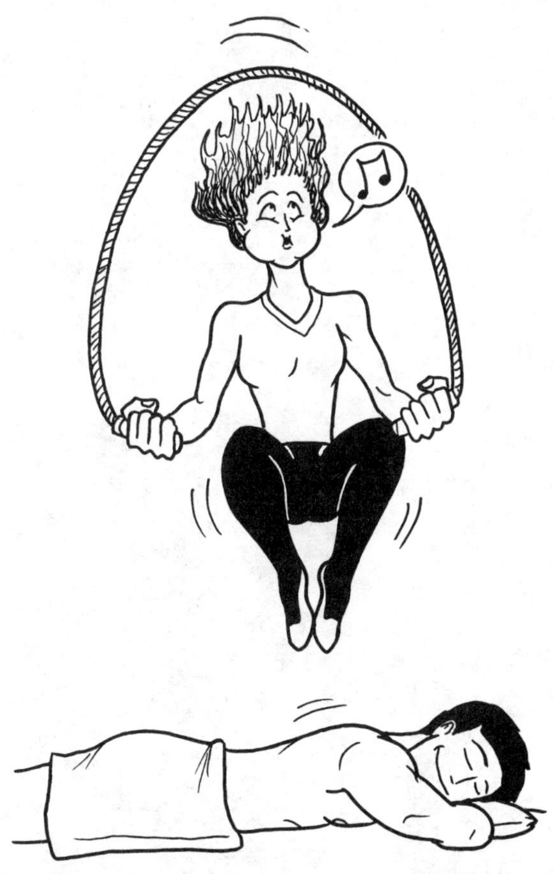

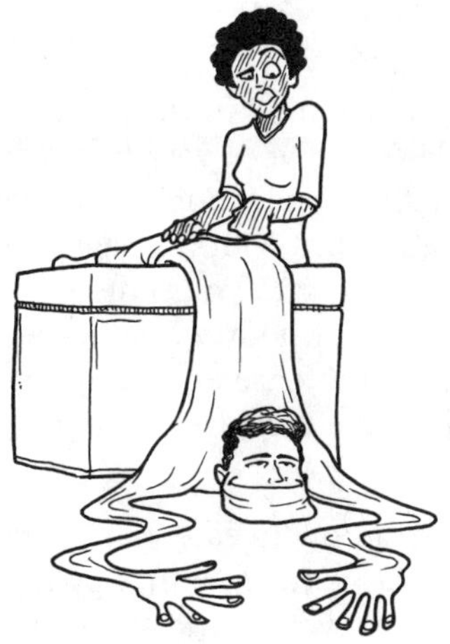

Chapter 13

Go with the Flow: Effleurage

In This Chapter

- Introducing effleurage: the long, gliding stroke
- Effleurage with the hands, thumbs, fists, and forearms
- Different effleurage techniques

If you've ever stroked a cat from nose to tail, you've had a little experience with *effleurage* (pronounced *eh-fluh-rajh*), one of the basic massage strokes in Swedish massage. Also known as a gliding stroke, effleurage involves long, smooth strokes over different parts of the body.

Light effleurage is great for preparing the body for deeper work, relaxing muscles, and spreading massage oil over the skin. Deeper effleurage, once muscles are relaxed and prepared, can facilitate blood and lymph flow, loosen muscle fibers, and improve organ functions.

Hand Over Hand Above the Rest

The full hand stroke is the basic effleurage stroke and the one used in the beginning of a Swedish massage session. Just imagine how you would feel at your very first massage session if you lay down on the table, unclothed, nervous, and feeling vulnerable, and your massage therapist began immediately to dig deep into your muscles with heavy, hard strokes. Ouch! Your body wouldn't be ready, and your muscles would tense up against the assault—the opposite of what a massage is supposed to do!

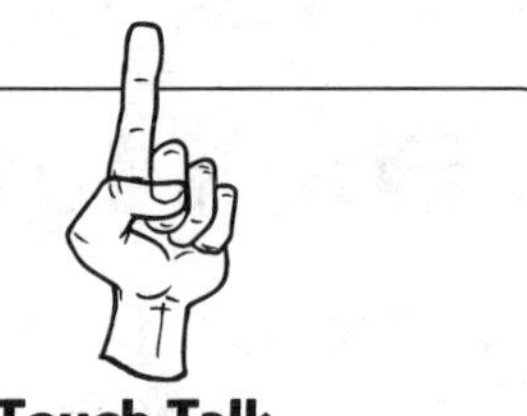

Touch Talk

Effleurage, from the French verb *effleurer*, meaning "to graze, to skim the surface of, or to touch lightly," is the term coined by Dr. Johann Mezger (1839–1909) to refer to a long, gliding massage stroke. Dr. Mezger was a Dutch physician who is credited with establishing massage as a scientific area of study for physicians.

Instead, massage therapists know to ease you in gradually by starting with a gentle, soft, smooth, flowing, gliding effleurage stroke. Now your muscles are warming up. Now you're feeling relaxed. Ahhh. Superficial or light effleurage strokes are also great for calming and relaxing a nervous massagee, especially when the strokes are rhythmic and slow.

In an effleurage stroke, the entire hand is placed on the body and gently glides across a long surface, such as the whole leg, arm, the back, or even from crown to toe. Full-hand strokes are most effective for larger body parts, such as the back and limbs. One hand may work best for smaller limbs, but both hands may work simultaneously on the back, the abdomen, the buttocks, or the legs (one hand on each side of the leg), for example.

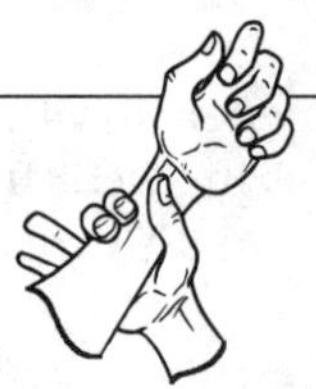

Your Finger on the Pulse

The light effleurage stroke may be used as a type of diagnostic tool. When a massage therapist first begins to work on a client, effleurage allows him or her to test muscles and other tissues for tight, loose, or particularly sensitive areas, helping to determine the format and techniques to be used during the massage session.

Effleurage strokes generally move toward the heart and in the direction of muscle fibers to best encourage productive circulation. Another technique is to maintain constant hand contact with the massagee, in which case the effleurage stroke would be applied from wrist to shoulder, and then a much lighter stroke would be used to return to the wrist or to the next area to be massaged. (The lighter return stroke is used to move away from the heart so that blood flow toward the heart isn't adversely affected.)

Deep effleurage is best accomplished with the full hand. Once the body is ready, the massager can apply firm, deep strokes in the direction of the heart to stimulate circulation and to help flush the organs and tissues with nutrients. Deep effleurage can be remarkably relaxing and renewing—a workout for your insides.

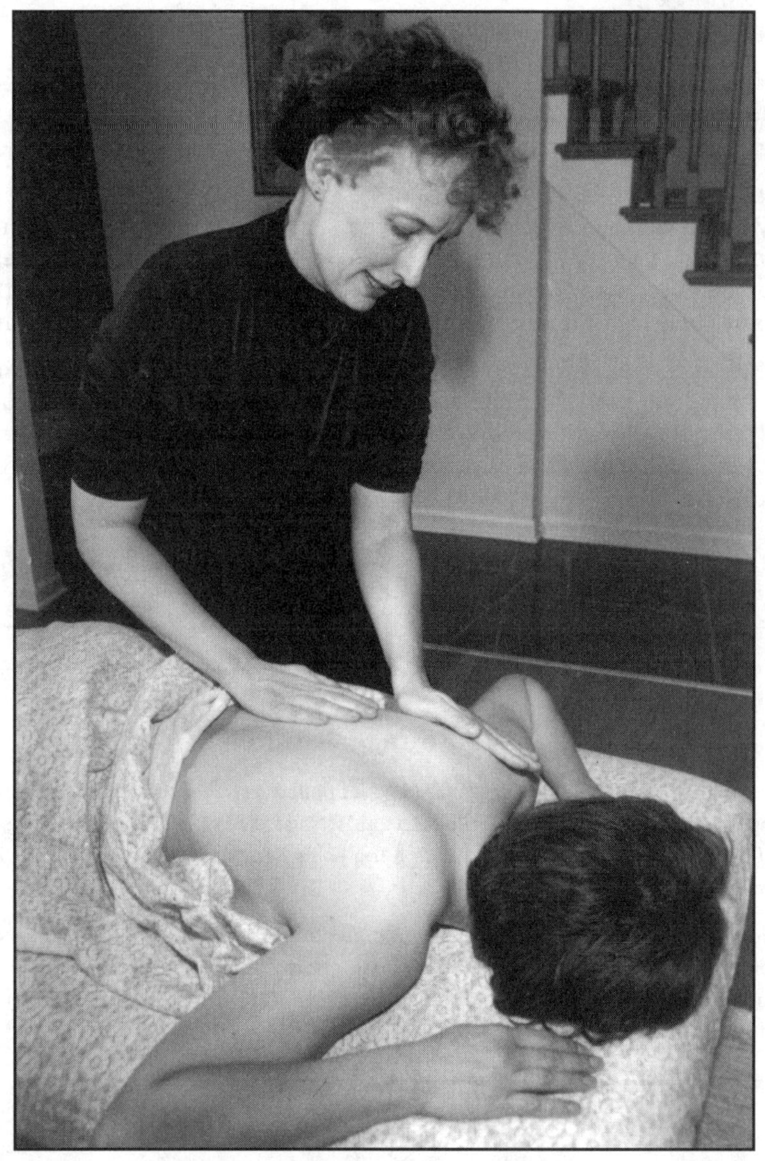

Joan demonstrates gliding hand over hand effleurage. Her hands glide up the back without losing contact with Melanie's skin.

All Thumbs

Although effleurage is generally performed with the entire hand, certain body parts are too small for your whole hand. Areas such as facial features (eyes, ears), toes, and hands can benefit from effleurage strokes performed with the thumbs and/or fingers.

Long, light thumb strokes over the face can be relaxing in a way you never imagined, especially if you've never experienced a face massage (rubbing your own temples in despair when you've got a splitting headache doesn't count!). Hands and feet can get a more targeted effect with thumb and finger effleurage, and long strokes with the thumbs on either side of the spine can be a great way to relax and loosen the back.

A basic effleurage stroke is performed with the full palm in contact with skin, fingers and thumbs together. An alternate version is the V stroke, in which the thumb is separated from the closed fingers to form a V. This stroke is particularly effective for the limbs because it allows the massager's hand to encircle the limb more fully during the stroke.

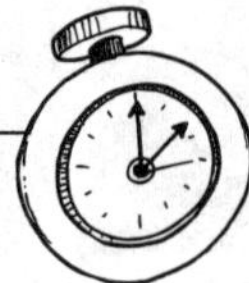

A Massage Minute

Aura stroking is a technique in which effleurage is applied just over the skin, without actually touching it. Some massage therapists use it to end a massage session. The purpose is to enhance energy flow by "massaging" the *aura*, which is the energy emanation surrounding the body like a whole-body halo.

Aura stroking is controversial because many people doubt the existence of the aura itself. A high-voltage photograph process known as Kirlian photography does reveal a luminescent halo emanating from the human body, and some people claim to be able to see auras, but skeptics abound nonetheless.

Open Fist of Peace

For a different effect, try doing effleurage with your fists instead of a flat hand. Not tight, clenched fists ready for a boxing match, but loose, open fists that gently glide over large areas of the body. The knuckles can go a little deeper into muscles and tissues, loosening them and relieving tension.

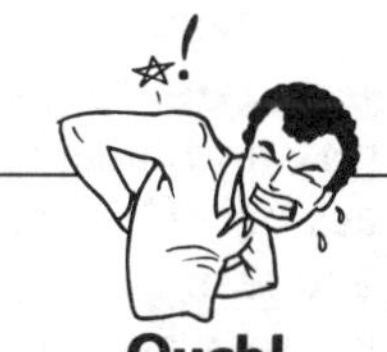

Ouch!

Never begin a massage too roughly. When you give a massage, remember to start out with slow, gentle, gliding effleurage strokes until the person you're massaging is clearly relaxed and ready for deeper muscle work.

Fist effleurage is good for stimulating blood and lymph flow because the stroke can move more deeply into the muscles. The lightest pressure stimulates lymph flow; deeper pressure pinches it off. Don't dig your fists in too deeply, though. The massager's fists should be relaxed, tension-free, and slightly open. You don't want to injure your own wrists and hands or cause the massagee pain.

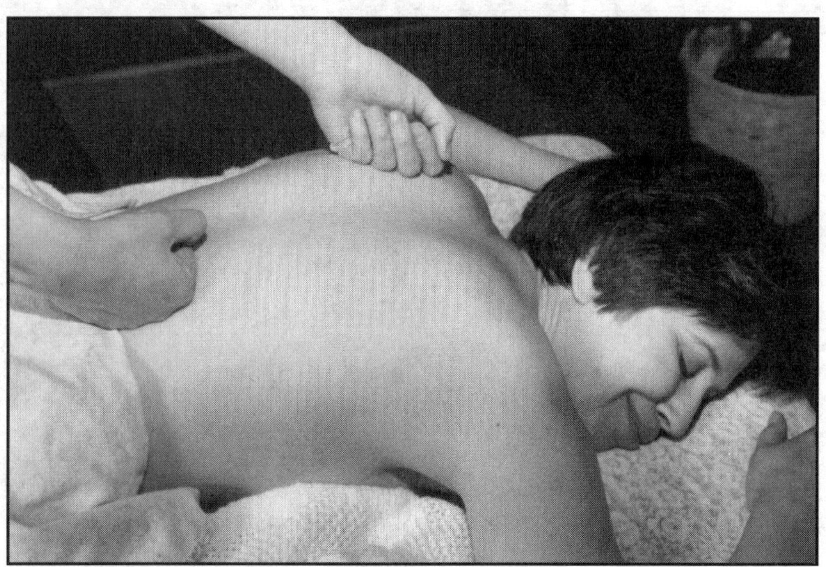

When gliding with loose fists, make sure the pressure is right. Joan checked with Melanie, who said, "It's great!"

Forearms: Prelude to an Elbow

Sometimes your palms aren't big enough to encompass an area satisfactorily. There's no sense in limiting yourself to the ends of your arms, though. Take a look at your forearms, and imagine them as rolling pins. Your forearms can be great tools to use on the back or other large body areas. Gently rest your forearm on the massagee's lower back and lean into it, just enough to exert gentle pressure. Now, slide your forearm, effleurage-style, up the back, on either side of the spine. (Stay off the spine, especially with the elbow, which can cause injury.) This stroke enables you to cover almost the entire back in one stroke. It feels great!

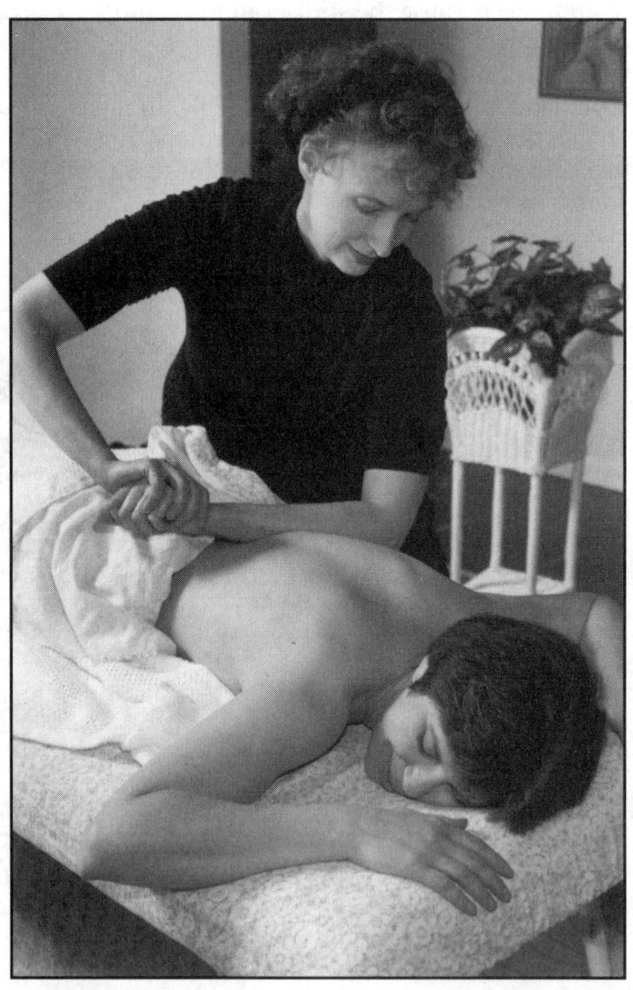

Use the soft part of your lower arm and lean into it. Pretend that your arm is a gliding rolling pin. We're just starting to cook!

Fanning: Summer Breezes

The fanning stroke is a lovely and creative variation of the effleurage stroke that covers a wider area than a closed hand and is a nice way to break up a routine of long, gliding strokes. Beginning with your hands placed next to each other, thumbs together and fingers fanned to the sides, fan the fingers over the body and back again. This stroke is calming and feels great. You can use it on any area of the body big enough to encompass the full hands; it feels especially good on the stomach and back. Plus, it's aesthetically pleasing, a beautiful stroke.

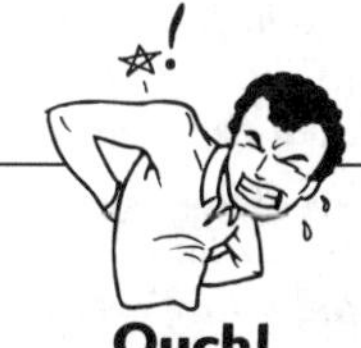

Ouch!

Deep effleurage mustn't be applied randomly. Always ask if the massagee has any injured or sensitive areas, and avoid directly massaging internal organs. You could cause serious injury if you press too hard in the wrong place.

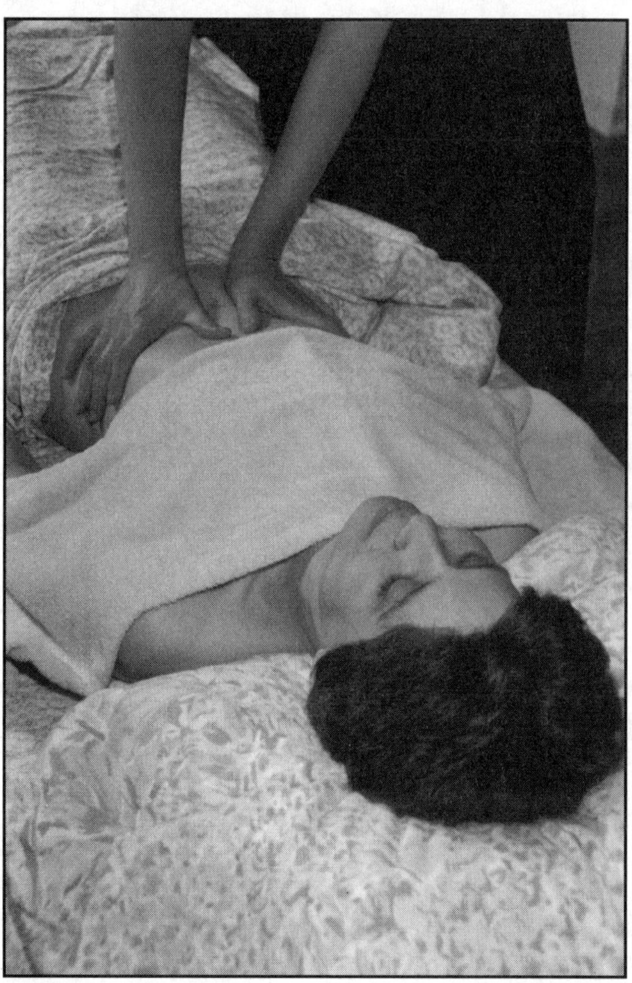

For a tummy fan, start with thumbs together and fingers fanned to the sides. Use light pressure on the stomach.

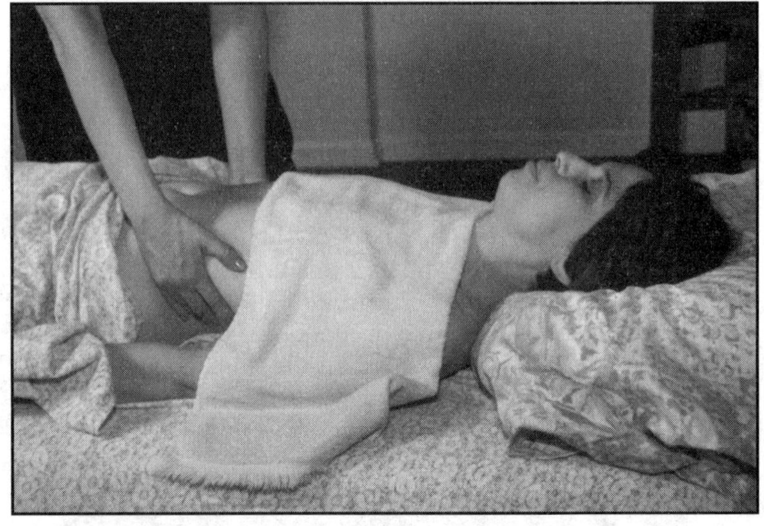

For the second part of the tummy fan, fan your fingers down the sides to the spine. Then, lift up back to the center of the tummy, providing a nice back release.

Feather Stroke: Goosebumps

When you were a little kid, you may have played a game where you and your friends wrote letters on each other's backs and tried to guess what they were or made X's and O's and other shapes that went along with sing-song rhyming games, such as "X marks the spot with a circle and a dot...." The purpose of these games seemed to be to watch the goosebumps pop out on someone's back. The person guessing the letters knew the feathery strokes felt good, too.

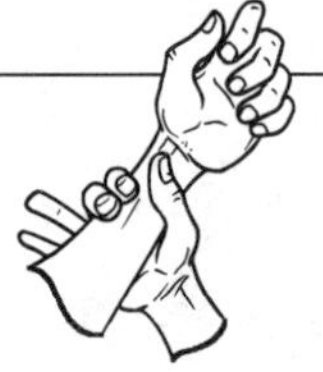

Your Finger on the Pulse

If you want to relax someone who is extremely nervous, jittery, or suffering from insomnia, a short massage consisting entirely of feather strokes can be quite effective. Run your fingertips very lightly over the back, arms, legs, head, and face and watch the nervous tension float away like feathers in the wind! If the person is ticklish, increase the pressure slightly so as not to increase nervousness.

Massage therapists are well aware of how good light, feathery strokes feel. These strokes are often used to end a massage, and although they don't have an effect on deep tissues and circulation, they do stimulate the nerves. If feather strokes are applied for an extended period of time, they are calming.

Feather stroking is easy. Run your fingertips or hands very lightly in long, flowing, wavy, or even tickly strokes over the skin. Watch the goosebumps pop out, and you'll know you're doing it right. If goosebumps persist, increase pressure just a bit to keep the nerves calm.

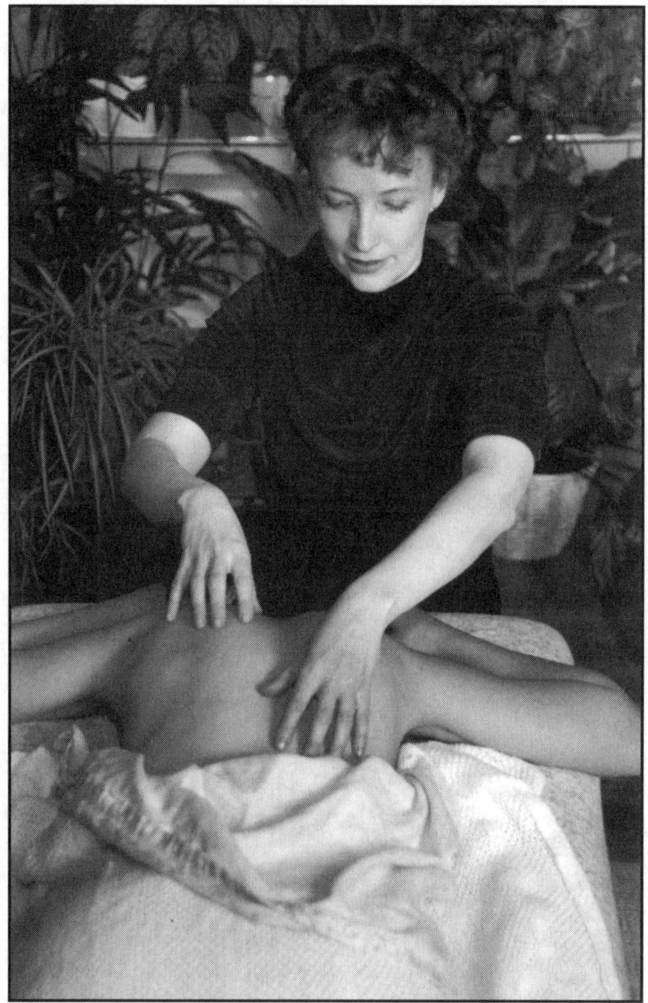

Vary your pressure with this feathery gliding stroke of the fingers.

The Least You Need to Know

- Effleurage is a French term referring to long, gliding massage strokes.
- You can perform effleurage with the entire hand, the thumbs and fingers, loose fists, or even the forearms.
- Effleurage strokes can be superficial, deep, or light as a feather. Each type of stroke serves a different purpose.

Chapter 14

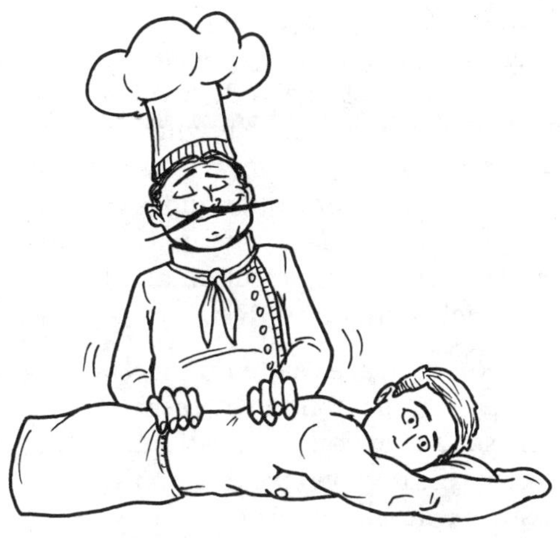

Oh, How We Knead You: Petrissage

In This Chapter

- The petrissage stroke: rolling, pinching, and pressing
- The effects of petrissage
- Various petrissage techniques

Petrissage (pronounced *pet-rih-sahj*) is another basic stroke used in Swedish massage, and it's quite different from effleurage. Unlike effleurage, in which large areas are covered in one stroke, petrissage is more focused. Performed on the fleshy areas of the body, the petrissage stroke involves picking up the skin and rolling, pressing, or squeezing it.

Petrissage is a great cleansing technique. It lifts the muscles away from the bones, allowing toxins and wastes to dislodge and enter the bloodstream, where they can then be eliminated. It's also good for jump-starting circulation by getting the blood and lymph flowing, breaking up muscle adhesions, and, in general, loosening, separating, and freeing your insides. Whether you're picking up and holding muscles or lifting and squeezing *fascia* (the connective tissue that supports your nerves and blood vessels), petrissage really gets you loose!

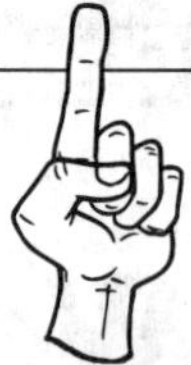

Touch Talk

Petrissage, a French noun translated as kneading or, figuratively, forming, is the term coined by Dr. Johann Mezger (1839–1909) to refer to a kneading massage stroke.

Fascia is the layer of fibrous connective tissue underlying and separating your skin from the organs, bones, and muscles beneath it. Your fascia supports your nerves and blood vessels. When kneaded and manipulated through massage, the fascia is loosened, releasing toxins and stimulating circulation.

Petrissage is particularly effective in a massage session when it follows a series of long, gliding, preparatory effleurage strokes; think of petrissage as the workout after the warm-up. The petrissage stroke is what many people think of when they envision a massage and what many try to do when they give someone a quick shoulder massage. Although some people are naturals at this type of massage stroke, the correct execution of a petrissage stroke isn't necessarily intuitive.

Have you ever received a massage that didn't feel very good, as though the person massaging you seemed to be merely pinching the surface of your skin without getting into the muscle? Petrissage involves picking up the skin and underlying tissue or muscle, and then rolling, squeezing, or applying firm pressure to it. To do petrissage effectively, you have to get right in there, not just work on the surface.

Petrissage shouldn't be painful. It has a deeply relaxing effect on the underlying muscle tissue. If you're having trouble finding a balance between a too-superficial stroke that isn't relaxing and a too-deep stroke that hurts, have the person you're massaging give you continuous feedback. Try different levels and depths of pressure until your massagee tells you you've got it.

A Massage Minute

Even though giving a massage can be a therapeutic experience, it can also be an exhausting and intense job. Massage therapists can suffer from burnout just like anyone else and may experience exhaustion, boredom, cynicism, detachment, and feelings of being unappreciated. Sound familiar?

Most massage therapists agree their job is a calling rather than a job, and they wouldn't trade it for a desk job in a million years; but just imagine giving eight one-hour massages every day all week! One of the best ways for massage therapists (and the rest of us, for that matter) to avoid job burnout is to get massaged regularly. Instant renewal!

Kneading Bread (or Muscle)

Performing the basic petrissage kneading stroke is a lot like kneading bread. To perform the kneading stroke, grasp the flesh (either the skin and underlying fascia, or the skin, fascia, and muscle) with one hand and gently but firmly press it into the cradle of the fingers of your other hand in a circular motion. As you work, squeeze the flesh as though you're milking it of its fluids—which, in a sense, you are.

Don't just pinch the top layer of skin—that hurts! Get deep into the tissue, but not painfully deep, either. Grasp the muscles gently, hold them, squeeze them, press them, and release them. For smaller areas, you can knead in a similar motion with your fingers and thumbs.

Another way is to compress the tissue with your palm and then lift it with your palm and the lower half of your fingers (the finger pads), as if you were fluffing a pillow. Alternate hands: compress and lift with the right hand, and then compress and lift with the left hand, rhythmically.

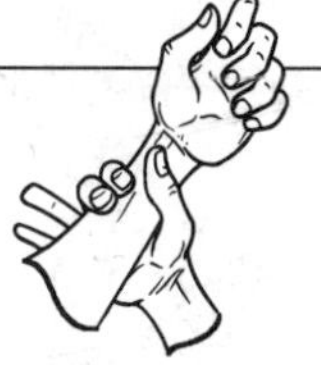

Your Finger on the Pulse

If you can't quite get the feel of the kneading stroke, or if you want more practice or want to build hand strength, try baking bread from scratch. In this age of convenience stores and bread machines, people rarely bake bread the old-fashioned way anymore, but it can be a great lesson in the technique of petrissage. Plus, it builds hand strength.

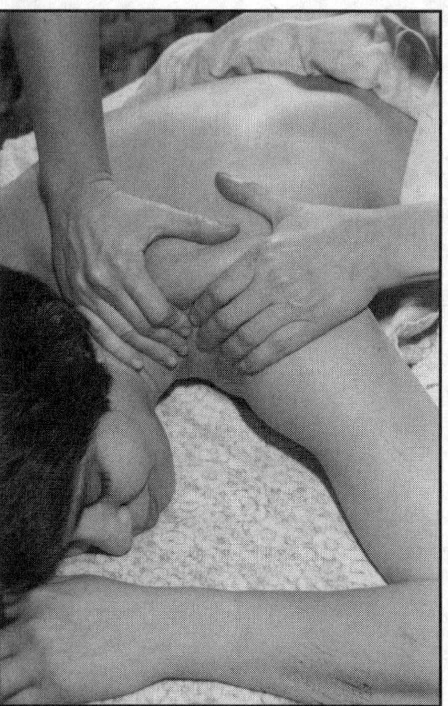

In kneading one hand feeds into the other. Don't pinch: work with full hands. As Joan finds that Melanie's shoulder is relaxing, she can begin to work the muscle more deeply.

Pulling: Give Me Some Muscle!

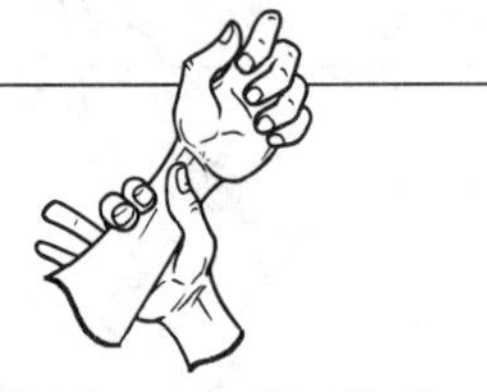

Your Finger on the Pulse

For those less-fleshy areas that seem unkneadable, perform the petrissage stroke using your finger and thumb rather than your whole hands. Kneading the face, feet, and hands in this way is very relaxing and great for increasing circulation, but be careful not to pinch! You still want to pick up the fascia along with the skin.

Just like effleurage, petrissagecan be performed with several different techniques. One of them is called *pulling*. Pulling involves grasping a muscle (see the following figure, in which Joan is grasping the trapezius muscle), lifting it up, and pulling on it, holding it there for several seconds.

Pulling the muscle accentuates the stretching and toxin-releasing aspect of the petrissage stroke. Lifting the muscle loosens adhesions and stiffness and creates space around the muscle for drainage and release. Sometimes, a particularly tight muscle will finally begin to release if you simply pick it up and hold it for a while. Tight muscles react well to being moved every now and then.

It helps to know something about anatomy to perform the pulling stroke, but many muscles are obvious if you feel around for them. Remember that the point isn't to pull the muscle right out of its skin, but to gently wrap your fingers around it, lift, and hold.

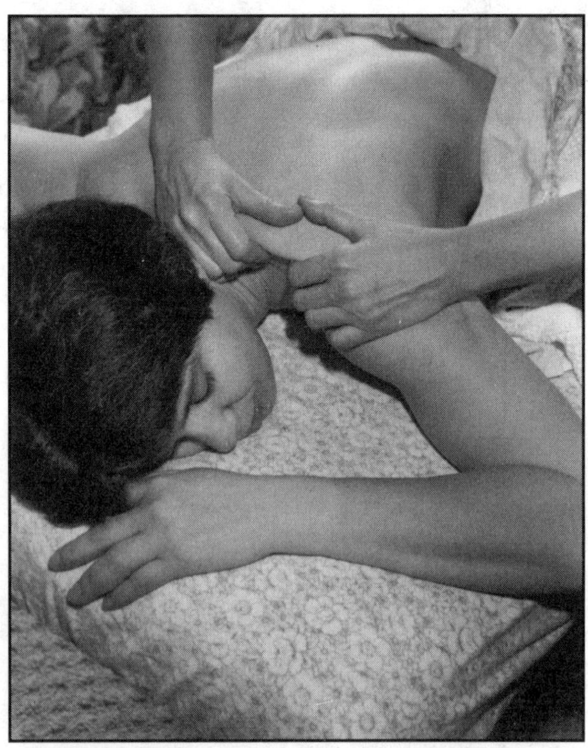

Joan is pulling Melanie's trapezius muscle toward her head and holding it there for a few seconds. Many people hold tension in the trapezius.

Wring in the New You!

Have you ever wrung out a towel that's filled with water? You hold the towel in a roll and twist, with one hand rotating in one direction and the other hand rotating in the other direction. Wringing a towel is the best way to get the bulk of the water out, and the wringing petrissage stroke is a great way to wring tension out of muscles.

Wringing is most easily performed on the legs or arms (which most resemble that rolled-up towel) because your hands can wrap around the limb. Wrap both hands around the area, next to each other, and then gently rotate one hand forward and one hand back. Alternate each hand's direction.

If you press too tightly or go too fast, manipulating only the surface of the skin, this stroke could cause a burning sensation on the skin. The wringing stroke doesn't burn. Instead, it should be gentle, gliding, and deep. Using massage oil will lessen the chance that you'll be pulling on the skin and creating the burning sensation, especially when your massagee's skin is sensitive or dry. However, don't use too much oil, or the tissue will be too slippery, and you won't be able to get a good grasp. The wringing stroke manipulates the underlying tissue, not just the skin's surface.

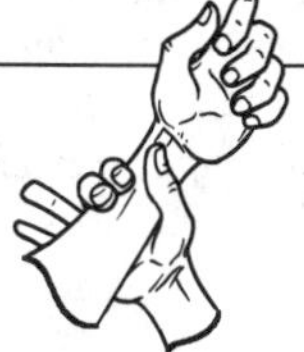

Your Finger on the Pulse

Massage oil has several purposes; one of them is to help the hands glide with less friction over the skin surface, lessening skin irritation, uncomfortable pinching, or burning sensations. Use just enough oil to keep the skin surface smooth so that your hands glide easily, and the massage experience will be more pleasant and comfortable for everyone.

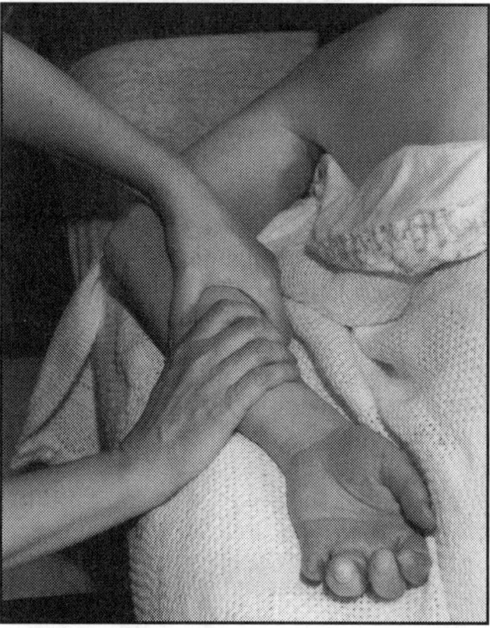

In wringing one hand rotates one way, and the other hand rotates the other way. Let your hands glide over the skin. Beautiful!

Rolling: "Roll, Roll, Roll Your Flesh..."

Rolling is a petrissage technique in which portions of the flesh are picked up and then rolled between the fingers and thumb. Unlike pulling, in which a muscle is lifted and held, the rolling stroke involves lifting and holding the skin and fascia only.

In a skin roll, you grab hold of some of the outer skin (the fascia) and walk your fingers up the back, sliding the skin up as you walk.

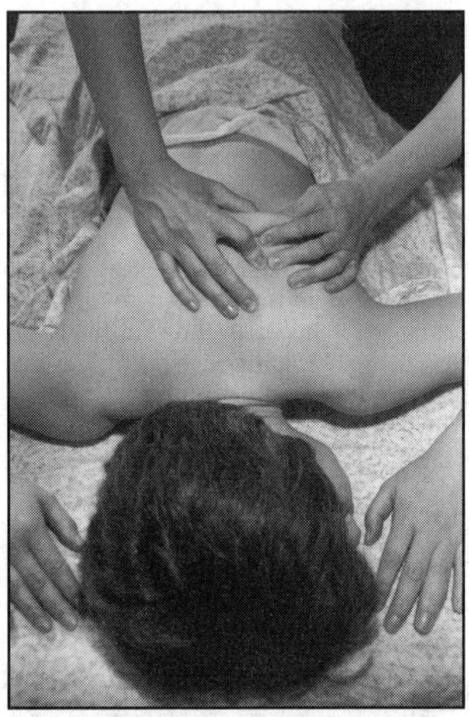

First, grasp the skin and underlying fascia between your fingers and thumb. Then, by moving your fingers and thumb in opposite directions, roll the flesh gently while holding it. Some people's skin lifts right up; others seem to have extremely tight fascia, making this stroke more difficult. Make sure the massagee knows to tell you if you're pinching. You may want to try this stroke on yourself first to get a sense of how the stroke feels as the massagee in relation to how it feels externally as the massager.

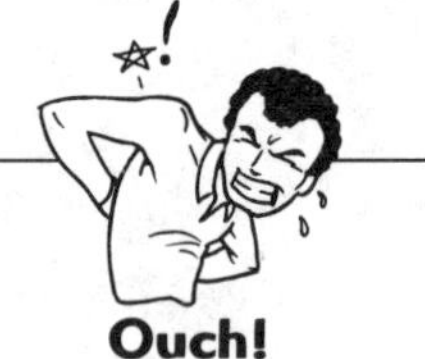

Ouch!

Avoid performing massage strokes directly on varicose veins or on or near bruises, broken skin, or broken bones.

Just like other petrissage strokes, this stroke creates space under the skin, helping to release stored toxins. The rolling stroke is unique, however, in that it concentrates on the fascia, which is a continuous network of tissue (like the skin) over the entire body. If you had the time, you could pick up an area of flesh, roll it, and keep rolling it until you've moved along the entire body without ever letting go.

Connecting to the fascia with the rolling stroke is relaxing in a different way than strokes that work directly on muscles are. When you work the fascia, you are working the underside of the skin, and such an all-encompassing tissue network, linked as it is to the blood vessels and nerve endings that travel throughout your entire body, may well deliver this message instantly over and through your whole being: "Feels so good!"

Pac-Man Petrissage

You probably remember the Pac-Man video arcade game, starring that big-mouthed circle that traveled through a maze gobbling up dots and flashing ghosts. In the Pac-Man petrissage stroke, which is a variation of the basic kneading stroke, one hand is the Pac-Man and the other hand, or rather the thumb, is the ghost. Moving over the surface of the skin, your Pac-Man hand repeatedly "swallows" the opposite thumb, which pushes up the skin surface around it so it can be most effectively kneaded by the Pac-Man hand. Just one more way to vary your massage routine, the Pac-Man stroke is fun, feels great, and may even spark some lively, nostalgic conversation about the good old days when video games were easy, quarters were plentiful, and you had nothing to do after school but see who was hanging out at the arcade.

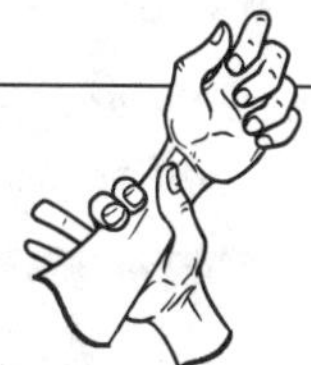

Your Finger on the Pulse

Because petrissage strokes are so cleansing, it's important for the massagee to drink a lot of water after a vigorous massage session. A good fluid intake (about 64 ounces of pure water per day is ideal) assists in the elimination of all those loosened toxins. Also, following petrissage with a smoothing, soothing effleurage stroke makes everything feel better.

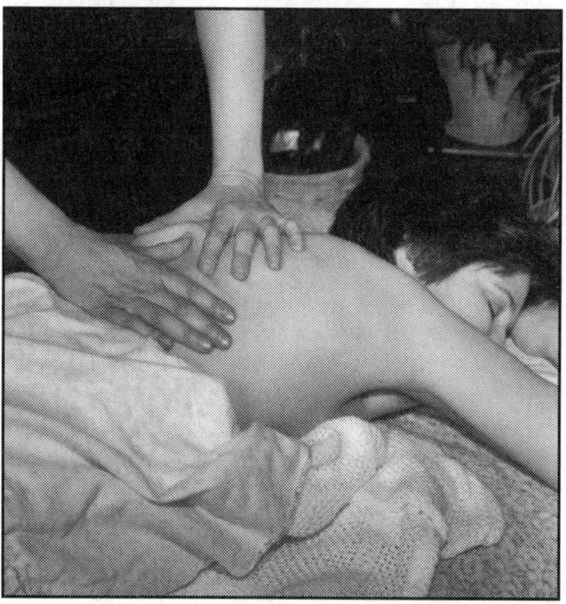

In the Pac-Man stroke, the thumb of one hand feeds into the C-shape of the other hand. Gobble up the thumb as you close the C around it. Do this all over the back.

The Least You Need to Know

- Petrissage is a French term referring to a kneading massage stroke.
- Petrissage is a great stroke for stimulating circulation and loosening tight muscle tissue.
- Different petrissage techniques include kneading, pulling, wringing, rolling, and the Pac-Man stroke.

Chapter 15

Groovin' to the Massage Beat: Compression and Percussion

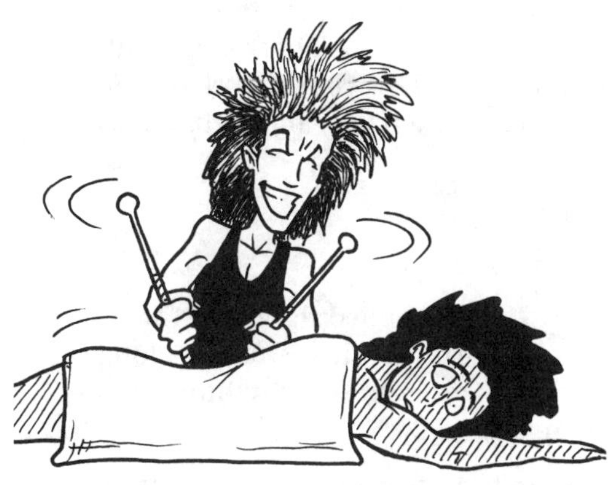

In This Chapter

- How to perform a compression stroke
- The effects of compression strokes
- What is a percussion stroke, and how do you do it?
- How percussion strokes affect the body

Compression and *percussion* (the latter is also known as *tapotement*) are two more types of classic Swedish massage strokes that have one thing in common: rhythm! They're both good follow-ups to petrissage, because they get even deeper into muscles to fully stimulate and activate muscle tissue. Plus, they're fun to do! If you're giving a massage with music in the background, you may find that your compression and percussion strokes fall right into the rhythm of the music, which enhances the massage experience for the massagee and helps you keep a consistent rhythm with your strokes.

Tapotement, from the French verb tapoter, is translated as "to pat, to tap, or to strum" and is the term coined by Dr. Johann Mezger (1839–1909) to refer to the percussion stroke. *Compression* is a type of friction massage stroke involving a rhythmic pressing motion performed with the hands or fingers.

The fact that Swedish massage employs French terminology (tapotement and effleurage, for example) is no accident. The French were the first to translate the ancient Chinese text *The Cong-Fou of the Tao-Tse*, which many believe was directly influential in the development of the techniques of Swedish massage. This classic work of Chinese health care described the use of herbal medicine, specific exercises, and certain massage techniques to treat disease and maintain health.

Pumping Muscle: Compression

The first type of rhythmic stroke is the compression stroke. Aimed right into the muscle tissue at an angle perpendicular to muscle fibers (rather than stroking along the direction of the fiber as in effleurage), compression strokes involve a rhythmic pumping movement, almost as if you were giving the muscle CPR.

Compression is often used in sports massage because it primes muscles for a workout, forcing nutrients such as oxygen into the muscles. The effect of compression strokes lasts long after the massage has ended, making it ideal for athletes about to compete. Even if your sport is taking an important test, dragging your kids to the grocery store, addressing the PTA for the first time, or proposing a radical new sales technique at the annual company meeting, priming your muscles and your mind via a pre-performance massage will have you performing at your peak.

Hand Over Hand

The full-hand compression stroke uses the entire surface of the hand to compress muscles. Because compression strokes are relatively firm, they can become tiring for the massager. Use your body weight and lean into the stroke, as Joan is doing in the photo, and your compression stroke will be more effective and less exhausting.

Press one entire hand, focusing on the heel of your hand, gently but deeply into the muscle tissue. Then press the other palm into the muscle just above the first hand. Work your hands along the body surface one after the other as if they were stepping across the body in a slow dance step. No music playing? Think of a slow "Row, Row, Row Your Boat."

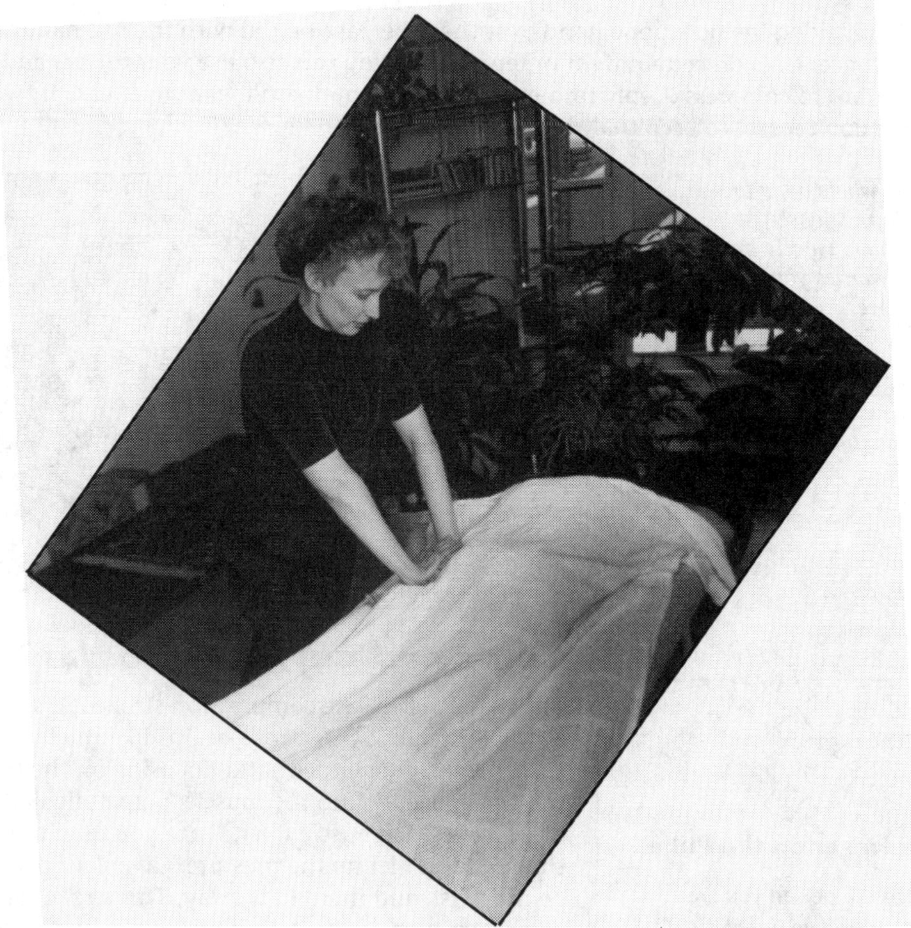

In this example of hand over hand compression, notice how Joan positions her body into a lunge. She uses the weight of her body, rather than brute arm strength. By using her body weight to compress, Joan's shoulders stay relaxed as she helps to relax Melanie.

Keep It Loose

Loose-fist compression strokes give a slightly different effect than full-hand compression strokes because the fist isn't a flat surface like the palm. Again, let your body help you with these firm compression strokes rather than trying to do all the work with your arms. Loose, open fists (don't ball them up like cannonballs, please—that's not comfy!) can get deep into muscle tissue because you are working the muscle fibers with your knuckles.

Travel along the body, one hand over the other, as you did with the full-hand stroke, or concentrate on certain tight or tense areas. You can also use your fingers and thumbs to compress deeply into muscle tissue that doesn't want to release its worries. But don't forget to keep that rhythm!

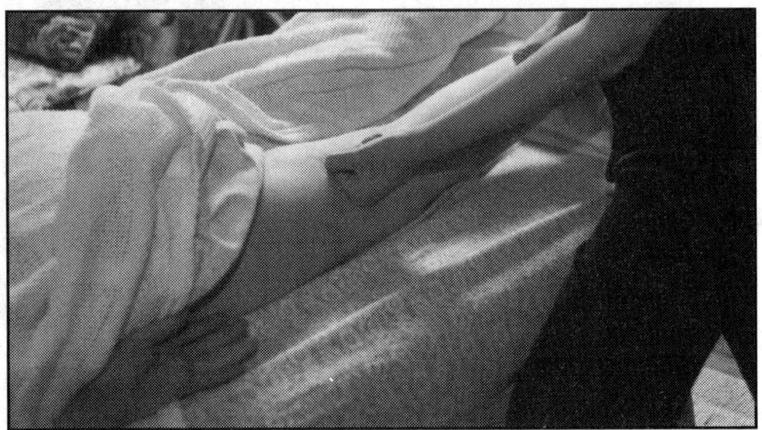

Use your whole body to lean into this loose-fist compression. Gently iron out any worries your friend might have.

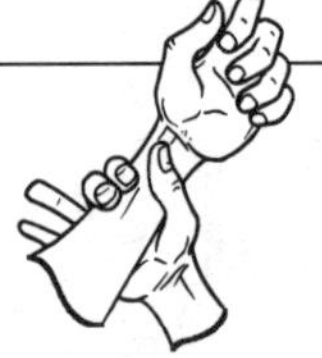

Your Finger on the Pulse

Encourage the person you are massaging to exhale deeply as you compress muscle tissue, particularly in areas where muscles are tight and resistant. Deep breathing aids relaxation, but it also helps make even more oxygen available to those muscles being deeply activated by your compression strokes.

Come on Baby, Let's Do the Twist

The twist-and-release compression stroke is a stroke with a twist—literally! This stroke begins like the full-hand stroke. Press your entire hand, focusing on the heel of the hand, deeply into the muscle, perpendicular to the direction of the muscle fiber. Once you're in there, though, don't let up the pressure. Give your palm a gentle twist, and then lift it away. This stroke further stimulates muscle circulation by giving the muscle fibers a little tweak. Soon, those muscles will be flushed with vital nutrients. Do this stroke to a slow song with a steady beat (think of your favorite slow blues song or spiritual, such as "Amazing Grace"). Each stroke takes a little more time, and you don't want to rush it, but you may still want to groove with the rhythm (how sweet the sound!).

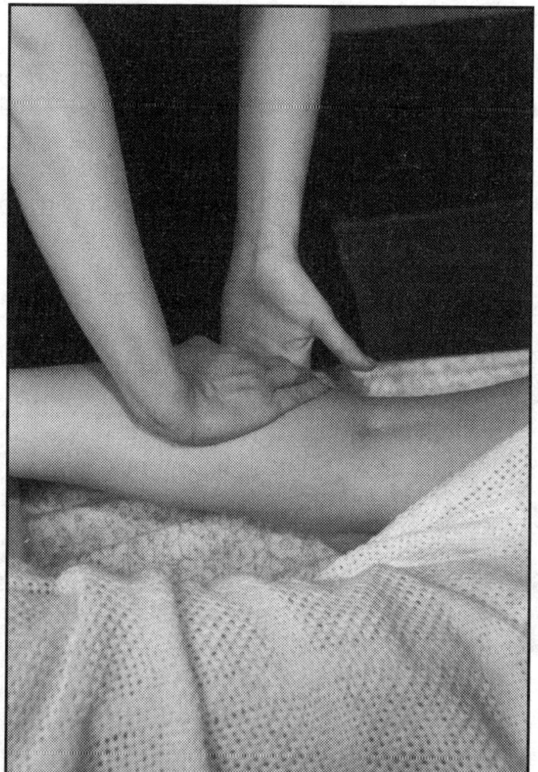

For a twist-and-release stroke, push down, twist the palm around, and then lift up. Let's do the twist up and down!

Percussion: Drum Roll Please...

The difference between compression and percussion strokes, or tapotement, is like the difference between a heartfelt ballad and a Sousa march. Percussion strokes consist of quick striking motions that bear little resemblance to anything you probably imagine when you hear the word *stroke*. They aren't rough or painful. Keep those wrists loose. The emphasis should be on the "upswing," and your hands will bounce off the skin of the person you are massaging. Percussion strokes should stimulate and activate muscles and skin, but they don't cause any bruises!

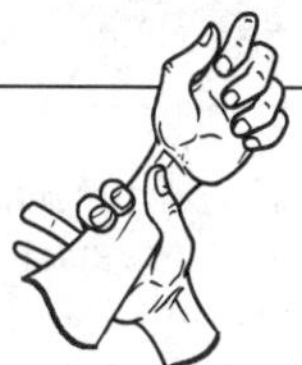

Your Finger on the Pulse

Listening to music isn't the only way to be inspired by rhythm. Next time you're outside, listen for the rhythms of nature: waves on the shore, the chirping of tree frogs, the midwinter call of a cardinal, rain, crickets chirping at dusk, the swell and fall of cicadas in midsummer. Then imitate these rhythms when you use compression and percussion strokes in massage.

Hacking: Chop! Chop!

Has your massagee dozed off? Wouldn't you hate for him or her to miss out on any aspect of the wonderful massage you are performing? Then try some gentle hacking—a wonderful way to be awakened! The hacking percussion stroke is great for stimulating the body. Although the mention of hacking may lead you to envision large Scandinavian women with deep voices beating some poor soul into submission with the edges of their enormous hands, hacking is more effective when performed gently.

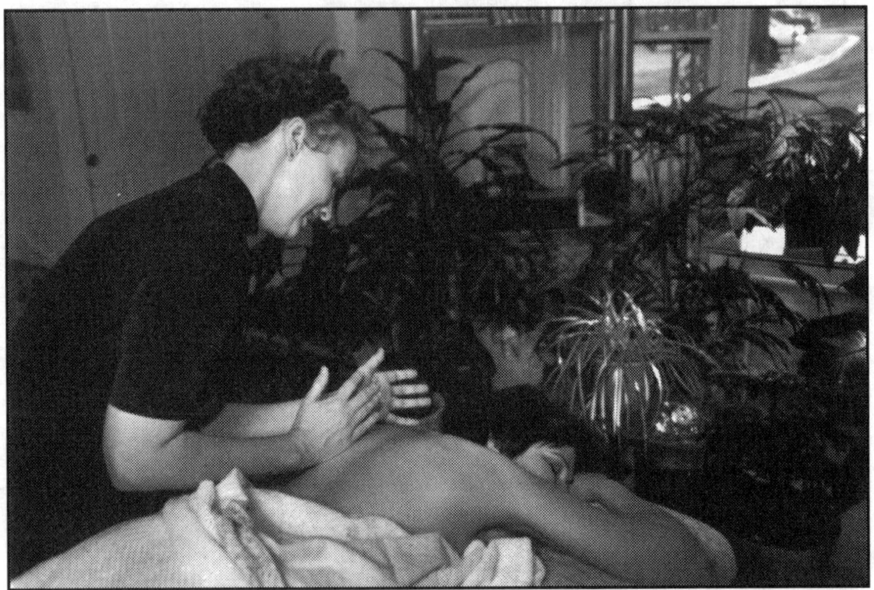

Keep your hand relaxed and vary the speed when hacking. This stroke is a gentle way to revive a sleeping friend.

Your hands are relaxed with fingers slightly apart so that, as you strike the skin surface, your fingers can transmit a gentle vibration when they come together (keep wrist bone off area of contact). Your rhythm can vary from quick to slow to quick again. Pretend the edges of your hands are drumsticks and you're doing a light drum roll. This stroke works on any part of the body that is relatively fleshy, such as the back, legs, and buttocks.

Avoid percussion strokes directly over vital organs such as the heart, stomach, kidneys, and liver, and delicate areas such as the backs of knees, underarms, and throat. Even when gentle, a misplaced percussion stroke could cause damage or pain. Stick to fleshy muscle areas where organ function is safely and indirectly stimulated, such as the buttocks, the backs of the thighs, and the upper/mid back (but don't pound on the back, and stay off the spine!).

Cup Your Hands

Like hacking, cupping uses only the edges of your hands, but it also uses the tips of your fingers. Cup your hands loosely and gently drum on the muscles. Keep those wrists relaxed so your hand bounces off the skin. Cupping is good for more sensitive areas and should be administered quickly and lightly. Cupping is also a great technique for relieving lung congestion from both the chest and back.

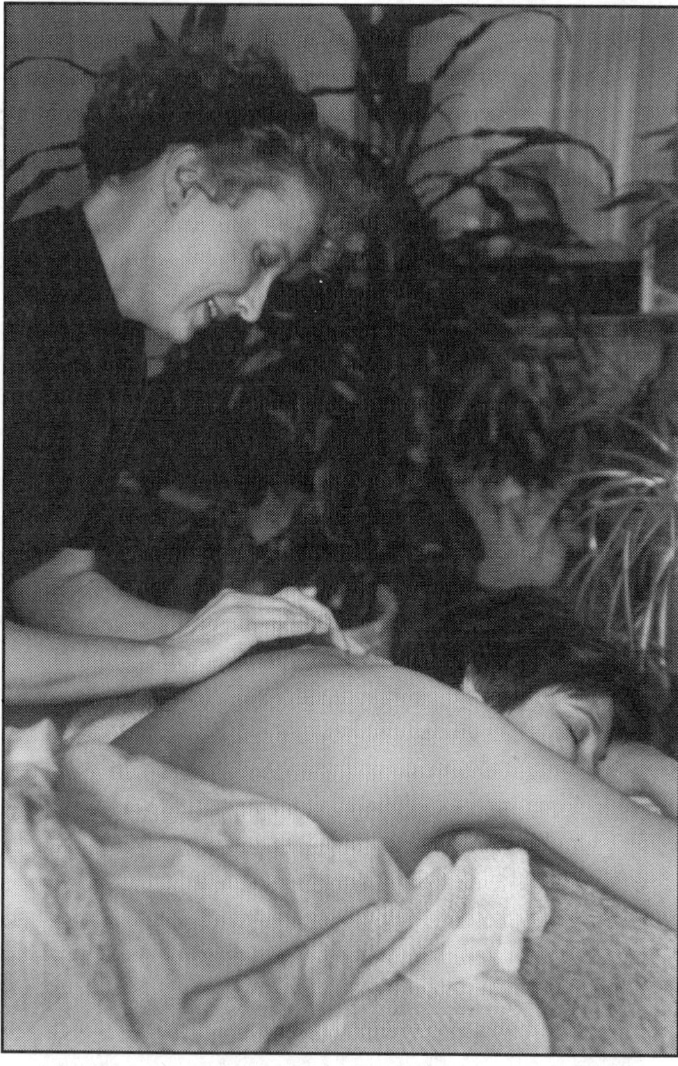

When cupping, don't slap! Keep the hands cupped. This stroke works especially well to bring circulation to sensitive areas.

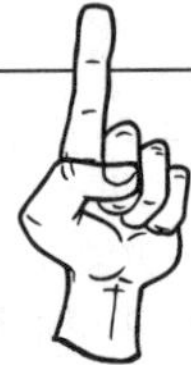

Touch Talk

Your **gluteus** muscles are the muscles of your buttocks, responsible for extending, abducting, and rotating the thigh (see Chapter 6, "The Body Made Easy"). One of the largest muscle groups in your body, they are a common place to hold tension. They are also a common focus of attention in our figure-conscious society. With all that pressure, your gluteus muscles could probably use a good massage!

Pounding: Tension Be Gone!

Some larger muscles really know how to hold on to tension no matter what you do. Lots of people hold tension in their *gluteus* muscles, for example (yes, those muscles you sit on!). Larger muscles, such as the gluteus muscles, are the best ones to target with the pounding percussion stroke because it can certainly get vigorous (although it still isn't rough enough to cause injury). Just to be safe, we recommend that you limit use of the pounding stroke to the gluteus muscle group.

To perform the pounding stroke, make your hands into fists (they can be tighter than the open fists used in the open-fist compression stroke), and then, still keeping your wrists loose, bounce those fists robustly against that stubborn muscle. Banish the tightness, the tension, and the stiffness with the pounding stroke and watch your massagee finally, truly, deeply relax, even visibly sinking more deeply into the massage table or floor.

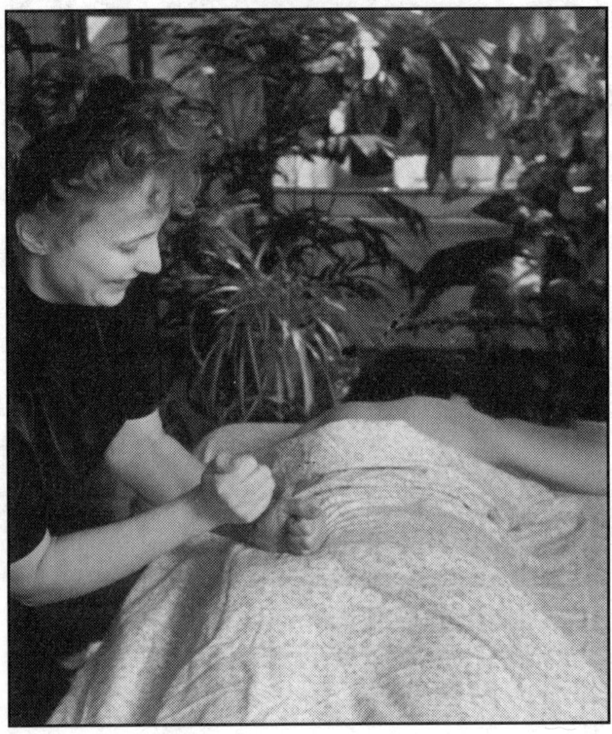

Pound away on those gluteus muscles. Lots of people hold and store their tensions here.

Happy Tapping: The Micromassage

After a refreshing interlude of pounding, you may want to bring your massagee out of the percussion mode gradually. *Tapping* is a great way to move into another type of stroke, such as friction or vibration. Tapping is a gentle percussion stroke that is stimulating, especially to the skin, but also highly relaxing. Like the other percussion strokes, it is performed with loose wrists; the fingers are also loose. For this stroke, you let your fingers do the walking…er, tapping.

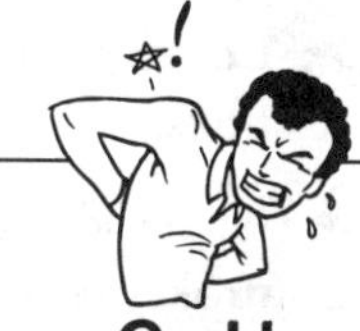

Ouch!

Never apply percussion strokes to injured or highly sensitive areas. Even though percussion strokes are gentle, they do stimulate muscles to contract and release. On healthy muscle tissue, the effect is toning, but on damaged muscles, the effect may cause or aggravate injury.

Tapping is more finely focused but less deep than other percussion strokes because the fingers are, obviously, smaller and less heavy than your entire hand. Tapping is, therefore, good for smaller, more delicate surfaces such as the face, neck, and hands, although it can also be used over larger areas such as the back and legs, for variety—it feels great anywhere. To perform the stroke, gently tap your fingers against the skin surface in the manner you would for the cupping stroke, but use only your fingertips, as if you're typing on a computer keyboard.

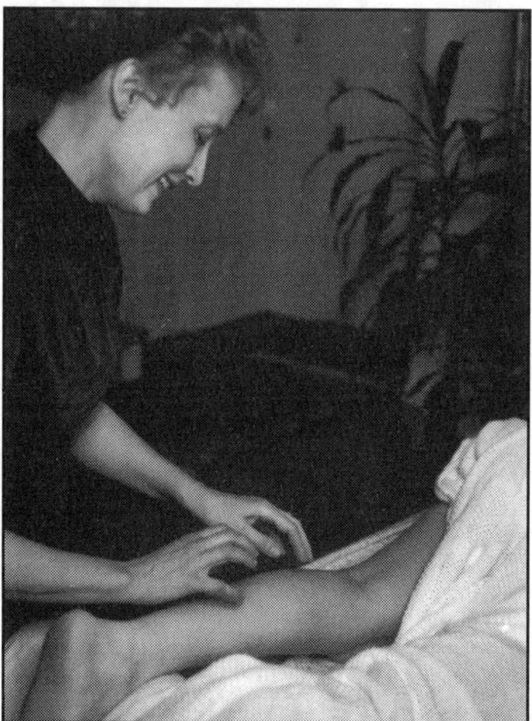

Try tapping with the fingertips as another way to activate circulation.

The Least You Need to Know

- ➤ Compression strokes are deeply stimulating to muscles, helping to flush them with nutrients and increase their performance.
- ➤ Compression strokes include full-hand, open fist, and twist-and-release variations.
- ➤ Percussion strokes, also called tapotement, are quick, light, highly stimulating strokes resembling the action used to execute a drum roll.
- ➤ Percussion strokes include hacking, cupping, pounding, and tapping.

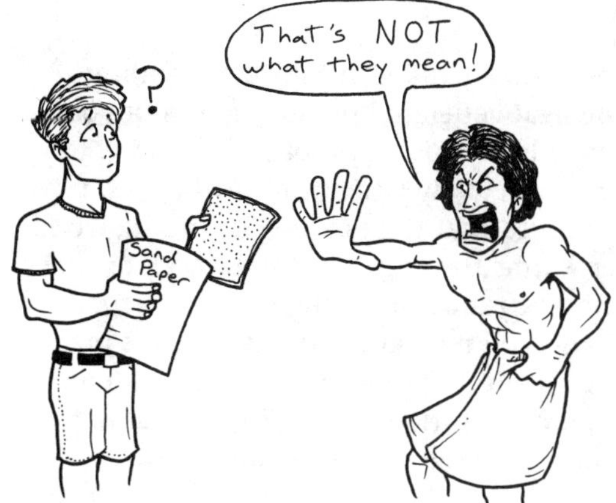

Chapter 16

Heat It Up and Shake It Out: Friction and Vibration

In This Chapter

- What is a friction stroke, and how do you do it?
- The effects of friction strokes
- How to perform vibration strokes
- The effects of vibration strokes

You've learned how to stroke, knead, compress, and percuss, but that's not all there is to know about Swedish massage. *Friction* and *vibration* add even more variety to your massage repertoire. These strokes really get things moving, heating up the body by rubbing tissue against tissue and by shaking every last bit of tension out of those stroked, kneaded, compressed, and percussed muscles. If you ever doubted massage could truly relax you, by now you're probably just about convinced that it can turn you into a happy mound of serenity. This chapter should banish any remaining reservations.

Friction: Turn Up the Heat!

Have you ever rubbed your hands together very quickly (like Pat Morita in healing mode in the movie *The Karate Kid)* and felt the heat generated by the friction of your palms? At the very least, you've probably rubbed your hands together instinctively when the weather is nippy. Maybe you've noticed that the process of sanding wood with sandpaper warms the paper and the wood, or that a bicycle tire is warm to the touch after skidding across the pavement, and you may know that your car's brakes get hot when you slam them on to avoid an accident. All these are examples of friction, and friction, as any Physics 101 student can tell you, generates heat.

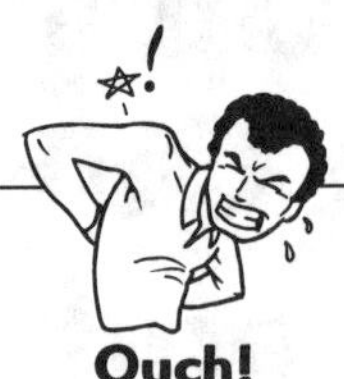

Ouch!

Muscles and tissues respond better to friction and vibration strokes when they are first warmed up with gentle effleurage followed by petrissage. Otherwise, friction and vibration strokes won't feel as good because your body won't be ready for such vigorous movement. After lots of effleurage and petrissage, however, friction and vibration strokes feel great and loosen, stretch, soften, and heat up the warmed-up muscles, skin, and fascia.

The purpose of friction strokes in Swedish massage is to use the body to help itself—to move tissue against tissue to soften and stretch the fascia, improve the circulation, break up muscle adhesions and tightness, boost your *metabolic rate* (the rate at which you transform food into energy), and promote movement of the *interstitial fluids* between cells and blood vessels. Friction strokes also generate heat in the body. Just as warm bread dough is easier to knead than cold dough, warm muscles are more pliable, flexible, relaxed, and less likely to be torn or injured than cold muscles.

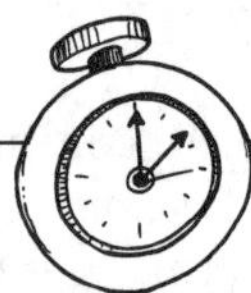

A Massage Minute

Friction strokes as a part of Swedish massage aren't the same as friction rubs, a bracing spa treatment popular in northern Europe in which the skin is vigorously brushed, sloughed, and scrubbed with a wet or dry brush, salt, or loofah sponges. Vigorous skin brushing and sloughing, both dry and wet, is also an important and popular hygiene and beauty treatment in Japan. These friction rubs increase skin circulation dramatically, improve skin texture, and seem to impart some of their dynamic energy to the person experiencing the rub. See Chapter 20, "The Spa Treatment: Spa-cial Pleasures," for more on friction rubs and how to do them yourself.

Friction is also great for increasing skin circulation; after a good friction rub, the skin will be rosy, warm, and flushed with blood. It even enhances the function of your joints by increasing circulation and fluid absorption in the areas around the joints. In other words, friction strokes are all-around, surface-to-deep tissue enhancers that help to put your body back into a warm, relaxed, stress-free state (and chances are good that your mind will come along for the ride).

You can apply friction strokes in various ways, but in all cases, your hand, fingers, or thumbs should move with the skin surface so that the underside of the skin moves firmly against underlying muscle, bones, or other tissues. One of the most common friction strokes is the circular stroke. Your full hand, palm, or fingers press deeply into the skin and move it in a circular motion over the tissue beneath. This stroke moves the superficial tissue over the deeper tissue. There is no sliding over the surface of the skin. This stroke works the underlying fascia and is effective for almost any area of the body, but be careful not to press too deeply on sensitive areas. You can apply deeper friction strokes over thick, fleshy areas of muscle.

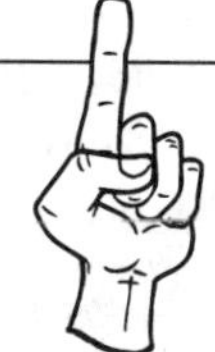

Touch Talk

Your **metabolic rate**, or "rate of living," refers to the processes within your cells that transform food into energy. Ideally, your metabolism is balanced (or in a state of *homeostasis*) so that you produce as much energy as you need. Friction strokes boost cellular activity, helping to maintain an ideal state of homeostasis, which is characterized by appropriate appetite and energy levels.

Hands Across the Muscle: Cross-Fiber Friction

Another friction stroke is called *cross-fiber friction*. In cross-fiber friction, the fingers or thumbs move the skin and fascia back and forth across a muscle, perpendicular to the muscle fibers. Start gently, and then gradually go deeper across the muscle, isolating your stroke to a single muscle or stiff area. As your fingers press tissue against tissue, the friction between the fascia and underlying muscle will warm the area, stretch and soften the fascia, loosen the muscle, and break up any adhesions, *fibrosis* (the presence of fibrous tissue where it doesn't belong), or general stiffness.

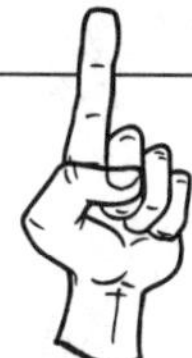

Touch Talk

Interstitial fluids are the fluids between cells and blood vessels within the body. Through various processes, these fluids are constantly transferred in and out of cells, helping to remove waste products and deliver nutrients. Friction strokes enhance the movement of these fluids.

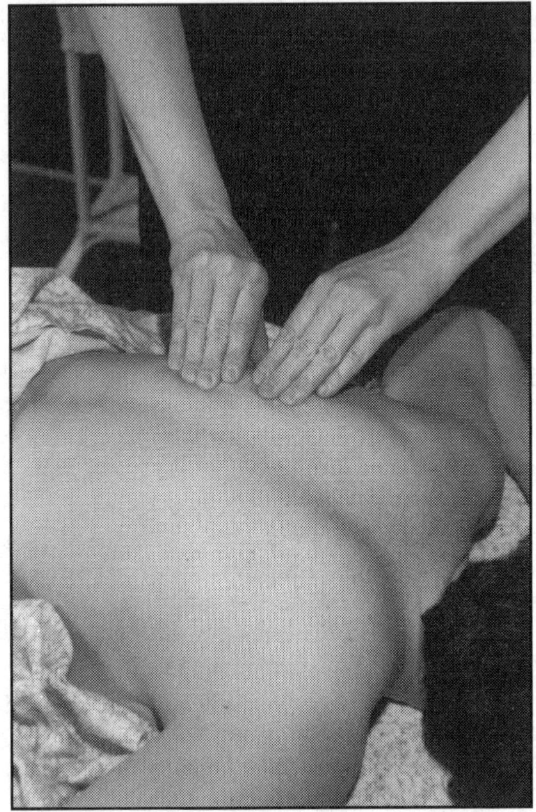

For cross-fiber friction, keep your hands on the skin as you move your fingers back and forth. Gradually begin working deeper. The fingers move counter to the direction of the muscle fibers. (Time for an anatomy review? See Chapter 6.)

This stroke is particularly beneficial for injured muscle tissue, regardless of whether the injury is recent or an old one. It breaks up the adhesions, scar tissue, and fibrosis that can occur when injured tissue is healing or has healed improperly, thereby restoring flexibility and suppleness to muscles, tendons, ligaments, and connective tissue. Even for noninjured muscles, though, cross-fiber friction loosens and stretches tissues, enhancing flexibility, decreasing chances of muscle injury, and giving the tissues (down to the tiniest capillaries) a sensational rush of nutrients.

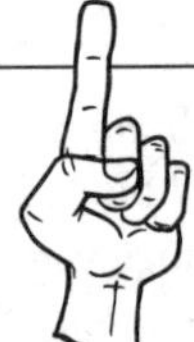

Touch Talk

Fibrosis is a process in which fibrous tissue forms in the body. When this fibrous tissue develops where it wouldn't normally belong, such as around the site of a muscle injury, it can limit function, causing stiffness or even pain. Friction strokes can help to break apart fibrous tissue and promote normal healing, restoring muscle function.

Go with that Muscle Flow: Longitudinal Friction

Sometimes, overworking muscles can cause them to contract and stay that way, especially if you aren't in the habit of stretching out after a workout. Contracted muscles "stick" in their shortened state of exertion and can cause pain, stiffness, and the muscle-bound look—you know, the hunky weightlifter who can bench-press 300 pounds but can't quite lower his arms all the way down to his sides.

The purpose of stretching after a workout is to remind the muscles that they aren't really short and bunchy, but long, strong, and supple. Longitudinal friction strokes can be an additional reminder to those stubborn muscles because these strokes work in the direction of muscle fibers, lengthening and aligning muscles to coax them back to their natural resting state.

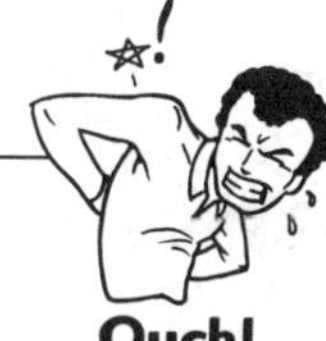

Ouch!

Although cross-fiber friction is an excellent therapy for injured tissue, the treatment of injuries via massage should be left to trained massage therapists. In other words, don't try fixing your friend's torn calf muscle or even your own sprained wrist unless you've received competent professional instruction and your doctor's okay.

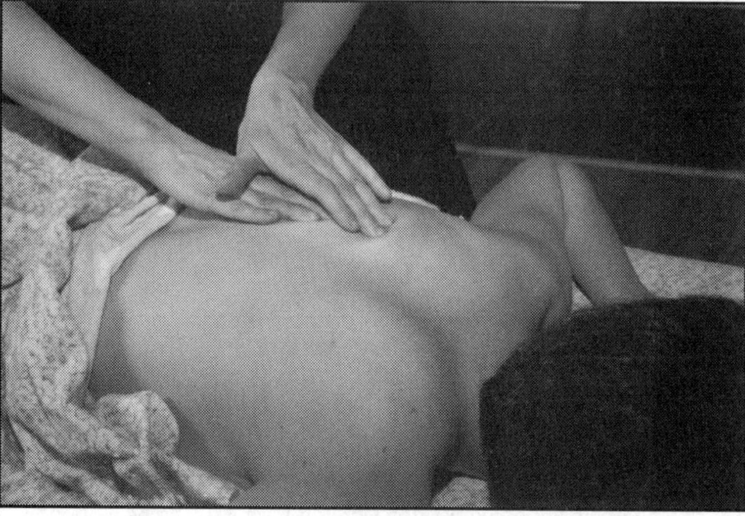

With longitudinal friction, the fingers are deeply gliding in the same direction as the muscle fibers, working out those trigger points (see Chapter 7).

Like the other friction strokes, longitudinal friction also involves moving the skin and underlying tissue along with the movement of your hand, palm, or fingers, rather than just moving your hand over the skin surface. Rather than in a circular or perpendicular direction, however, the longitudinal friction stroke moves in the direction of the muscle fibers, smoothing out the contractions experienced under exertion. You can

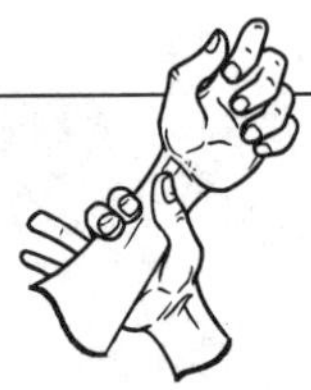

Your Finger on the Pulse

If you're not sure what the proper friction technique is, try this: Put your hand on your opposite forearm and brush your hand back and forth over the skin. That's not the classic friction stroke, though it is skin-skin friction and can be nicely warming. Now place your finger pads on your arm and let them sink in. Then move the underlying tissue over the deeper tissue. Your fingers shouldn't move from their place on your skin. That's the classic friction stroke.

also use longitudinal friction to locate trigger points, or sensitive areas in muscles that are a source of pain (see Chapter 11, "Welcome to the World of Massage"). Longitudinal friction strokes are a great complement to cross-fiber friction strokes, so try it both ways to get Maximum Friction Impact (the newest blockbuster movie?).

Shake that Booty (and Everything Else): Vibration

Remember all those movies and sitcoms that parodied the old weight-loss spas by showing a scary-looking machine with a belt that the "victim" put around his or her buttocks or back, only to be vibrated into oblivion? In Swedish massage, *vibration* is neither so complicated nor so violent. Vibration also doesn't melt away fat, increase muscle, or work any other miracle on the body. It does, however, activate, stimulate, or relax the body, depending on the intensity and duration of the vibration.

You can implement vibration the good old-fashioned way, with your hands, palms, and/or fingers, or you can use a variety of vibration equipment (see Chapter 9, "Getting, or Giving, a Massage at Home," for more on vibration equipment). Whatever the method, vibration feels great, especially after a long session of effleurage and petrissage. It revs you up, calms you down, and gets you really, really loose.

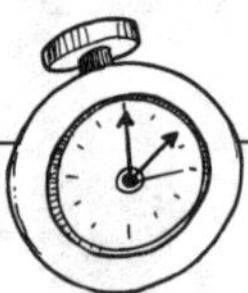

A Massage Minute

Mechanical vibrators use various types of motion. Oscillating vibrators move back and forth, orbital vibrators move in circles, and percussion/compression vibrators have a thumping motion. Vibrators range from small, hand-held models limited to a single type of motion, to expensive floor-standing models that have a variety of interchangeable heads. An additional benefit of vibration equipment is that it gives the massage therapist (and the amateur, too) a break from the strenuous workout of manual massage.

Let's Shake Hands: Palms

The easiest, cheapest, and often most gently effective method of vibration can be performed with the palms. Although you can't vibrate your hands as fast as a mechanical vibrator (which can move up to 100 vibrations a second), you can accomplish somewhere between 5 and 10 vibrations per second with practice. Besides, faster vibrations aren't necessarily preferable.

Technically, vibration is a form of friction, and just as in the friction stroke, your hands stay connected to a single area of the skin and then vibrate, either quickly or slowly, creating friction between fascia, muscle, and bone. Vibration is quicker than the classic friction strokes, of course, and has a rhythm to it that friction strokes don't necessarily have.

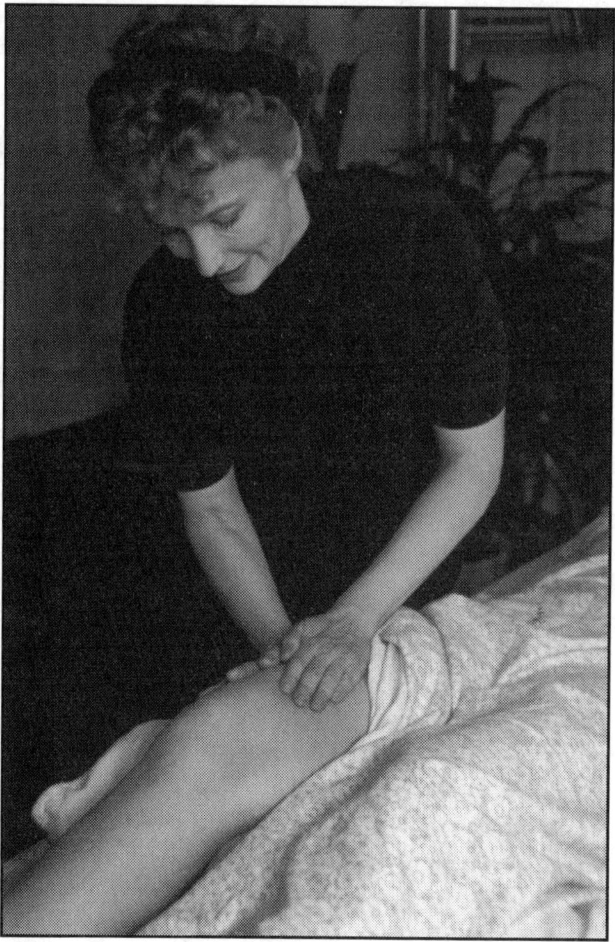

For palm vibration, stay connected to the skin and vibrate those hands.

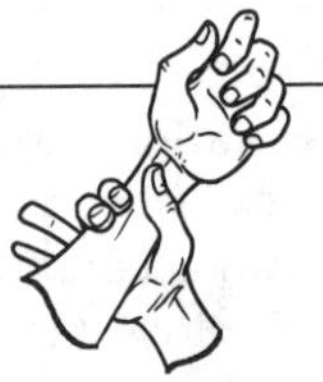

Your Finger on the Pulse

Vibration massage applied deeply for up to about 30 seconds is stimulating. More lightly applied, vibration is incredibly relaxing. When administered for extended periods (say, longer than a minute), vibration can numb the area as the nerves react against the vigorous movement, but this technique can be helpful for areas that need to be exhausted because they're experiencing muscle spasms.

To try vibration with your palms, place your hands on the body over a fleshy area such as the thigh, buttocks, or upper back. Then, keeping your hands in place, vibrate them quickly, shaking the skin and underlying tissue all the way to the bone. Imagine you are riding in a car over a bumpy road or shivering with cold. The vibrations of your hand should travel through the muscle of the person you are massaging, shaking the muscle loose and giving nerve endings a wake-up call. It is helpful to use your arms and shoulders to help with the movement. For a change, try finger vibration, great for smaller areas such as the hands, feet, and face. Place your fingers firmly on skin over muscle and vibrate them quickly but gently.

Jiggle All the Way: Grasping

Another vibration technique is to pick up the muscle before vibrating it. Similar to the pulling petrissage technique but with more jiggle, *grasping* really shakes the tension out of a particularly tight or stubbornly stiff muscle.

To administer this technique, wrap your fingers around the targeted muscle (such as the calf muscle, see the following figure) and gently lift it off the bone. Then vibrate the muscle with your hands until it releases—it won't take long. Don't worry if you can't feel the release. Just vibrate the muscle for 10 seconds or so, release it, and if it is still stiff, repeat the process. Ask the person receiving the massage if the muscle feels less tight. For larger areas, try jostling the entire muscle group side to side or up or down for a period of time.

Grasping vibration is good for large muscles you can feel, but it is too rough for sensitive areas. Instead, try jostling or shaking, which works well for larger areas. Jostle the entire muscle group side to side or up and down for a minute or so.

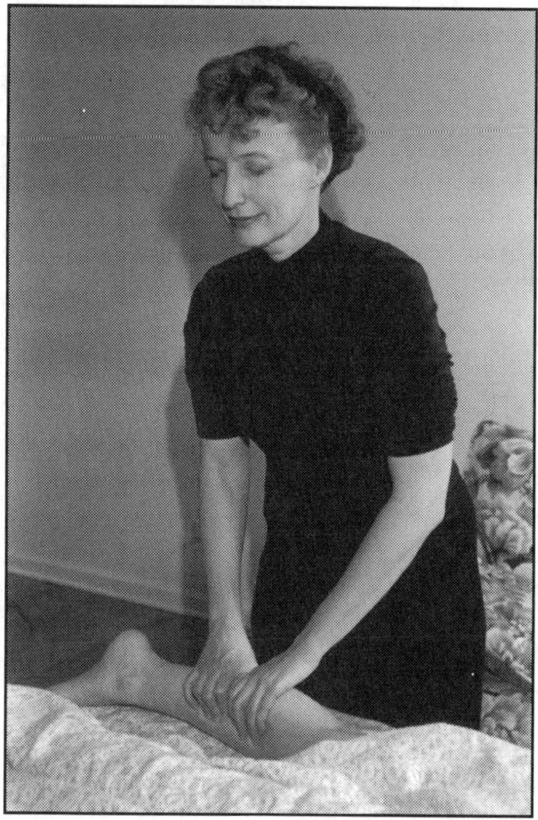

For a grasping vibration, pull up on the muscle and vibrate your hands. Every once in a while, close your eyes as Joan is doing here. Let your sense of touch guide you.

The Least You Need to Know

- Friction strokes move skin against underlying muscles and other tissues to increase circulation and to loosen and soften connective tissue, making it more pliable and functional.
- Friction strokes include circular, cross-fiber, and longitudinal friction.
- You can implement vibration with the hands, fingers, or with special vibration equipment. Vibration can stimulate, relax, or numb an area, depending on how you apply it.
- Vibration strokes include palm vibration, finger vibration, grasping, jostling, and shaking.

Chapter 17

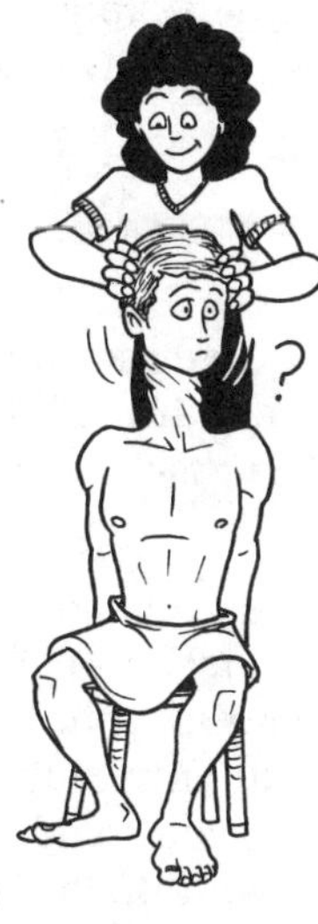

Goin' Round and Round: Increasing Range of Motion

In This Chapter

- What is range of motion?
- What can range of motion exercises do for you?
- Lower-body range of motion exercises you can try
- Exercises for the upper body

If you were to lift your right arm out to your side, then draw huge circles in the air, as large as your shoulder joint would allow, you would be moving your shoulder joint through its range of motion (ROM). Flexing your foot as much as possible and then pointing the toe as far down as possible moves your ankle joint through a ROM. If a massage therapist held your lower leg, then moved it down and up as far as your knee would allow, that would be working the knee joint through its ROM.

"So what?" you might be thinking. "What good does that do?" Range of motion bodywork can be of great benefit. It can help a massage therapist see where you're particularly stiff or lacking in flexibility. It can reveal areas of tension you hadn't noticed. It can also help to loosen and relax your joints, making them more flexible

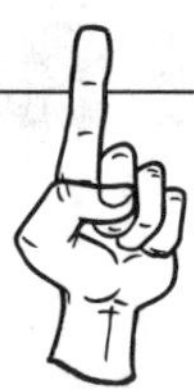

Touch Talk

Hard end feel refers to the limit of a joint's range of motion because of bone prohibiting further movement. **Soft end feel** refers to the limit of a joint's range of motion because of soft tissue such as skin and muscle prohibiting further movement. **Springy end feel** refers to the limit of a joint's range of motion because of tendons, ligaments, or other connective tissue prohibiting further movement.

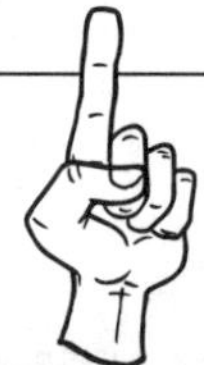

Touch Talk

Active ROM movements are movements of a joint through its range of motion that you make yourself, without assistance, such as circling your arms. **Passive ROM movements** are movements of a joint through its range of motion made by someone else without your assistance, such as a massage therapist circling your arm for you while you stay relaxed.

and exposing them to movements they'd forgotten they could make! This chapter will show you how to explore, and increase, your range of motion.

Out of Your Range

How do you know when you've reached the end of your range of motion? Joints let you know when they're at their limit in three ways: *hard end feel, soft end feel*, and *springy end feel*.

Hard end feel occurs when the bones of the joint can't go any further. To discover hard end feel, straighten your leg as far as you can. At some point, your lower leg stops extending upward because your knee only allows the joint to extend so far. Otherwise, you could fold your lower leg back over the top of your thigh! The point where your lower leg can't raise any more is an example of hard end feel. Bone limits the movement, and bone, of course, is hard, hence the name.

Soft end feel occurs when soft tissue stops the range of motion. For example, bend your arm in at the elbow so your hand comes toward your shoulder. At some point, your skin and biceps will get in the way and you can't get your lower arm any closer to your upper arm. That point is soft end feel.

Springy end feel is limited by ligaments, tendons, and other fibrous tissue. Most joints are limited by springy end feel. For example, try to bend your fingers back towards the back of your hand. They'll only go so far, but they spring back and forth around the limit of their range.

The two ways to assess range of motion are through *active ROM movements* and *passive ROM movements*. Active movements are movements you make on your own, such as when you make circles with your arms. Passive movements are made when someone moves the joint through its range of motion for you, without any exertion on your part. Both are helpful in different situations, but in this chapter, we'll focus on passive ROM movements as a part of the massage process.

A Helping Hand to Assist Flexibility

Range of motion refers to what your joints can do, but doesn't necessarily refer to what your joints *usually* do. Most of us have set patterns of movement and don't fully utilize every joint's complete range of motion. The result? Certain movements are more difficult, even painful. When you never move your body in a certain way, the area may atrophy or stiffen; if you do suddenly decide to start moving in this new and unexpected way, your body will cry, "foul!"

Say you've never tried yoga before, but one day you decide to sit in the lotus position, just to see what it's like. You sit, you pull one ankle onto the opposite thigh, and then you try to pull the other ankle over the first ankle and onto your other thigh—pull, pull, puuuullllll! Ouch. No, your hips aren't used to bending that way, and neither are your knees. You might accomplish the feat, but you'll probably feel it the next day as sore muscles and achy joints.

Just as massage can activate muscle tissue you don't normally use, it can also remind joints of all the ways they could move if only they tried. Yet your massage therapist won't try to force your joints into a painful position (and you shouldn't try that at home, either). Instead, joints should be moved gently to test the area around the end of each joint's range of motion. How far feels good, and how far is too far? How big a circle can your leg make without hurting? How far forward can you bend your head to feel a gentle stretch in the neck muscles and vertebrae? Through these gentle and persuasive movements, you'll feel your joints opening and becoming more flexible, comfortable, and loose.

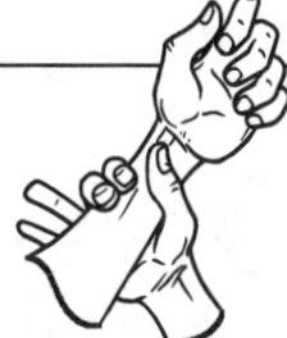

Your Finger on the Pulse

Between massages, you can keep your joints limber with active range of motion exercises. Try this one after a long day at the computer: Gently circle your hands at the wrists, first clockwise, then counterclockwise. Bend each finger back until you feel a slight stretch. Spread fingers out as wide as possible, and then clench them into fists as tightly as possible. Repeat the exercise a few times.

Feet First

Let's start at the bottom—the bottom half of your body, that is. Try each of these range of motion exercises on the lucky person you are massaging. Go slowly and stay in close communication with your massagee so you don't move a joint where it doesn't want to go.

You're Pullin' My Leg

Gently and slowly grasp the leg at the ankle and pull it straight out. Imagine you're trying to make your massagee just a little bit taller. The pulling sensation should feel pleasant. Be sure to do both legs. This exercise loosens and stretches the hip joint.

Leg Pull. Pull the leg at the ankle. Slowly… Firmly… Watch the stretch go all the way up the body. Joan pulls both legs one at a time and then together so Melanie will feel balanced.

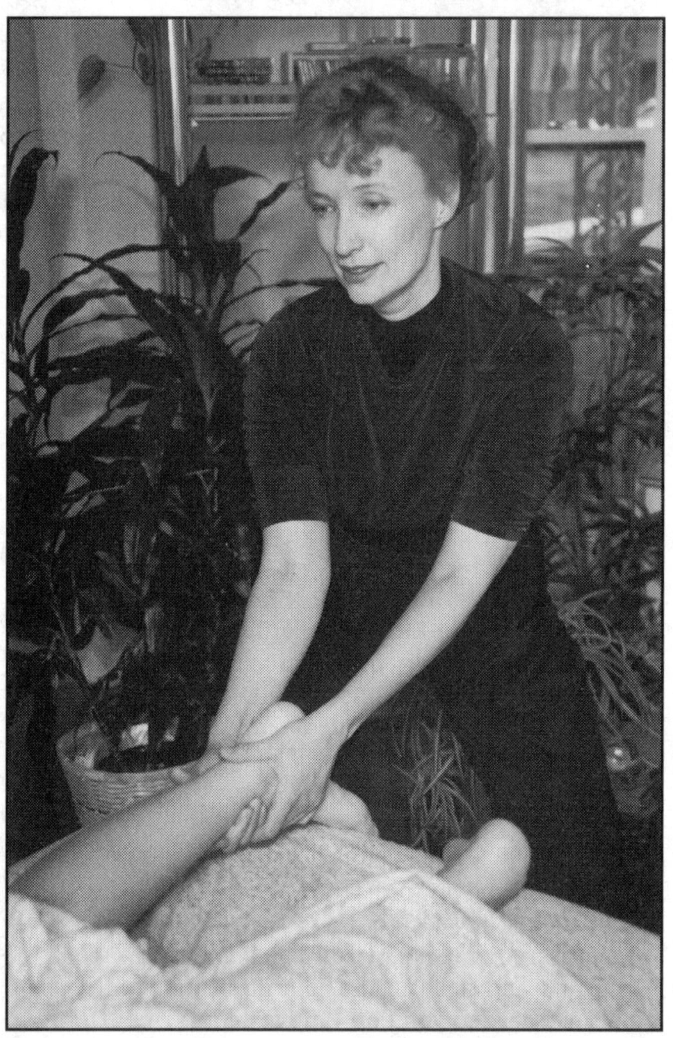

Loosen Those Hips

People who sit at a desk all day tend to have stiff hip joints because their hips are usually stuck in one position and aren't experiencing a full range of motion. As your massagee lies on his or her stomach, bend the legs up at the knees, cross the knees, and gently push each foot toward the floor. Go very slowly. This exercise could hurt if you go too far or too fast.

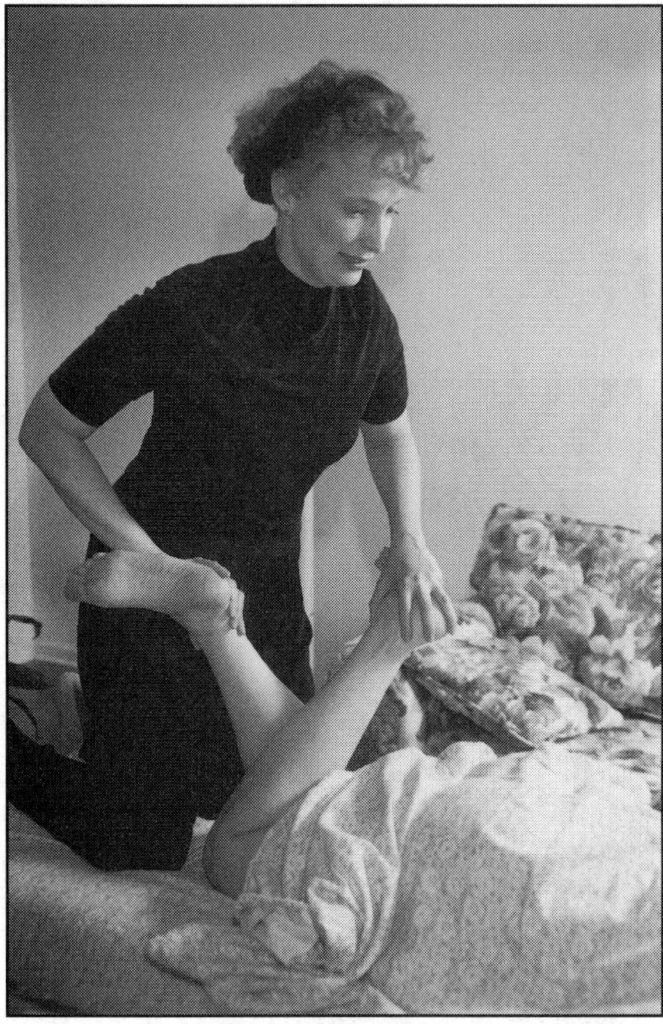

Loosen the Hips. This is a fine stretch for tight hips. (If you sit a lot, it's a must!) Be gentle and move slowly. Continually check with your partner to see that the stretch is comfortable.

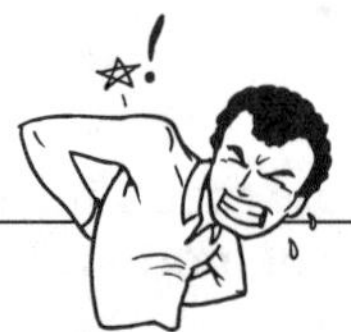

Ouch!

If you live a sedentary lifestyle, sitting for long periods each day at work and then going home to a night of television on the couch, all your joints will suffer. Make an effort to get moving whenever possible. Walk, play sports, romp with your kids, take an exercise or yoga class. Your joints, and the rest of you, will work a whole lot better.

Hip Figure Eight

Again with the hips! Chances are, they need exercise, and hip stretches feel really good, so your massagee probably won't object. For the Hip Figure Eight, have your massagee lie on his or her back. Pick up one leg, keeping the knee joint straight. Then, rather than drawing a figure eight with the foot, as you might guess, imagine the entire leg is drawing a figure eight whose loops extend outward toward the foot and inward into the hip joint. Yes, it will be a little figure eight, but it will do the big job of getting into that joint and loosening it.

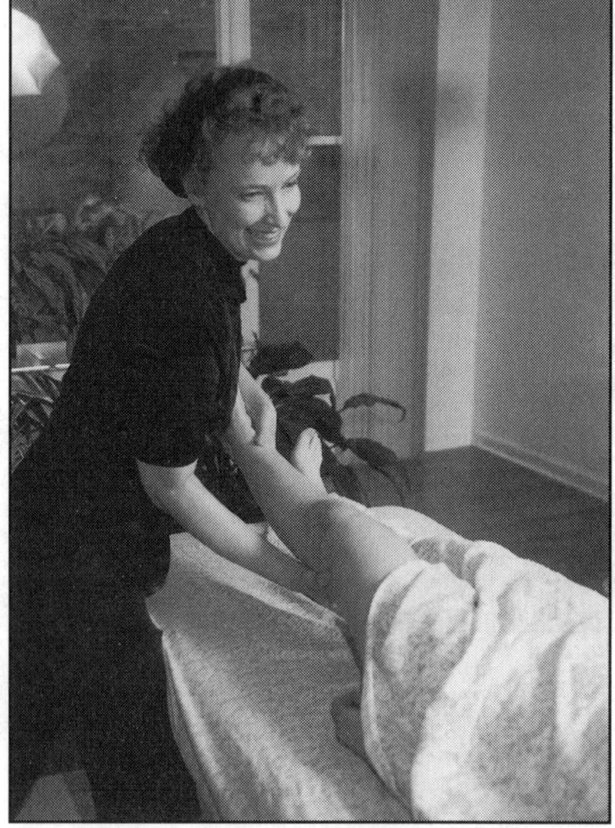

Hip Figure Eight. Lift the leg slightly up, hold it straight, and slowly draw a figure eight into the hip joint. Push the leg in and pull it out. Joan's having fun. Melanie is too as her hip loosens up!

Loosen Those Ankles

Ankles can get stiff, too, when you sit for long periods of time. Rotating them yourself under your desk can help, but having someone else do it feels even better! Hold the massagee's foot and gently move the foot in large circles, rotating the ankle joint. The calf muscles also stretch and contract with this movement—two exercises for the price of one!

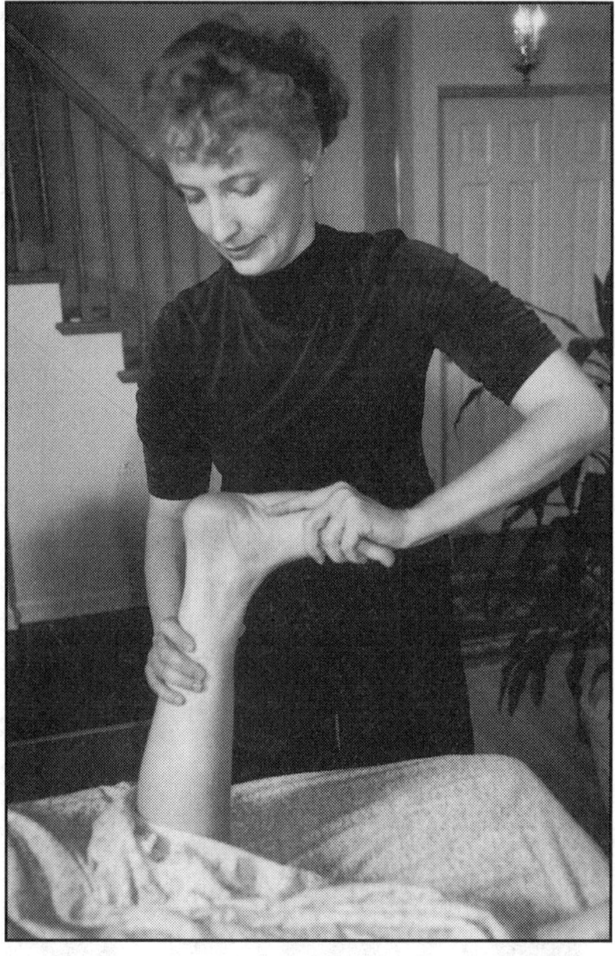

Loosen the Ankles. Slowly rotate the ankle joint by moving the foot around. Use your other hand to steady the leg. This rotation not only loosens the ankles, but stretches the lower leg muscles too.

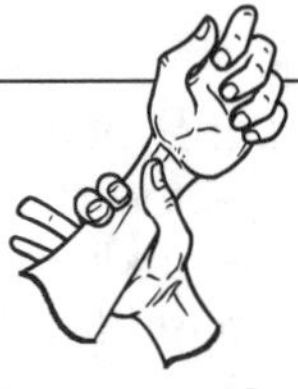

Your Finger on the Pulse

Try this yoga spinal twist, which also happens to be a great range of motion exercise: Sit with both legs straight in front of you. Cross your left leg over your right so your left knee is raised and left foot is on the floor. Place your bent right elbow on the outside of your left knee. Twist your spine and try to look behind you. Repeat on the other side.

The Torso with Moreso

You might not imagine that your torso could have a range of motion, because it isn't exactly a joint. It's full of vertebrae, though, which are all joints, and it can get plenty stiff, especially when it isn't used very much. You know that stiff feeling when you wake up in the morning? That's from not using your body all night long, and the desire to stretch is your body's way of moving itself through a range of motion to wake up those joints and muscles.

For this torso stretch, as your massagee lies on his or her stomach, place your hands on the back, one towards the upper back, the other towards the lower back. Then, gently push your hands in opposite directions, subtly stretching and lengthening the back.

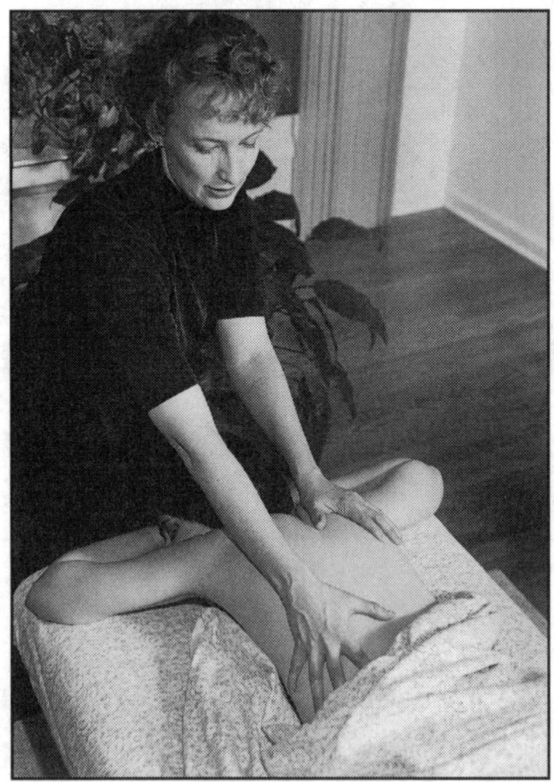

Torso with Moreso. Push one hand forward, the other one back, to stretch out the torso. Alternate to stretch both sides of the back.

Neck and Shoulders Above the Crowd

To top it off, let's not forget the top half of your body, which we teased just a bit with that last torso stretch. In general, the joints in your top half are smaller than those in your bottom half, but they can get just as stiff and painful, as anyone who has ever experienced tennis elbow, carpal tunnel syndrome, or a bad shoulder from too much racquetball can attest.

Shoulder Swing

Shoulders hold a lot of tension, especially when we hike them up around our ears in response to stress, or use them to hold a phone against our impossibly bent necks so our hands can stay free to do three other things at the same time. Sound familiar? A lot of shoulder tension is muscular, but when you continually hold your shoulders in one position, the joints can suffer, too.

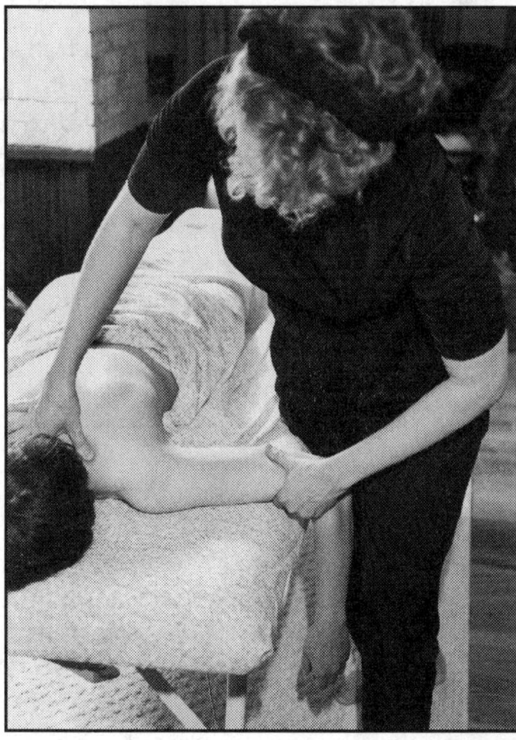

Shoulder Swing. Massaging the thumb across the top of the shoulder, Joan swings Melanie's arm slightly back and forth. This relieves the tension in the shoulders.

To loosen shoulder joints, hold your massagee's arm above the elbow as your massagee lies on his or her stomach. Place your opposite hand on the area between the neck and shoulder joint. Then, move the upper arm up, down, in circles, and all around, working it through its entire range of motion. As you move the arm, press with your opposite thumb into different areas of the muscles between the neck and shoulder to help loosen the muscles stabilizing the shoulder joint.

Shoulder Cha-Cha

For this shoulder exercise, put one hand over the shoulder joint and cradle the shoulder blade with your other hand. Then, moving the hands in opposition (one goes up while the other goes down, and vice versa), coax that shoulder joint back into action with a gentle cha-cha-cha!

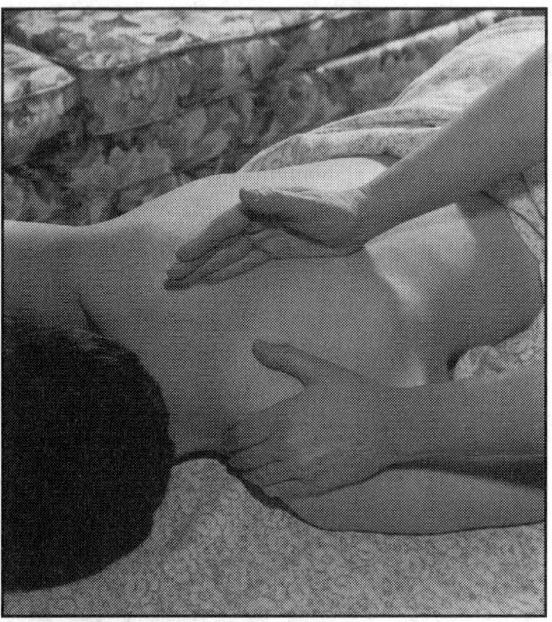

Shoulder Cha-Cha. Slide one hand toward the neck as the other hand pulls down. The hands move counter to each other—back and forth. Work all around the shoulder blade where there are lots of muscles (and so, lots of tension!). Cha-cha-cha!

A Massage Minute

One of the most common and most painful joint disorders is arthritis, which is characterized by inflammation of the joint. In rheumatoid arthritis, the joint lining swells, causing pain and the erosion of cartilage around the joint. Calcium deposits build up around the joint and eventually the joint is unable to move. The disease is progressive, and many joints are often affected.

Osteoarthritis is a degenerative disease that is a function of aging and usually occurs in joints that have been periodically overused or injured. Joint cartilage erodes away, and the bones thicken and become less mobile. Massage is particularly helpful in cases of osteoarthritis because it can help to relieve pain and keep joints mobile.

Neck Rollin'

Who doesn't hold tension in the neck? Those relatively tiny neck vertebrae not only have to hold the weight of your great big, heavy, brain-filled head, but they have to keep it upright and moving in whatever direction you want it to go, all day long. Then, at night, your neck may get assaulted further as you crank it around in awkward positions while you sleep. You probably know how miserable it feels to wake up with a stiff neck that won't go away all day—sometimes not even for several days. Give someone's neck a little TLC with a nice, slow neck roll.

For the neck roll, take the weight of your massagee's head completely in your hands. A lot of people have trouble completely releasing the weight of their head. (Subconsciously, we want to hold on!) Let your massagee know if you feel he or she isn't completely releasing the neck. Then, very slowly and gently move the head in small circles. Whenever you sense the neck muscles grabbing for control again, encourage your massagee to relax and let go. Assure him or her that you've got the head and you won't drop it! (And then, of course, don't drop it!)

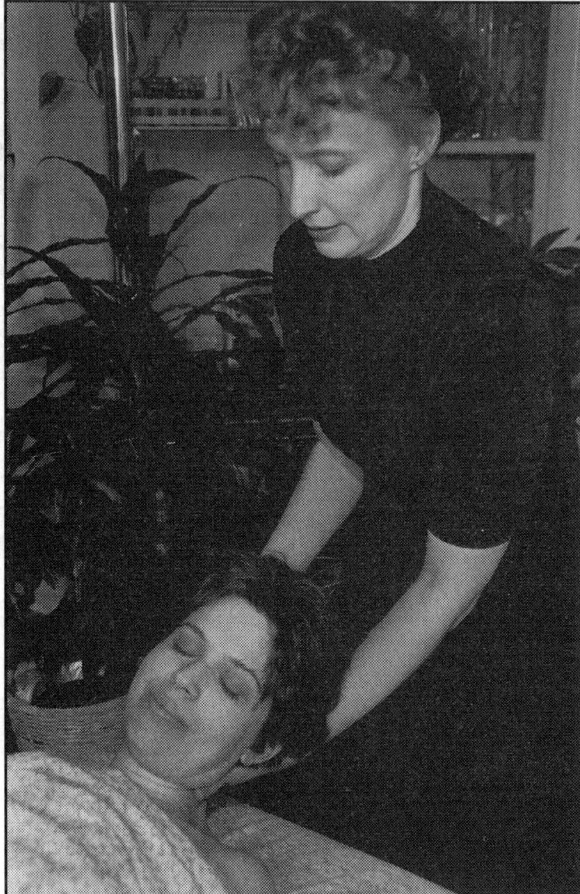

Neck Roll. Melanie rests the weight of her head completely in Joan's expert hands. Joan slowly moves Melanie's head in a circular motion to loosen neck muscles.

Neck Stretch

Remember how you stretched those hip joints by pulling on the leg? While you've still got your massagee's head in your hands, very gently but firmly pull the head towards you. Make sure the head is on straight, so that the neck vertebrae are in line with the spine, for maximum stretch and minimum stress on the entire spinal column.

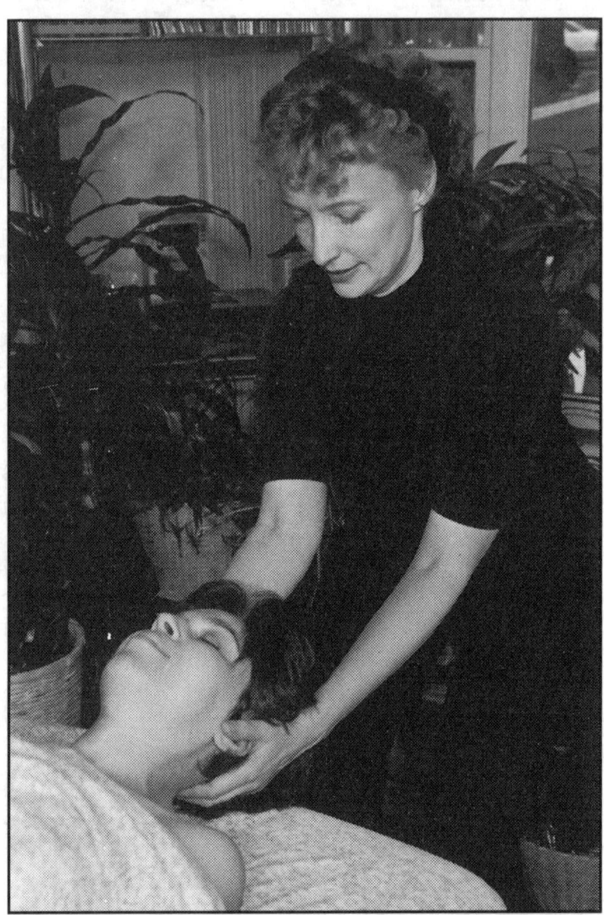

Neck Stretch. With the weight of Melanie's head resting in Joan's hands, Joan gently supports and stretches the neck.

Cradle Relief

It's difficult to release the neck muscles to anyone else's control, and it's just as difficult to release the neck muscles for a massage if you have to lie on your stomach but have to twist your head to the side. The solution? Professional massage tables are often equipped with head cradles so the client can lie face down with the entire spinal column in line, for better access to neck muscles and a more comfortable and relaxed position.

Gentle range of motion massage can increase anyone's range of motion, helping to increase flexibility and mobility of all your muscles and joints.

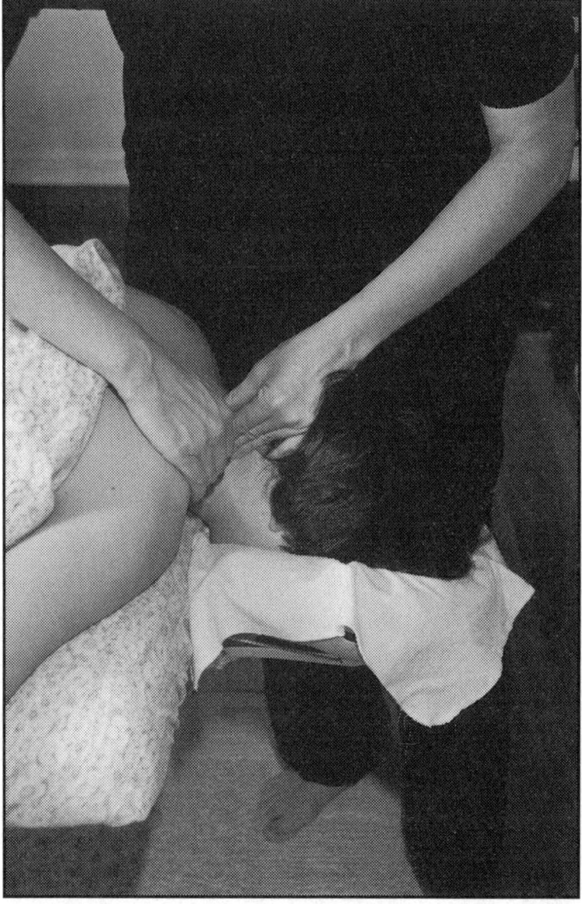

Cradle Relief. Professional massage tables often have "head cradles" that allow the massage therapist greater access to those tight neck muscles.

The Least You Need to Know

- Range of motion is the scope of movement of a given joint.
- Range of motion exercises can be active—performed by you—or passive—performed on you by someone else without any exertion on your part.
- Passive range of motion exercises as part of a complete massage can enhance flexibility and relieve tension.

Part 5

Massage the Senses

Time for some specialization. This part introduces you to some truly sensual pleasures, although we can hardly call them luxuries, because they are so beneficial to your health.

What do you do when you can't find anyone to give you a massage? Give one to yourself! We'll show you how to relax with some easy but incredibly rejuvenating self-massage techniques for your face, your jaw, your head, and those poor, overworked feet.

Next, we'll introduce you to the "scentuous" world of aromatherapy: what it is, where it came from, and what it can do for you. Learn how to add an aromatic component to your massage. Your skin will glow, your mind will relax, and your body will respond to the therapy of essential oils.

For some real indulgence, we'll introduce you to the spa experience. If you like the idea of visiting a health spa, complete with professional massages, saunas, steambaths, herbal soaks, mud packs, and body wraps, we'll fill you in on what to expect. We'll also give you some great ideas for creating your own oasis: a customized home spa for the ultimate in self-indulgence at the drop of a hat (and for a fraction of the cost of a spa vacation).

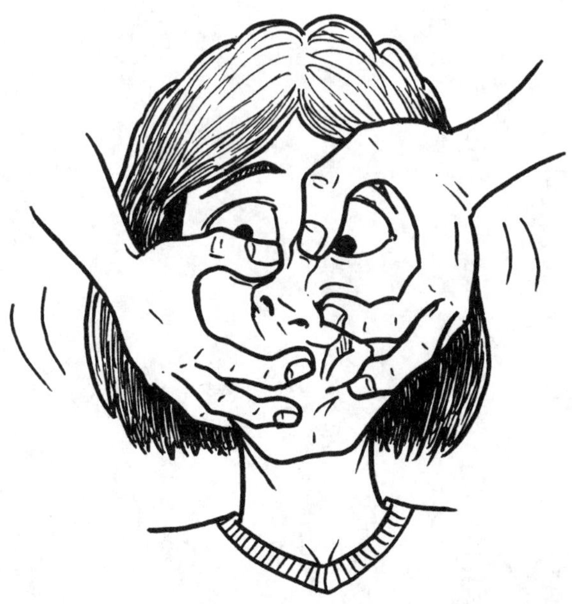

Chapter 18

Give Yourself a Hand: Self-Massage Techniques

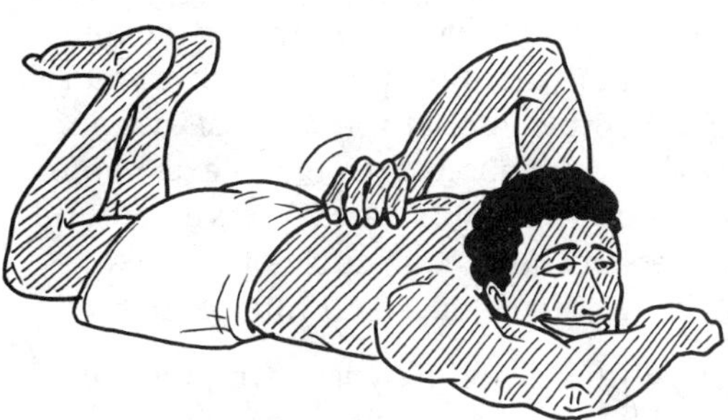

In This Chapter

- How can self-massage help you help yourself?
- Self-acupressure
- Self-massage for the head, face, neck, and feet
- Why self-massage is the ultimate convenience massage

How can you be your own best friend? Learn the great art of self-massage—and practice often! Self-massage is really just common sense. When something hurts, your impulse is to touch it, right? When you accidentally leave the upper cabinet door open and then bump your head into the corner (don't you just hate that?), what's the first thing you do (besides let out a stream of expletives)? You rub the sore spot on your head. When you bump your funny bone, you rub your elbow. When you have a headache, you may rub your neck, or your temples, or your forehead. Humans know instinctively that touch helps to alleviate pain and stress. However, we may not know the best way to help ourselves through the power of our own hands. That's where massage comes in!

Push Yourself: Self-Acupressure

Although this book focuses on the techniques of Swedish massage, we'd like to take a little time out to talk about self-acupressure, a good way to relieve pain and discomfort. Self-acupressure involves pressing your pressure points to relieve pain, stiffness, discomfort, or blocked energy. You can often find your own pressure points by feeling around for sensitive, sore, slightly raised, or slightly sunken areas (not injuries). Get to know your body, and you'll be more in tune to where your pressure points are. (They may not be exactly where someone else's pressure points are.)

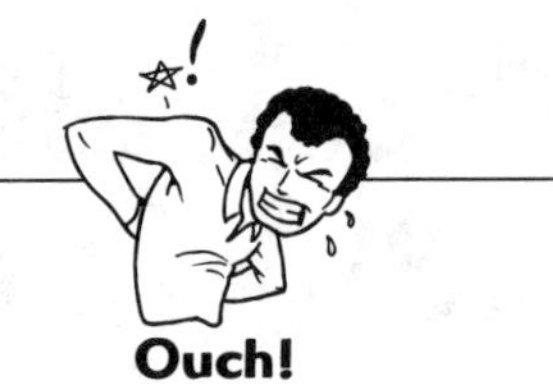

Ouch!

When practicing self-acupressure (or any massage stroke), never press directly on injured areas, broken skin, pimples, cysts, broken bones, sprains, varicose veins, or any place that really hurts. When we say pressure points are sensitive spots, we don't mean injured spots. You can press around injuries, but never directly on them.

When you press a pressure point, don't worry about pressing too hard. But you don't want to bruise yourself, either! Firm, gentle pressure that's just shy of discomfort is the ticket. Don't worry about getting the exact point, either. When you find a sensitive area, press all around it with your fingers or thumb in a circle of approximately two inches in diameter. You'll hit the spot.

If you're not comfortable finding your own pressure points and would like a nice, concise, clear guide showing where you should press for problem A, disorder B, or mild annoyance C, there are many books that explain the details of different acupressure points and how to perform acupressure on yourself. Keep in mind, however, that different acupressure systems and practitioners have different ideas about where pressure points are located. Most agree on some of the spots, but if you look at all the books out there, you'll see quite a range of ways to relieve, say, a headache or insomnia.

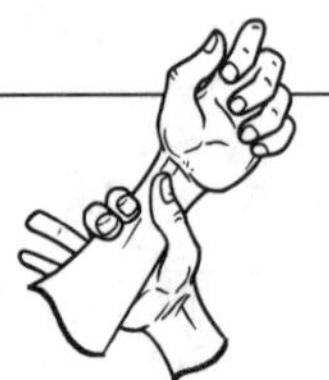

Your Finger on the Pulse

Although we won't go into too much detail about specific self-acupressure techniques in this book, here's one to try: Lie on your back and press with your fingers alongside each nostril. Sinuses will clear and drain. To energize yourself, close your eyes and tap with your fingers all around the face and head.

Knowing this, you can then decide to find a book you like that gives you a detailed map of the body's pressure points, and get pressin'! Or, as we've just suggested, you can try to map your own body's pressure points by intuition and exploration.

Let's Face It!

This section details some specific self-massage techniques that can make you feel like you've given yourself a supreme indulgence (but without any calories or fat!). One of the best places for self-massage is your head, because you can reach every part of it. Most people also carry a lot of tension in the head, neck, and face, so self-massage to the head is a "no-brainer."(The following techniques can really make a difference in your daily comfort level.)

Headache Haven

Who hasn't had a headache? If you never have, you're certainly in the minority. Headaches are one of the most common minor health complaints and also one of the hardest to diagnose because they can be caused by so many things.

Most of the time, even if you don't know the exact cause, you can relieve a headache fairly easily. You can pop over-the-counter painkillers, of course. But wouldn't it be nice to be able to relieve your headache without taking so much aspirin, acetaminophen, ibuprofen, or whatever you typically use? Not every headache can be relieved with self-massage, but many can be, so why not try it before rushing off to your stash of pill bottles?

Often, a headache that occurs around the forehead can be traced to tight muscles around where the base of the skull meets the neck. You should be able to feel a ridge at the base of your skull. Massage the ridge with your fingers; massage around and under it, and then move your fingers all around the scalp as though you were giving your hair a good shampoo to help release overall scalp tension and tension headaches.

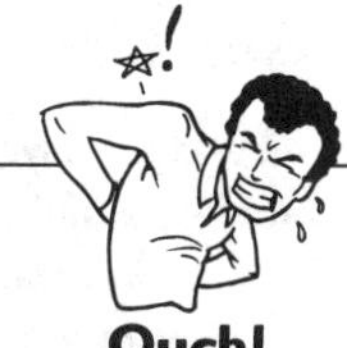

Ouch!

Most headaches are caused from tension, stress, muscle strain, or other temporary and mild conditions. However, if your headache persists for more than a couple of days, is so severe you can't function, is accompanied by vision changes, or occurs in any sort of discernible pattern, such as only at night, see your doctor to rule out a serious condition.

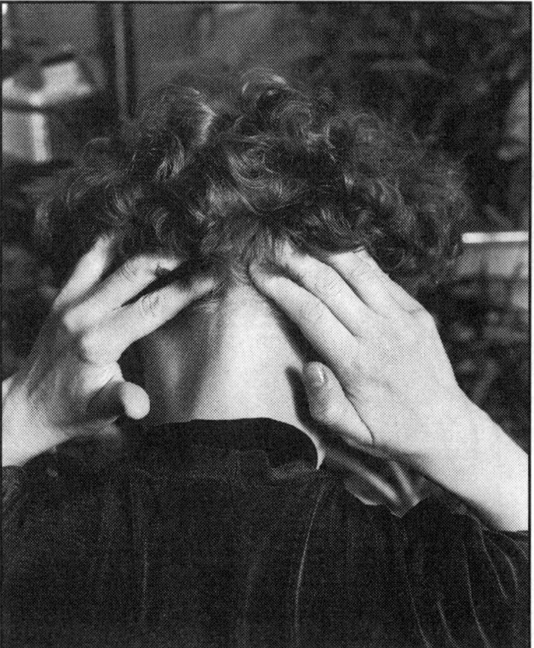

Headache Haven. Got the headache blues? Massage the base of the skull (occipitalis) to help relieve pent-up head strain.

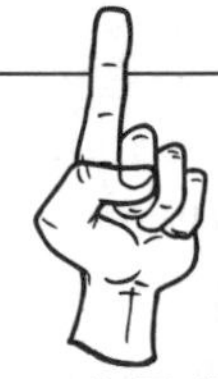

Touch Talk

Temporomandibular joint syndrome, or **TMJ,** is a chronic, painful condition usually resulting from jaw trauma, such as a car accident or a major dental procedure. Temporo means skull bones, and mandibular refers to the jaw bone, or mandible. TMJ can be characterized by clicking or other jaw noises, pain, and dysfunction of any of the jaw muscles.

Jostle that Jaw

Jaws carry lots of tension, too. When you're particularly irritated with that person in the apartment above you who likes to practice aerobics at 3:00 in the morning, for example, you might clench your jaw. Some people grind their teeth in their sleep, which is not only bad for their teeth, but a big stress on their jaws. *Temporomandibular joint syndrome*, or *TMJ*, is another common problem that causes chronic, sometimes debilitating jaw pain. Massage can help in all cases.

While opening and closing your mouth, feel with your fingers the area about an inch or two in front of each ear. Can you find the jaw joint? Pressing this point or rubbing it gently in a circular motion, à la acupressure, can bring immediate relief to a stiff and painful jaw.

Another good way to relieve jaw tension is to massage the jaw with your fingers, kneading and moving in small circles over all the jaw muscles. Begin at your chin and work your way up to your ears, covering the entire jaw region. Don't forget to massage beneath the jawline. You'll feel so relaxed afterwards, you may not want to talk for awhile. Let your jaw bask in its relaxed state.

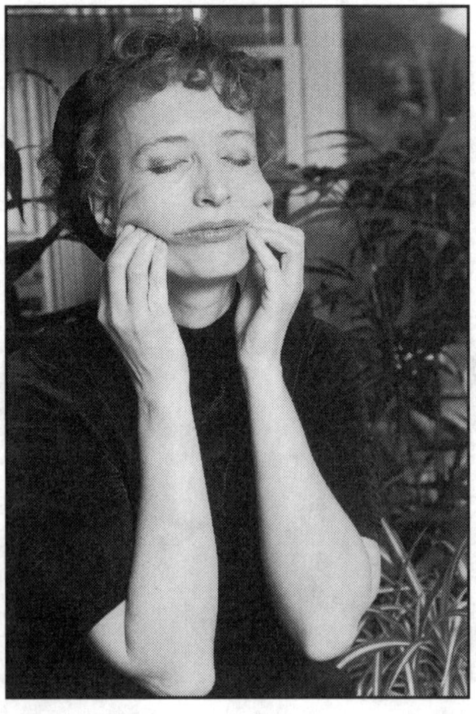

Jaw Jostle. Circle and knead your fingers into the muscles of the jaw. Start at the chin and work up to the ears. Then, circle back down again. Try it a few more times.

Forehead Scissors Stroke

Ah, the furrowed brow—sign of deep thought, concentration, and major stress! Next time you find yourself dwelling on that stack of bills or that employee evaluation you just received or that disturbing note from your son's teacher about the seriousness of plagiarism, check to see whether your brow is furrowed. Chances are good that it is. So take time out every so often to give your forehead a good massage.

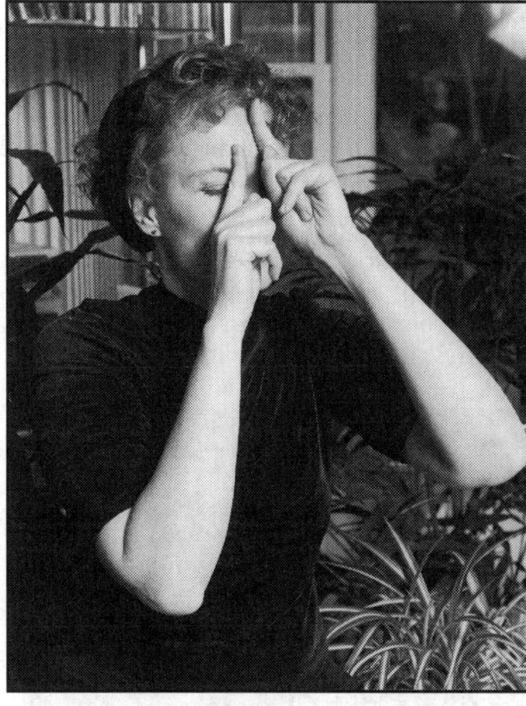

Forehead Scissors Stroke. Cross the fingers up and down, back and forth across the forehead. This loosens up the scalp muscles (frontalis).

For the forehead scissors stroke, place your index fingers, one over each eyebrow, on your forehead. Then move them alternately up and down, massaging the skin and underlying tissues. Move your fingers apart and together, covering your entire forehead. This stroke loosens the face and scalp muscles, and it feels great! Once you've tried it, you'll probably find yourself practicing it all the time. In fact, we'll take a break and do it right now! Ahh! (It feels great after a day at the computer screen, too!)

Get Off Your Feet and Out on the Dance Floor

We tend to carry lots of tension at our very tops, and at our very bottoms, too—in other words, in our feet! No wonder. Our poor little (or big, as the case may be) feet carry our entire weight around all day long, enduring all that walking, running, pacing, tapping, and pounding. And when our feet hurt, the rest of us hurts. Foot problems can result in posture problems, headaches, backaches, muscle aches, and even fatigue.

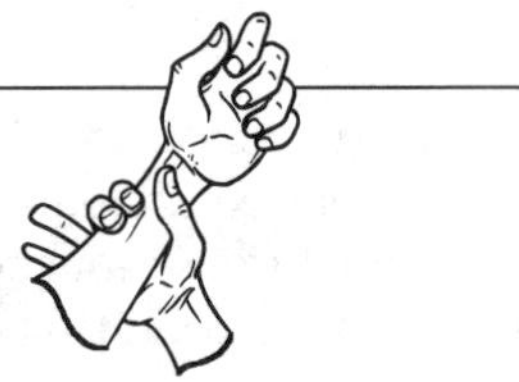

Your Finger on the Pulse

Gravity works against our feet. Blood pools in them, and weight sits on them; they are the workhorses of our bodies. Once every day, turn things around. Prop your feet on a stool at your desk, or better yet, lie on the floor against a wall, scoot up to the wall, and rest your legs against it so your feet reign supreme, even if just for five minutes.

Reflexology works on the feet, and you can practice reflexology techniques on yourself (see Chapter 11). Some of the following general Swedish massage techniques applied to your feet have reflexology effects, too, and give those tootsies the break they need.

Spread Those Toes

One way to relieve foot tension is to separate your toes, which tend to stick together like a junior high clique, probably in an effort to endure all that stress—united we fall, divided we stand, and all that. What you need to "explain" to your foot (via massage, of course) is that the toes can use an occasional break from each other.

Sit comfortably on the floor and interlace your fingers between your toes. At first, you may find it surprisingly difficult to fit a finger between each pair of toes, but as your toes become used to occasional trial separations, this refreshing toe stretch will become easier.

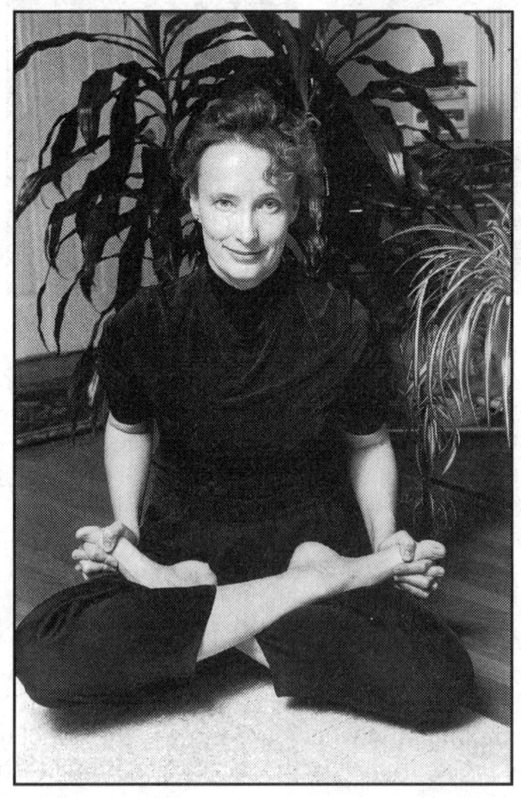

Spread Your Toes. Okay…if it's not comfortable bringing both feet up into yoga's Lotus pose like Joan, try bringing up just one foot at a time. Interlace your fingers with your toes. Grow into the pose.

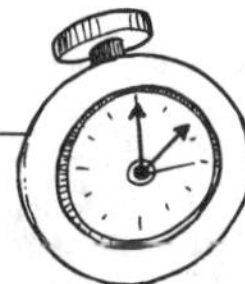

A Massage Minute

Your feet contain 19 muscles, 26 bones, 33 joints, and over 100 ligaments. That's a lot of stuff that can hurt if it isn't treated properly! Well-fitting footwear can be crucial. Wearing high-heeled shoes, for example, often results in a flattening of the foot's crosswise arch, a condition more prevalent in women who wear heels often. The primary symptom of fallen crosswise arches is pain in the instep of the foot. The only way to treat this condition is to stop wearing high-heeled shoes or, less ideally, to wear arch supports in the shoes.

Expand Those Arches

Your foot contains two arches, one lengthwise and one crosswise, which are supported by the foot bones, ligaments, joints, tendons, and muscles. These arches can take a lot of use. When they are abused, however, by chronic strain or by trauma, they may collapse, resulting in flattening feet and fallen arches.

For foot arch relief after a long day, expand those arches! Sit comfortably, bend one leg, and hold your foot bottom-side up. Place your loose fist into your foot's arch and gently rock it back and forth so that your knuckles massage your arch. According to reflexology, this movement will also improve digestive system functioning, so if your hard day has resulted in sore feet *and* indigestion, you know what to do!

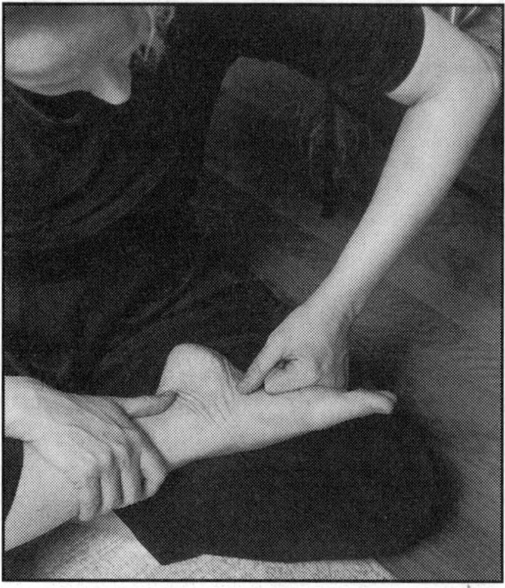

Expand Your Arches. With a loose fist, rock and roll your hand up and down the arch. In reflexology, this massages the reflexes for the digestive system.

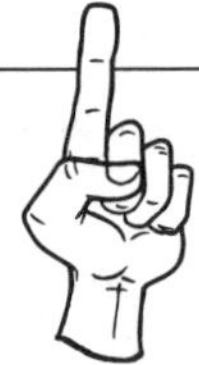

Touch Talk

Metatarsals are the five bones that extend from the area of the heel toward the first bones of the toe, almost like pre-toes. They can be likened to the metacarpals in the hands. **Phalanges** are the toe bones; the word also applies to the finger bones.

Do a Spinal Twist on Your Foot

No, your foot doesn't have a spine—it actually has five spines, or long bone chains that run through it to support it and help it move. These chains consist primarily of the *metatarsals* (five bones that extend from the heel area to the toe area) and the *phalanges* (toe bones).

To give your foot's spine a nice release, hold your foot out in front of you. Place both hands on the sole of the foot near the ankle. Keep your bottom hand steady and twist your top hand up and down the foot along the arch. Move up towards the toes then back towards the other hand. Don't forget to do both feet! According to reflexology, this stretch also works the spinal reflex, helping to develop a more supple spine.

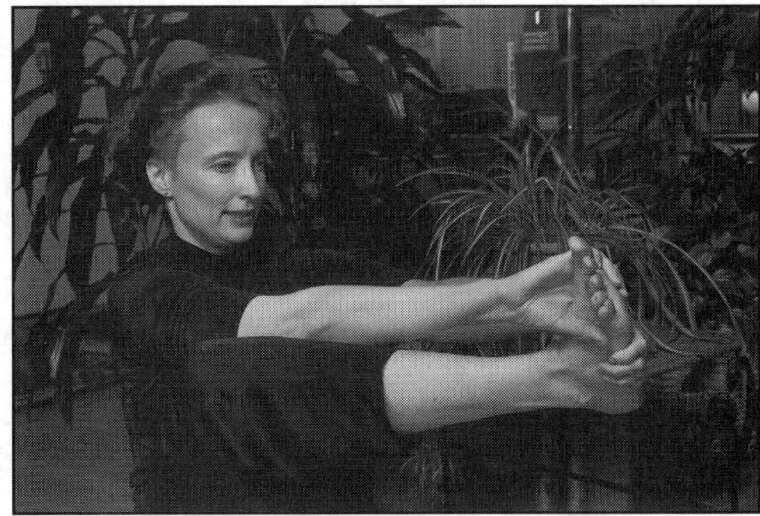

Foot Spinal Twist. Keep your bottom hand secure. Walk your top hand up and down the inside of the foot. Gently give a slight twist to the foot as you walk the hand. The inside of the foot is the spinal reflex, according to reflexology.

Anywhere, Anytime

Perhaps the best thing about self-massage is that you can do it anywhere, anytime. You don't have to persuade someone that you need a massage, and you don't have to pay for it after it's finished. It's the ultimate convenience. Although it feels great to get a massage from someone else, it also feels great to give yourself the love and support any best friend would be glad to offer.

The Least You Need to Know

- Humans know instinctively that self-massage dissolves tension and helps alleviate pain, so self-massage makes sense and should be practiced often.
- Because many people tend to hold tension in their faces, necks, and feet, self-acupressure and self-massage of these areas are superb tension-dispellers. And they feel sublime!
- Self-massage can relieve headache, jaw, and foot pain.
- Self-massage is a great way to reap the benefits of massage whenever and wherever you need to—it's the ultimate in convenience!

Chapter 19

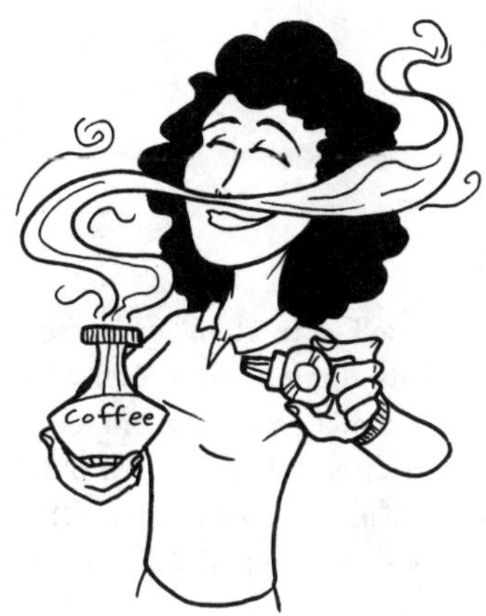

Aromatherapy Is Scent-sational!

In This Chapter

- What good does it do to smell stuff?
- The distinguished history of aromatherapy
- What can aromatherapy do for your health, your massage experience, your skin, and your brain?
- Is aromatherapy safe?
- Which essential oils are best for you?

Imagine the scent of freshly mowed grass, the seashore, warm cinnamon rolls, hot chocolate, fresh coffee, peppermint tea, a pine forest, spring rain, tilled earth, a bubbling stew, baking bread, roses, peonies, honeysuckle, lilacs. Chances are, when you think of these aromas, you do more than recall the thing that causes the scent. They probably evoke vivid memories or at least specific feelings you might not even be able to describe.

No doubt about it, your nose is a powerful sense organ, even though its primary function is to direct, warm, and filter air into your lungs. Along the nose's air passageways are 5 to 10 million olfactory cells sensitive to thousands of different aromas. Once crucial for our survival, our sense of smell has been largely replaced by our senses of sight and hearing, but we still retain it—and wouldn't want to do without it.

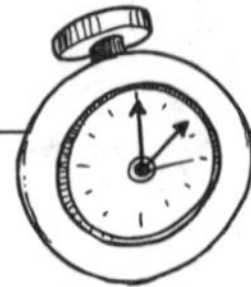

A Massage Minute

If you think you can smell well, compare the human sense of smell (5 to 10 million olfactory cells) to our fellow creatures in the animal kingdom. Rabbits have approximately 100 million olfactory cells, and sheepdogs have 220 million. A dog's nose is a million times more sensitive than a human's, and some dogs can track scents for miles, even when the trail is days old. Dogs have been used to sniff skin cells and breath samples to detect skin and lung cancer with an amazing degree of accuracy. They are also able to alert their owners of impending epileptic seizures, possibly due to the smell of pre-seizure chemical changes.

Lead by a Nose

Although we don't depend on our noses to warn us of impending danger anymore, research suggests that our noses tell us a lot. Scent plays a large part in what makes us choose a mate, according to several studies. You know that feeling of chemistry between two people who are mutually attracted to each other? A lot of that feeling is based on scent, undetectable to our conscious minds but strongly influential nonetheless.

During ovulation, a woman's sense of smell becomes more acute, and smell plays an even larger role in sexual attraction for women than it does for men. A woman's sense of smell becomes distorted and more sensitive during pregnancy, resulting in strong food aversions designed to protect the fetus. For example, java lovers may suddenly be sickened by the smell of a brewing pot of coffee, alcoholic drinks may smell awful, the scent of hot dogs on the grill (or other nitrite-laden foods) may cause nausea, and less-than-perfectly-fresh foods a woman may once have eaten may now seem repulsive. Newborns, too, are particularly "scent-sitive," and can distinguish their own mothers' scents from other people within a few hours after birth.

Scent also retains a strong psychological hold on us. Many people believe, for example, that pleasant odors are healthy and unpleasant odors are unhealthy. This makes "scents" because our noses help us survive by keeping us away from bad-smelling substances that could be toxic, such as rotten food or polluted environments, and directing us towards healthful, fresh food or fresh air or clean water.

Even the impression of a bad odor can change our perception of ourselves and our environments. In one experiment, subjects were put in a room without any odors and asked to list their physical problems. Next, they were told a bad odor was infiltrating the room, even though it wasn't. They were then asked to list their physical problems again. The subjects listed more problems when they believed a bad odor was present, even though nothing in their environments had changed.

A Massage Minute

The human sense of smell is approximately 10,000 times more acute than our other senses. Although we can see and hear things that are too far away to smell, seeing and hearing are more recent evolutionary developments, which we can use to our advantage because we stand upright. Organisms lower to the ground can't see or hear as far from their non-erect vantage points, so their very survival depends on an acute sense of smell. Humans have retained this acute sense even though our survival no longer depends on it.

Other studies have shown that, in the presence of pleasant aromas, human creativity is heightened and mood is elevated; unpleasant aromas tend to depress moods. But what's pleasant and unpleasant to one person might be different to another. Most people find the smell of lavender or spiced apple pleasant, but someone who once got the flu after eating apple pie or was raised by an unkind person who always wore lavender perfume will find those odors distinctly unpleasant.

The Nose Knows: Aroma and the Brain

Aromas seem to be particularly powerful in evoking emotional sensations and vivid memories. Unlike our other sense impressions, which first travel to higher, thinking regions of the brain where they are analyzed and interpreted, olfactory impressions travel straight to the more primitive emotional center in the brain, the limbic system (see Chapter 8, "Putting Your Mind to It").

A Massage Minute

According to some sources, our sense of taste is up to 90 percent reliant on our sense of smell. That's why you can barely taste things when you are congested with a head cold and, possibly, why food that smells great usually tastes great, too. If you are a literature buff, you may have read Marcel Proust's *Remembrance of Things Past*, in which the main character takes one bite of a madeleine (a French cookie) and is vividly transported back to his forgotten childhood, which he then proceeds to relate at length. The pastry's aroma, more than its taste, probably transported the main character into his remembrance.

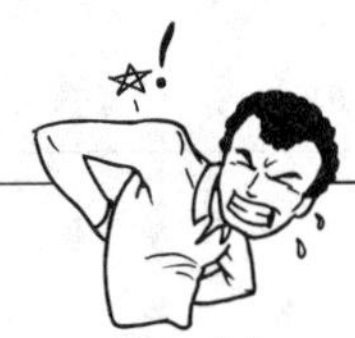

Ouch!

Essential oils are potent substances and should not be inhaled, applied to the skin, or especially ingested without an awareness of potential effects. Although many essential oils have been inappropriately maligned, a few are toxic. The following essential oils are just a few that can be toxic and should never be ingested without medical supervision, *especially during pregnancy* (always check with your doctor before ingesting any essential oil): basil, boldo, calamus, clary sage, horseradish, hyssop, mugwort, mustard, pennyroyal, rue, savin, tansy, thuja, wintergreen, wormseed, and wormwood.

This action center causes an immediate feeling before the sense impression is analyzed, so if you smell, for example, ocean air, you may suddenly recall the feeling you had as a child on a family vacation to the beach before you even consciously realize that you are smelling the ocean. Or, when you smell a strong, unpleasant odor, such as a skunk or rotting eggs or a sewage treatment plant, you may immediately react by backing away or closing the car window before your mind processes the likely source of the foul odor.

Why does the nose have a direct line to the limbic system, whereas your eyes and ears have to deliver their sensations through more indirect routes, first being subjected to thought before action? It probably has to do with evolution again. At one time, when we relied so heavily upon our olfactory systems for survival, we had to react quickly in the event of danger or to secure something desirable, such as a fresh piece of food. We've had no reason to refine or further develop this method of reaction, so we retain it.

Aromas continue to evoke in us sudden and intense memories and emotions. They are part of a more primitive intelligence that is nonetheless a meaningful part of our existence.

A Massage Minute

So-called "sick building syndrome," a condition in which office workers suffer from vague physical complaints with no apparent cause, may be caused by the body's reaction to the scent of a large mixture of artificial chemicals present in poorly ventilated buildings. Although these smells are too subtle to detect consciously, evidence has shown that the body can react to aromas detected only on a subconscious level, and that unpleasant or unnatural aromas can cause symptoms of depressed mood and ill health.

So what does all this have to do with aromatherapy or, even more to the point, with massage? Aromatherapy takes advantage of our sense of smell to heal us in many ways. Aromatherapy massage is a subcategory of aromatherapy, and it can be a powerful physical and emotional experience, whether administered by a professional massage therapist or an amateur at home.

What Is Aromatherapy?

Strictly speaking, *aromatherapy* is the therapeutic use of pure essential oils. Pure essential oils are extracted from plants via steam distillation and are considered to be the "soul" of the plant, containing not only powerful vitamins, antiseptics, antibiotics, hormones, antivirals, and antifungals, but also the plant's vital energy. These substances and energies can be inhaled or absorbed through the skin, the aspect most relevant to aromatherapy massage. (Although some health practitioners, particularly those practicing Chinese medicine or Indian Ayur-Veda, may prescribe medicines or remedies containing essential oils, always let your physician know about any essential oils you are using, and don't ingest essential oils unless under direct supervision of a knowledgeable practitioner.)

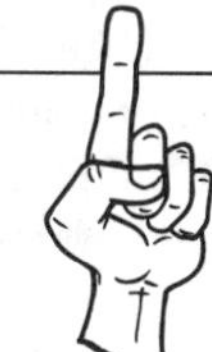

Touch Talk

Aromatherapy is the therapeutic use of pure essential oils, either applied to the skin or inhaled through various methods. This term is also used to describe scent-oriented therapies that use plant oils. **Steam distillation** involves passing steam through plants and collecting the vapors and is the only way to extract a plant's pure essential oil. **Cold pressing** presses oil from the plant. **Decoction** obtains an extract by boiling plant parts. **Infusion** involves pouring boiling water over plant parts and steeping them or soaking plants in vegetable oil. Some plants require solvents such as alcohol to release their essences.

Aromatherapy is sometimes used more loosely to encompass a wide range of scent-oriented therapies that use plant essences attained through various methods. Pure essential oils can be derived only through *steam distillation*, but plant oils can also be obtained through *cold pressing* or other forms of pressure, *decoction*, oil or water *infusion*, or by using solvents.

Different from herbal medicine, which uses the whole plant in various ways, aromatherapy is a more subtle, even spiritual, way to adjust the mood and heal the body because it uses only the purest, lightest, most essential part of the plant. According to aromatherapists, the plant's most powerful healing properties are retained and concentrated in the essential oil.

If It's Good Enough for King Tut...

Evidence of aromatherapy techniques exists as far back as civilization itself. The ancient Chinese pharmacopoeia lists certain herbs whose scents were thought to have therapeutic effects. The ancient Hindu scriptures list hundreds of aromatic substances for religious and therapeutic use. But the first civilization to really take aromatherapy and run with it was the ancient Egyptians.

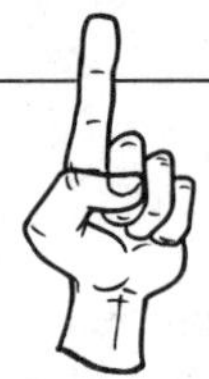

Touch Talk

Aromatics is both a practice and a product. The practice of aromatics involves the use of plant fragrances in general, not limited to essential oils. Before the invention of steam distillation, oils were typically infused with a plant's essence by soaking the plant in the oil. These oils are more appropriately called aromatics than essential oils.

The Egyptians were using infused oils in 3,000 B.C. for massage, surgery, food preservation, and mummification. Because essential oils kill bacteria, they are effective preservatives and digestive aids for food and, as evidenced by the well-preserved bodies of ancient Egyptians, effective at preserving just about anything that might otherwise tend to decompose.

From China, India, and Egypt, the art of aromatherapy spread to Greece and Rome, where it was further refined. By fumigating Athens with *aromatics*, Hippocrates was able to stave off a plague. In Persia, the famed physician/philosopher Avicenna developed steam distillation to create flower waters and essential oils, and the process was introduced to Europe in the 13th century by Arnald de Villanova, a physician. However, essential oil production was not widely practiced in Europe until the 16th century, when a German physician, Hieronymous Brunschweig, wrote a two-volume book describing steam distillation.

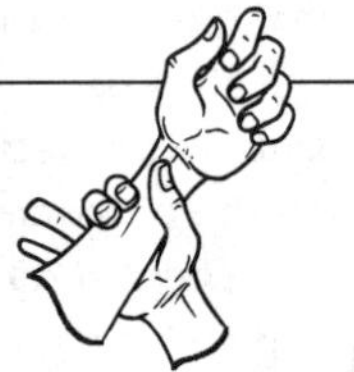

Your Finger on the Pulse

Lavender essential oil is one of the all-time great, all-purpose healers. If you like its scent, use it whenever you can because it is sure to address almost any healing needs your body may have.

Aromatherapy (which wasn't called aromatherapy yet) died down in Europe until the late 1920s, when a chemist, René-Maurice Gattefossé, coined the term *aromatherapy* (or to him, aromathérapie) to refer to his work with essential oils. Gattefossé's family owned a perfumery, and during a lab explosion, he immediately immersed his severely burned hand in lavender oil. The hand healed with amazing speed and without any scarring, prompting Gattefossé's interest in and work with essential oils as antiseptics.

Aromatherapy massage began a bit later in France with Marguerite Maury, a French biochemist who revived the ancient use of essential oils as an integral part of massage, rather than as substances to be taken internally. Maury also proposed that certain mixtures of essential oils be tailored to balance an individual's spiritual nature.

Aromatherapy massage is now an increasingly popular bodywork-of-choice for many in the United States. Not a specific massage technique in itself, aromatherapy massage involves using essential oils to enhance any massage technique. It is often used in Swedish massage.

What Aromatherapy Can Do for You

We've already mentioned a little about what aromatherapy can do for you, but the possibilities are endless—especially because the applications of aromatherapy are endless! Aromatherapy can involve inhaling or being massaged with essential oils, and each method has its own benefits.

Do some research to discover which essential oils are best for what and which methods of application work best for particular ailments. The following brief list of common ailments and which essential oils can help is certainly not comprehensive. Books exclusively devoted to aromatherapy contain more detailed and inclusive guidance.

- Acne: chamomile, clove, juniper
- Anxiety: basil, cedarwood, jasmine
- Arthritis: angelica, carrot seed, frankincense
- Asthma: basil, clove, black spruce
- Bloating: mandarin, marjoram, rosemary
- Bruises: bay laurel, everlasting, lavender
- Burns: chamomile, geranium, lavender, rosemary
- Colds/flu: angelica, cinnamon, eucalyptus, garlic, lavender, myrrh, black pepper, peppermint, pine, tea tree
- Constipation: fennel, ginger, rose, rosemary
- Cough: cypress, eucalyptus, ginger, jasmine, juniper
- Depression: chamomile, frankincense, grapefruit, lemon, orange, sandalwood, ylang ylang
- Diabetes: cinnamon, eucalpytus, geranium
- Fatigue: basil, lavender, peppermint
- Grief: marjoram, rose
- Headache: ginger, lemongrass, peppermint, rosewood
- Hypertension: garlic, juniper, yarrow, ylang ylang
- Insect bites/stings: eucalyptus, lavender, patchouli, tea tree
- Menstrual pain: bay laurel, carrot seed, chamomile, myrrh
- Migraine: basil, chamomile, eucalyptus, lavender
- Nausea: cardamon, chamomile, fennel, ginger, peppermint
- Panic: clary sage, jasmine, lavender
- PMS: carrot seed, chamomile, fennel, patchouli, ylang ylang
- Sinus trouble: eucalyptus, peppermint, pine, tea tree

Most, but certainly not all, essential oils are safe, but all are extremely potent and need to be used only in very small amounts.

Rub It in: Aromatherapy Massage

Because aromatherapy can be used in conjunction with just about any type of bodywork, it can enhance and heighten any massage experience. In addition to conveying antibacterial, antiseptic, and other therapeutic properties through the skin to enhance the cleansing effects of massage, essential oils deliver aromas that add a deeply personal, emotional element to the massage experience.

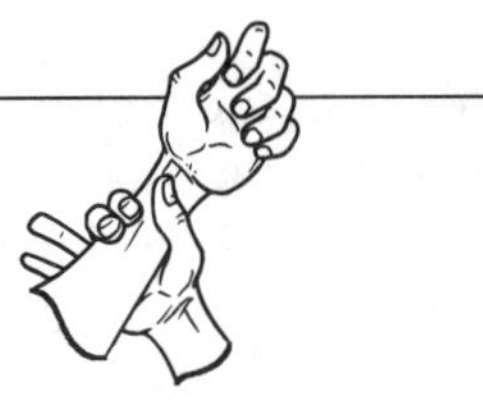

Your Finger on the Pulse

An aromatherapy massage that concentrates on the face can be an incredibly relaxing experience. Use a massage oil containing an essential oil (try juniper or chamomile) and stroke the face firmly but gently. Strokes with fingers from either side of the nose back towards the ears help to facilitate lymph drainage, flushing toxic waste products from the face.

Different massage therapists have different preferences for which essential oils work well and which techniques work best in conjunction with essential oils, but many tend to use aromatherapy while assisting the lymphatic system in its drainage processes. The lymphatic system's cleansing mechanisms are augmented by the cleansing effect of essential oils. Other methods may focus on facial massage or on certain areas of imbalance or injury.

In general, aromatherapy massage works the body and the senses inside and out. The action of massage increases the absorption of essential oils, manually and aromatically stimulating circulation, flushing the body of waste products, calming the nervous system, toning the digestion, normalizing glandular function, and bringing the emotions into balance. Plus, after an aromatherapy massage, your skin will glow like never before.

Rubbing It in for Beautiful Skin

Your skin is your largest organ and serves many purposes, from protecting your internal organs to serving as a highly effective organ of excretion, eliminating waste products through sweat, oil, and the skin's own special brand of respiration (see Chapter 5, "Massage Keeps All Systems Go"). Obviously, because the skin excretes, it must be somewhat permeable, but it doesn't let just anything soak in. Skin is water-resistant and multilayered. It is picky about which substances it will allow entrance to, which it will chemically alter first, and which it will reject. Some areas of your body are more permeable than others, especially those areas with lots of sweat glands, hair follicles, and pores.

Gender differences exist, too. Women's skin is thinner and more permeable than men's, and women's sweat is less acidic and bacteria-busting. In other words, women may absorb things more easily, but they may also be more subject to the ill effects of absorbed toxic substances than men.

When it comes to essential oils, however, the skin is pretty friendly. These natural oils are absorbed readily, especially when they are slightly warm (heating essential oils too much may destroy their properties) and accompanied by the friction of massage strokes. Covering oiled skin with a sheet or blanket can minimize the oil's absorption into the air and encourage its absorption into the skin, as well.

What does aromatherapy massage do for your skin? Sometimes skin goes untouched and inactivated for too long. It builds up dead skin cells, circulation is sluggish, and the skin may retain a dull, grayish appearance. Aromatherapy massage vigorously stimulates circulation to the skin, removing waste products and encouraging the delivery of vital nutrients to the skin surface. The warm oil and the massage action draws blood through the capillaries towards the skin's surface, and on the surface, essential oils cleanse pores and sweep the skin surface clean. Afterwards, skin is rosy, energized, bright, and clear. What a wonderful gift to such a valuable part of your body!

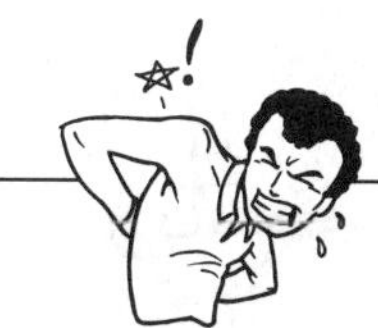

Ouch!

Essential oils penetrate the skin quickly and effectively. However, they should always be mixed with a carrier oil (a vegetable or fruit oil such as canola oil) because their potency could make them irritating to the skin if used full strength.

One exception is in the case of insect bites, stings, and cuts. For relief and antiseptic benefits, put a few drops of pure tea tree, lavender, or rosewood essential oil on a cotton ball and apply gently to the bite, cut, or sting. However, use essential oils directly on the skin with caution. A little goes a long way, and lower doses are more effective. Too much may burn or irritate the skin.

It's in the Air: Diffusers

Diffusers, or small air pumps attached to glass nebulizers, efficiently spread pure essential oils into the air and are probably the best way to permeate a room with the scent of essential oils without altering the delicate nature of the oils. Many claim that this method of inhalation can profoundly affect mood and can calm, relax, or energize you as needed.

For other easy do-it-yourself aromatherapy methods, try using bath oils that contain essential oils or substituting essential oils for your regular cologne (a dab or two will do the trick). You can also buy a ring that's made to be filled with essential oil and fit around a lightbulb. As the lightbulb warms, the oil warms and gently diffuses through the room.

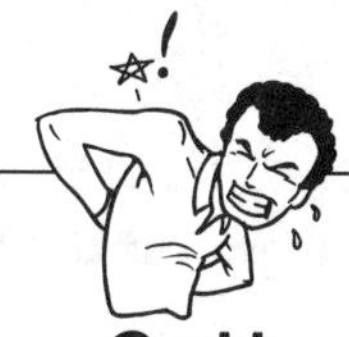

Ouch!

Never put anything into your diffuser but pure essential oil. Anything else may gum up the works. Semi-thick oils, such as patchouli and sandalwood, can be mixed with lighter essential oils. Periodically clean your nebulizer by detaching it from the pump and rinsing it in alcohol. Be cautious about using a diffuser around infants and pets; some diffused oils may be too strong for small lungs.

Natural Medicines for Your Health

All forms of *phytotherapy*, or plant-based medicine, including aromatherapy and herbalism, could be

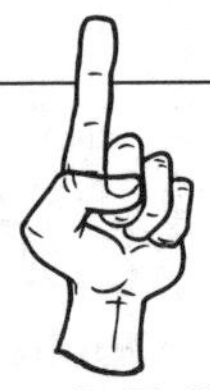

Touch Talk

Phytotherapy is the use of plants for therapeutic purposes. It includes herbal medicine, which uses whole plants or plant parts in various forms, from tinctures and teas to powders and pills. It also includes aromatherapy, which uses essential oils that are either inhaled or applied to the skin. The ancient art of phytotherapy has been practiced since the beginning of humankind in every civilization and on every continent.

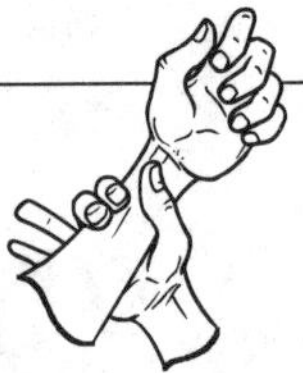

Your Finger on the Pulse

Incense, though not technically a practice of aromatherapy because it may not always contain pure essential oils and the burning process alters the oils, is an ancient way to use aroma that is still available today. Burn incense sticks (use an incense burner for safety) to fill a room with intense scent. Experiment with different aromas to see how they affect your mood, concentration, and energy level.

termed "natural." Phytotherapy is, therefore, distinctly and essentially different from drug therapy and even from the use of artificial essential oils. The whole point of phytotherapy is to capture the natural essence of life and use it to support life. Artificial substances aren't life. They are simply often-expensive imitators of substances in nature.

Why are natural substances better? Because plant essences come from life, they can communicate with life. Researchers have discovered the amazing ability of certain herbs and plant essences to normalize bodily functions, rather than reverse them.

For example, consider the popular herb *gingko biloba*. This leaf extract dramatically enhances circulation by dilating constricted blood vessels and is frequently used to treat heart and stroke patients. Whereas vasodilating drugs used for the same purpose tend to dilate blood vessels across the board, gingko biloba only dilates the blood vessels that are constricted, leaving the normal blood vessels alone. (For an excellent reference, see Glenn Rothfield, M.D., and Suzanne LeVert's book *Gingko Biloba*.) It's as though this leaf extract meets the body, asks it where it needs help, and then proceeds to offer help only where needed.

Essential oils, like herbs, interface with the body, normalizing, balancing, and equalizing it where it has fallen out of homeostasis or balance (see Chapter 6, "The Body Made Easy"). Essential oils contain vital energy as well as measurable therapeutic properties and can therefore go further in returning the body to its natural, homeostatic state than any artificial chemical can. It's like the difference between a fresh salad and a vitamin pill, a field of grass and a lawn of artificial turf, a good friend and a television program about *Friends*. Sure, one will sometimes do in the absence of the other, but isn't it nicer, healthier, and more life-bestowing to experience the real thing?

Aromatherapy Safety

Innocuous as a simple aroma may seem, aromatherapy can pose a few risks, which we've already briefly mentioned. Here's a recap:

- Never ingest any essential oils without the supervision of a qualified physician or other health practitioner.
- Never apply essential oils directly to the skin without first diluting them in a carrier oil, except as directed by a physician, or in the case of certain oils for insect bites and stings and as antiseptics for small cuts.
- Never permeate a room with essential oils by way of a diffuser or other methods when an infant or pet is present unless you use very diluted amounts.
- Always test skin products containing essential oils on a small area of skin before applying to large areas, especially if you have skin allergies or sensitive skin.
- Trust your instinct. If a certain essential oil scent is unpleasant to you, don't use it, even if it's supposed to cure some condition you have. Your emotional response to the scent will likely subvert any health benefit. If you are attracted to a certain essential oil's aroma, it will do you good, even if it isn't on some list of appropriate oils for your particular ailments.

The practice of aromatherapy is relatively harmless, and chances are, it will improve your health and well-being in a wonderful and enjoyable way that artificial chemicals will never quite capture. Aromatherapy balances your internal systems as it lifts your spirits. Combined with massage, it's a "scent-sual" experience you won't soon forget.

The Least You Need to Know

- Aromatherapy is the use of pure essential oils, inhaled or applied to the skin, for therapeutic purposes.
- Aromatherapy is an ancient art practiced since the beginning of civilization.
- Aromatherapy is natural medicine as opposed to medicine based on artificial substances and chemical reproductions of natural substances.
- Aromatherapy is good for your skin, your brain, your internal organs, and your emotional well-being.
- Aromatherapy is almost always safe, but a few precautions are in order.

Chapter 20

The Spa Treatment: Spa-cial Pleasures

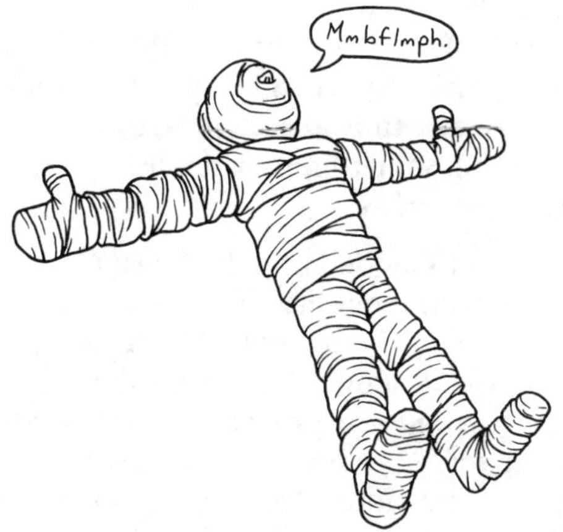

In This Chapter

- Are you a hedonist, and is that good or bad?
- A spa vacation instead of a week at Grandma's?
- How to create your own spa at home
- The true benefits of spa treatments

Would you consider yourself a voluptuary, an epicure, a sensualist, a downright, no-holds-barred devotee of *hedonism*? In other words, do you devote your life to the pursuit of pure pleasure?

Probably not. In this day and age, few of us have the time or the money to spend on much pleasure-seeking beyond an occasional bubble bath when the kids are at soccer practice, a decadent dessert after a grueling final exam, or a rare Sunday afternoon doing nothing but watching football and eating nachos. That's hardly hedonism—that's just stress relief.

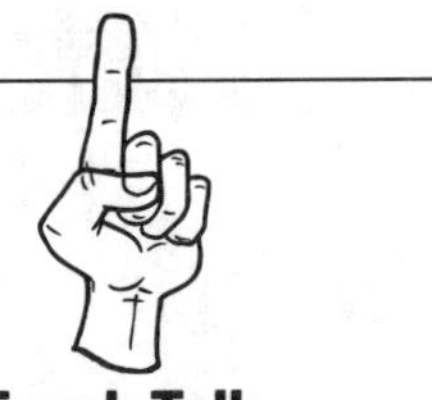

Touch Talk

Hedonism is a philosophy that states that pleasure is the principal good and all action should have pleasure as its aim. In psychology, hedonism refers to the idea that all human actions have pleasure as their purpose.

Plus, our culture tends to view pleasure-seeking as somewhat, well, hedonistic! Maybe it's the Puritan in all of us, but we feel pretty guilty when we spend too much time on ourselves—or any time at all, for that matter. Shouldn't we be getting something accomplished, or doing something for someone else?

What we forget is that in moderation, hedonism is anything but bad. It's self-renewal. Why shouldn't you spend your life being happy and enjoying your pursuits? Why shouldn't you spend some of your time doing something just for you and no one else? You can hardly give to others when you've got no inner resources left to give! The fact is, you'll be more effective and available to others if you indulge yourself now and then. If you look at it that way, hedonism can be downright selfless! Even a little hedonism goes a long way.

What's Your H.Q. (Hedonism Quotient)?

Some of you may find complete and total pleasure time for yourselves a little more often than others. How hedonistic are you? Take our test and find out how much you need a little pleasure in your life, then read on to learn more about the super self-pampering luxury of the spa (and how to create one at home!).

1. When you have a weekend without any scheduled plans, what do you typically do?
   - A. Clean the house or do yard work.
   - B. Ask your partner, the kids, or a friend what they want to do.
   - C. Unplug the phone; pull the blinds; order in; and spend the day bathing, reading, watching television, or napping.
   - D. Find something new and exciting to do—rock climbing, a road trip to a nearby city, dinner at an exotic ethnic restaurant, parasailing....

2. You won $500 in a local raffle. What do you spend it on?
   - A. Overdue bills.
   - B. A nice gift for someone who deserves it or a favorite charity.
   - C. Silk sheets, a velvet chaise for the bedroom, as much expensive wine or champagne as you can buy (you've always wanted to start a collection), or a mini-Jacuzzi for your bathroom.
   - D. An exciting weekend getaway to somewhere you've never been.

3. What causes you the most stress?
   A. Fulfilling all your obligations each day, whether work-related, family-related, financial, or just keeping your desk in order.
   B. When someone you love is having problems and you can't find a way to help them.
   C. Not having enough time for yourself. You need some private decompression time each day.
   D. Not having something to do. You get fidgety and bored if nothing fun is on your agenda.

4. Your friends would probably say the following best describes your personality:
   A. Organized, efficient, and practical.
   B. Social, giving, and empathetic.
   C. Easy-going, relaxed, and self-aware.
   D. Exciting, confident, maybe a little eccentric.

5. What is your favorite way to pamper yourself?
   A. Sitting down to a nice dinner and being able to enjoy it without distractions—a rare luxury in your life!
   B. Spending time with your friends by chatting over coffee, shopping at the mall, or just talking on the phone.
   C. Drawing a scented bubble bath, lighting some candles, playing soft music, and soaking for an hour with the bathroom door locked.
   D. Traveling somewhere far away from your daily life, such as a spa resort or one of those adventure tours.

RESULTS:

If you answered mostly As, you've probably already guessed that you could pamper yourself a lot more than you do. Sure, you're the one people count on to get the job done. Your house is clean; your boss is satisfied; your personal life is in order. But what about you?

You may feel proud of your accomplishments and your ability to handle life, but you often neglect your personal need to de-stress and are more focused on getting things done than on how you feel. It might be difficult, but try to start indulging in little acts of hedonism, say once a week. Take a hot bath on a Saturday night. Get a professional manicure and pedicure. For heaven's sake, go get a massage! You'll find that you become even more efficient and ready to take on life's challenges, and you'll feel better doing it, too.

If you answered mostly Bs, you're very oriented toward the needs of others, but seldom focus on your own needs. You are a great shoulder to cry on, but whose shoulder do you cry on when life overwhelms you (and we all get overwhelmed now and then)? You need to remember that meeting your own needs will make you more effective in meeting the needs of others. If you are the type of person who depends on the opinions of others for self-esteem, you could benefit immensely from cultivating some of those buried inner resources.

Force yourself to meet your own needs now and then. You're worth it! It might be easier to start with some friends—a group of you indulging yourselves at a day spa, for example, with facials, body wraps, mud baths, and massages. Eventually, though, practice some hedonism on your own: yoga classes, a monthly massage, a movie that interests you but not your spouse or kids. Getting to know, trust, and care for yourself on your own terms and in your own space will help you to grow as an individual and to be a better partner, parent, and friend.

If you answered mainly Cs, you are fairly adept at the art of self-indulgence. But when we say "self-indulgence," we don't mean that in any negative light. You recognized somewhere along the line that you need time for yourself, and darn it, you're going to take that time, no matter what! And you should. De-stressing by paying attention to yourself makes you a more relaxed and effective person. People envy your stress-free soul and wonder how you're able to put up with all that you do.

But maybe you are getting bored with your standard bubble baths and pedicures. Try something new and different. Visit a spa, or make your bathroom into one. Try some pampering treatments you haven't tried, such as body wraps, mud baths, or different herbal soaks. And don't forget massage—the bodywork options out there are endless.

If you answered mainly Ds, you're a mover and a shaker. You have no problem with hedonism because you love to have fun, and you believe it makes you a better and more interesting person. And you're right! Your fun is usually action-oriented, based on unique adventures, excitement, and breaking away from your daily grind. You have the wonderful gift of a courageous spirit.

But sometimes, you may push yourself too hard in an effort to outdo yourself or others. Don't let your spirit of adventure get in the way of real self-care. After rappelling down that cliff face, your body probably needs a little attention. What about a massage? Can you lie still for that long? In other words, as you live on the edge, don't forget to step back now and then, look inward, and reacquaint yourself with stillness, peace, and the quiet voice of your body telling you that just for today, it would prefer an aromatherapy massage and an hour of meditation. After all, what good is all that excitement if you never sit back and reflect on what it has taught you?

Feel Spa-ctacularly Pampered

What do you do for your annual two-week vacation? Visit your parents? Take the kids to Disney World? Tick off your list of social obligations? Or maybe you spend your vacation on the chores of life that wouldn't normally get done, such as painting the house, redoing the roof, balancing your checkbook, or enjoying some peaceful down time while the kids are at camp.

But have you ever considered taking a spa vacation? No, they aren't just for the rich and famous. A wide range of spa options exist in every price range, and the types of spa experiences vary drastically, too, from lush and expensive to down-home.

Spas typically offer a wide range of massage and bodywork options, pampering beauty treatments, and classes on everything from yoga to meditation techniques to high-impact aerobics. The food is usually superb, and the focus of the experience is you, you, all you! In the morning, you might go on a quiet nature walk, take a sauna, relax into a mud bath, be thoroughly scrubbed until your skin glows, and then enjoy a Swedish massage that melts you into a person who doesn't remember the meaning of the word stress—all before lunch!

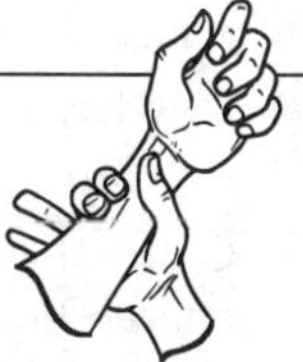

Your Finger on the Pulse

Deciding you'd like to visit a spa and finding your ideal spa experience are two different matters. Where do you start? Your massage therapist might know of spas that focus on bodywork. Your travel agent should have information on spa vacation packages. Look for books on spas, and/or scan the Internet for information. Many spas have Web sites that give you all the information you need.

Live in Luxury: The Home Spa

Maybe a spa vacation just isn't in your budget, or you have too many obligations when it comes to your precious vacation time. Or you'd like a little spa time on a more frequent basis—say weekly, or even daily. It's easy to enjoy the spa experience in your own home. Creating a home spa is a lot of fun and well worth it when you consider all the benefits of re-energizing yourself and banishing your stress.

First, though, you'll need a plan. Where will your home spa be? Your bathroom is an ideal setting. All you need is a little storage space, a bathtub, a shower, and some supplies. The following sections will fill you in on some of the pampering procedures of professional spas, as well as how to try them at home. To equip your home spa, keep any or all of the following in stock, depending on which treatments you'd like to try:

- Aromatherapy candles in scents you love, for ambiance. Try lavender, vanilla, citrus, cinnamon, or pine for starters.
- Essential oils in scents you love to mix with bathwater or lotions or to diffuse through the air.
- Essential oil diffuser and/or incense with holder.
- A selection of herbs and dried flowers, such as rose petals, lavender, and citrus peel, for use in the bath or for herbal wraps.
- A pound of sea salt and a pound of dried seaweed for the bath.
- Cider, wine, or rice vinegar for the bath.
- A comfortable (but waterproof) chair, for a homemade steam tent (we'll explain how to create one later in the chapter).
- A large woolen blanket for a homemade steam tent.

- A large bowl or pot that holds about a gallon of water for a homemade steam tent.
- Powdered clay or purchased mud-based facial treatments for mud facials, packs, or wraps.
- Clean sheets, towels, and a rubber sheet or other waterproof covering or purchased body wrap kits for body wraps.
- A variety of scrubbers: loofah sponges, sea sponges, scrubbing mitts, body brushes, face brushes, or anything else you can find that looks luxurious.
- A manicure/pedicure tool set: nail scrub brush, nail files, emery boards, buffers, and polish, if you use it.
- Scented foot and hand cream, body lotion, and face lotion, or unscented lotion to which you can add essential oils (about 15 drops per ounce of lotion).

Keep your bathroom clean (or at least clean before your spa sessions), so you aren't distracted by soap scum in the crevices when you're trying to relax, and keep lots of fresh linens on hand. Dim the lights, put on your favorite peace-inducing music, light a few candles, make sure the door locks, and get down to the business of serious pampering! Even though the previous list looks long, remember that it's not the amount of stuff in your spa that matters, but the state of relaxation you can achieve (and sometimes, all that takes is a bathtub, hot water, and a towel!).

The Soak

Remember when you were a kid and you hated taking a bath? Now, it is probably a rare and superindulgent luxury. But soaking in an aromatic tub can also be a sensual and profoundly rejuvenating experience. At professional spas, you may get to soak in aromatherapy baths, herbal baths, mud baths, or whirlpool baths. In many cultures, bathing is an art.

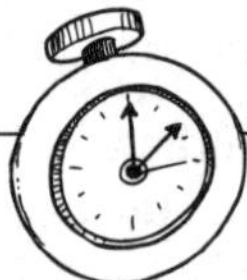

A Massage Minute

In Japan, bathing is serious business. Bathtubs are beautiful and dramatically deep (often crafted of wood) and filled to the brim with water, allowing a comfortable full-body soak. Flowers, leaves, citrus peel, herbs, and even rice wine are mixed into the water. Baths are preceded by vigorous scrubs to remove toxins and ready the skin for the soaking experience. Sometimes, scrub and soak sessions are alternated several times for a penetrating clean that gives a new, almost spiritual meaning to good hygiene.

Each bathing method has its cleansing and relaxing benefits. At home, however, you can get many of the same effects:

- For an aromatherapy bath, add a few drops of essential oil to your bathwater, and then soak and savor the aroma, allowing it to relax and heal you. (See Chapter 19, "Aromatherapy Is Scent-sational!," for a list of aromatherapy oils to try.)
- To add herbs or other substances to your bathwater, make a bath tea bag out of a square of muslin or cheesecloth. Tie it securely and hang it over the faucet so the water runs over it before running into the bath. What to put in your bath tea bag? Try fresh or dried pine needles, lavender, rose petals, citrus peel, pieces of seaweed, or rice bran. Or try your own favorite herbs, roots, and flowers (but first be sure they aren't irritating to the skin).
- You probably don't want to attempt the mess of a mud bath in your own bathroom, and you probably don't have the equipment to keep the mud heated to the ideal temperature. For a similarly primal experience, add sea salt and/or powdered seaweed to bathwater.
- Add 16 ounces of vinegar (apple cider, wine, or rice vinegar are types to try) to bathwater to tone and cleanse the skin.
- For itchy skin, pour a pound of corn starch mixed with a little water to make a paste into warm bathwater. Or grind up a pound of oatmeal in your blender until it is the consistency of flour, mix with a half pound of baking soda, place the mixture in a muslin or cheesecloth bag, and let it soak along with you.
- For the Jacuzzi experience, consider installing a few whirlpool jets in your bathtub. Hydrotherapy and massage all at once in the privacy of your own bathroom! Not cheap, but oh, so worth it.

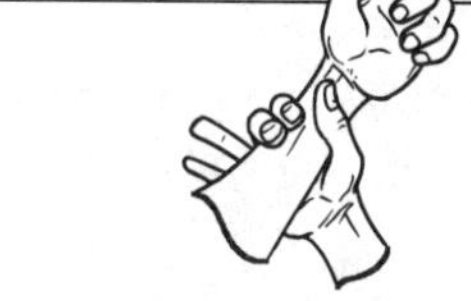

Your Finger on the Pulse

To get the most out of your bath experience, drink plenty of pure water, herbal tea, or fresh juice beforehand. Scrub your skin thoroughly in the shower and rinse well. While running your bath, add aromatic or other beneficial ingredients to the bathwater. Soak for at least 20 minutes, preferably 30. Then, get out slowly, dry yourself well, and relax quietly for at least another 30 minutes. If you have relaxed to the point of grogginess, rinse off in a cool shower for a bit of a vascular workout, and to tonify.

Sauna Versus Steam

Saunas and steam baths are two popular forms of body cleansing you can now find in just about every major health club and hotel in town Some spas are located in areas with natural hot or cold springs, but most have constructed saunas and steam baths for your heat-seeking pleasure. The main difference between saunas and steam baths is that saunas—wooden rooms that contain heated rocks—contain dry heat, and steam baths—rooms or body-sized boxes with holes for your head to emerge—contain wet

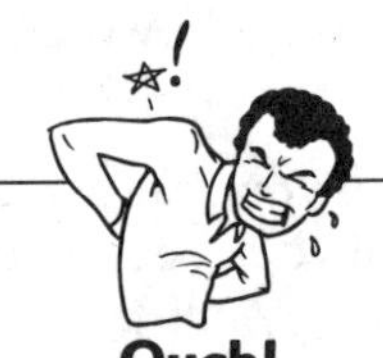

Ouch!

Never stay in a sauna or steam bath for more than 20 to 30 minutes. If you start to feel dizzy sooner, listen to your body and come out early. People with high blood pressure or heart disease should exercise extra caution, and pregnant women shouldn't engage in any activity that raises the body temperature above 100 degrees.

heat. Saunas are typically 180 to 190 degrees Fahrenheit; steam baths are typically 120 to 130 degrees Fahrenheit because the body is less able to sweat in an environment where the air is already saturated with moisture.

In either case, you'll sweat plenty, purging your body—via your skin (that excellent excretory organ)—of all the junk you've been filling it with over the years (and all the junk your body naturally produces, no matter what you fill it with).

Can you replicate the sauna or steam bath in your own home? Well, you can build your own sauna, but if that's not in your budget, you can certainly create your own steam tent. Heat about a gallon of water to the point where it is almost simmering—steaming, but without bubbles. Carefully pour the water into a large bowl or pot placed on a thick towel in your home spa. For the aromatherapy effect, add a few drops of your favorite essential oil.

Next, take off any clothing you don't want to get sweaty. Place a chair over or directly behind the bowl, sit, and drape a large woolen blanket over your head, the chair, and the bowl. Relax and breathe deeply for 10 to 20 minutes. Then, for that extra kick, remove the blanket and immediately jump into a cool shower.

A Massage Minute

During an intense steam bath, heavy smokers will sweat tar out of their bodies, leaving telltale stains on the steam bath seat. During body wraps, smokers may also turn the sheets in which they are wrapped a yellow color as they sweat out those toxins.

Down and Dirty: Mud Masks

Time for a mud pie in the face—a grown-up mud pie, that is! What good is mud? It isn't a magic formula, but it is a great way to heat the body, which relaxes muscles and nerves, and to draw toxins and waste products from the skin, which cleanses the system. Skin can also absorb nutrients and minerals from mud.

Mud can be applied in a variety of ways. At a spa, you can treat yourself to a mud bath, where you'll be immersed up to the neck in a tub of mud. Mud wraps and packs are other forms of application in which mud is applied to the whole body (a wrap) or just to injured, arthritic, overworked, or just plain achy areas. The body or body part is then wrapped in cloth and then plastic (or some other covering that keeps the heat and moisture in), swaddled in blankets, and left to bake for awhile.

Can you obtain the benefits of mud at home? Probably the least messy way is to purchase a mud-based facial treatment, which can tighten, tone, and draw impurities from your skin. Try one while soaking in an aromatherapy or herbal bath for multiple benefits in one home spa session. Slather it on according to directions.

Or mix purchased powdered clay with water to make your own mud. For extra luxury, add a couple drops of essential oil to your mud mixture. Apply it to your face or body, let it dry, and then rinse gently with plain water. (Be careful not to get "mud in your eye," and remember that some essential oils can be irritants—test first or make sure you are using a non-irritating oil.) For an at-home mud pack, wrap the area you've covered in mud with a warm, wet towel and then with something to prohibit evaporation, such as plastic wrap. Relax for 20 minutes, and then rinse off the mud.

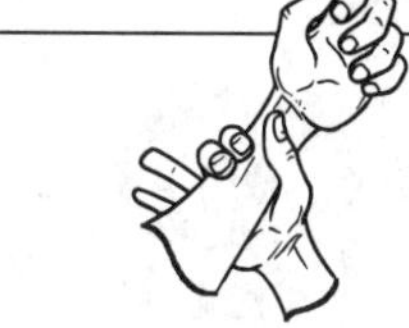

Your Finger on the Pulse

A mud facial is just one of many facial options. You'll find a wide variety of natural facial products available in stores. Or raid the kitchen and make your own. Apply these masks before a bath and then rinse them afterwards: try warm cooked oatmeal and honey, fruit puree thickened with flour, cucumber slices, mashed tofu, almond or sesame butter, or whipped egg white. Or invent your own!

Oompah Loofah! (and Other Scrubbers)

Nothing makes a bath work to your advantage like a pre-bath scrub. Talk about invigorating! You've got lots of options beyond your basic washcloth, and each is worth exploring if you're interested in clear, luminescent, glowing skin. Scrubbing before a soak cleanses the skin of oils and pollutants, sloughs off dead skin cells, massages the skin surface to increase circulation, and generally prepares the skin to best absorb and utilize the nutritive and/or therapeutic substances you've added to your bathwater, whether essential oils or seaweed.

Scrubbing tools are many and largely a matter of preference, but you might try the following:

- **Natural loofah sponges.** Loofah sponges are dried gourd fibers that soften and become more flexible when wet. They are still fairly abrasive, however, and are best reserved for areas of thicker skin such as the feet, knees, elbows, buttocks, and back. After your skin is more accustomed to scrubbing, loofah sponges are also good for the arms, legs, and stomach. In addition to its natural sponge shape, loofah is also available in scrubbing mitts.

- **Natural sea sponges.** These sponges are soft and best for delicate areas such as the face and neck. They won't have much of an effect elsewhere, unless your skin is ultrasensitive.
- **Natural bristle brushes.** These brushes come with a handle or a band to go across the back of your hand. The brush should be comfortable to hold and aesthetically pleasing. Avoid synthetic bristles. Small, very soft brushes are best for the face.
- **Pumice stones.** These stones are made from volcanic material and are for very thick, stubborn skin areas such as the bottoms of your feet and heels.

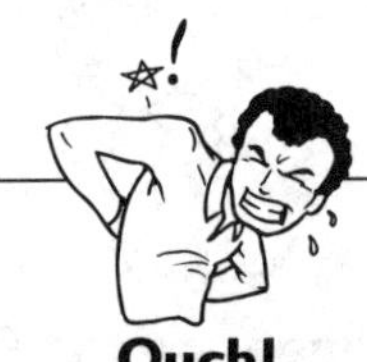

Ouch!

Scrubbing feels great, but if your skin is used to a slather of soap and a rinse in the shower, you'll have to break it in to scrubbing gradually. Start with very gentle circular motions and softer scrubbers. As your skin adjusts, you can scrub with more vigor, and the experience will become more massage-like.

Check your local bath store every so often. New products emerge all the time for your scrubbing pleasure.

Once you've got your scrubbing tools ready, start at your feet and scrub upwards. Never scrub so hard as to irritate your skin, especially at first, before your skin is used to a hearty scrubbing. Scrub in a circular motion and always move towards your heart (just like in massage): up each leg, up the torso, from hand to shoulder, and then (with a very soft brush or sponge) over the face and neck.

"It's a Wrap": Body Wraps

One of the more popular treatments at a spa is the body wrap. You can also purchase quite elaborate body wrap treatments for use at home. Body wraps are, essentially, strips of fabric or large sheets soaked in herbs, minerals, or other substances and then wrapped tightly around the body. Next, the body is wrapped in a type of covering to prohibit evaporation. Then, it's time to sweat it out (literally!). The traditional body wrap covers the entire body, but smaller-scale wraps are also available for spot areas, such as the often troublesome expanse between the knees and waist.

You'll hear lots of claims concerning body wraps, such as absolute 100 percent guarantees of inch loss and/or weight loss. However, the fact is that body wraps don't dissolve fat, although you might sweat out some water weight (which you'll quickly regain). Some people also claim body wraps draw out the fluid between your cells in which toxins are deposited. You may hear a variety of explanations for why body wraps work, depending on the body wrap manufacturer or the spa where you receive one.

But do they work? According to many, they sure do. Because the skin is absorbent, it can draw in nutrients from herbal infusions. In addition, body wraps are profoundly relaxing, cleansing, and you'll certainly feel cleaner, lighter, firmer, fresher, and more toned after you've experienced one. Whether you know exactly why you feel that way may not matter. The effects of a body wrap aren't eternal, however, and to keep that cleansed and toned feeling, you'll have to get wrapped regularly.

The best way to try a body wrap at home is to recruit a friend, because you can't wrap your whole body yourself (you can take turns wrapping each other). Cook a couple of clean white cotton sheets in a tea-like mixture of your favorite herbs steeped in boiling water, then wring out the sheet or cloth very well so it will wrap more securely and maintain the warmth more effectively. (Also fold the sheet somewhat systematically before boiling so it is easier to wring out and wrap without getting twisted and tangled. If you take too much time to untwist the sheet, it will cool off too much by the time you get to the wrapping.) Have your friend wrap you tightly in the sheet. Before the heat escapes, have yourself wrapped again in a rubber sheet, plastic, or any other evaporation-proof covering. A blanket is nice for a third layer. Relax for 20 to 30 minutes, but don't let your friend leave—you'll need someone to unwrap you!

The other option (for the less ambitious) is to purchase a body wrap kit. These kits can be expensive, but they give you everything you need for partial or full wraps. You can do the partial wraps yourself, but for a full wrap, you'll need a friend. You'll feel like mummies at first, but once you emerge from your cocoons, you'll feel as fresh and beautiful as butterflies!

Manicures and Pedicures, Too

How could a little attention to those insignificant-looking sheaths of *keratin* on the ends of your fingers and toes possibly qualify as a hedonistic experience? An afternoon spent being manicured and pedicured can be ultimately relaxing and leave you feeling quite pampered, even regal.

Small sheaths of keratin though they may be, our fingernails and toenails are attached to our hands and feet, and that's no insignificant attachment. Because our hands and feet correspond to the systems and structures throughout our entire bodies, attention to these extremities is like attention to the whole you in microcosm.

No, manicures and pedicures aren't the same as reflexology or acupressure or any other type of bodywork. They are smaller in scope—but we all know about the value of small packages! When you receive a manicure and a pedicure, even if you give one to yourself, it is almost as if time has stopped. Suddenly, your attention is focused on the minutiae of you, and that can make you feel good, and important, and worthy.

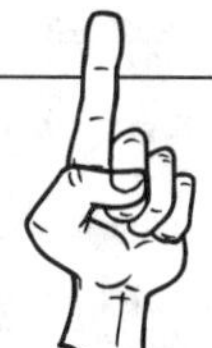

Touch Talk

Keratin is the substance out of which your nails and hair are primarily made, and keratization is the process by which living cells (such as those in the hair roots and nail bases) become dead, tough material without nerves or blood vessels.

Manicures and pedicures by professionals are the ultimate, often accompanied by long hand and foot soaks; lotions; oils; and lots of detailed care with brushes, files, emery boards, buffers, polishes, and even mini-massages! But you can give yourself a great manicure and pedicure in your home spa (or take turns with a friend) with the right equipment and a spare 30 minutes or so.

Manicures and pedicures are perfect for a post-bath ritual because the hands and feet have just soaked and softened. Alternatively, soak your hands or feet for 5 or 10 minutes in a bowl of warm water to which you've added essential oils, fragrant herbs, or flower petals. Scrub your hands or feet and nails with a nail brush to encourage blood flow and get any residual dirt out of the crevices. Rinse well and apply lotion or oil. Gently push cuticles back with a cotton swab, trim and shape nails, and then buff until your nails glow.

Personally, we prefer nails that aren't too long, especially if you give massages. If you like the polished look, wait until the lotion or oil has completely soaked in, and then rub nails with a towel so no oily residue remains. Polish won't stick as well if there's residue.

Remember: The best part of the spa experience, whether at home or away, isn't only the final product (you looking spectacular), but also the loving process of taking care of yourself by giving your body and mind a mini-vacation with maximum impact. You've got a life to attend to, people to care for, and you do a great job. Conclusion? You deserve to be a hedonist every now and then!

The Least You Need to Know

- A little hedonism is good for you!
- Spa vacations may seem self-indulgent, but they are a great way to recharge.
- You can create your own at-home spa with some basic equipment.
- No matter where your spa, you can enjoy soaks, saunas, steam baths, mud packs and masks, invigorating body scrubs, body wraps, manicures, and pedicures—and you deserve it!

Part 6
Massage for Your Life

This last section personalizes massage even further. No matter what your situation, we've got a massage for you! If you have minor or major physical problems, we'll show you what massage can do for you. Even if you've experienced a tragedy, a trauma, or if touch has been used against you, massage can help, but the approach is a little different—slower, at your own pace, and sometimes in conjunction with psychological care.

For those athletes out there, we'll go into lots more detail about the benefits of sports massage. We devote a whole chapter to women in which we hope to inspire you about the true nature of beauty, then show you how massage can help you with the pains and discomforts of PMS, pregnancy, childbirth, and menopause. We'll also show you how to give a great massage to your infant and offer tips on how to make massage fun for kids. For you men out there, we also offer our views on how massage can help you. For seniors, we have a special section on the many ways massage can enrich your life.

Last of all, we haven't forgotten our fellow creatures in the animal kingdom. Reward your loyal companion with the health-bestowing benefits of pet massage. Animals can derive great benefits from massage, just like humans. We'll give you some great techniques for massaging your dog, your cat, and some of the more unusual pets you might share your life with.

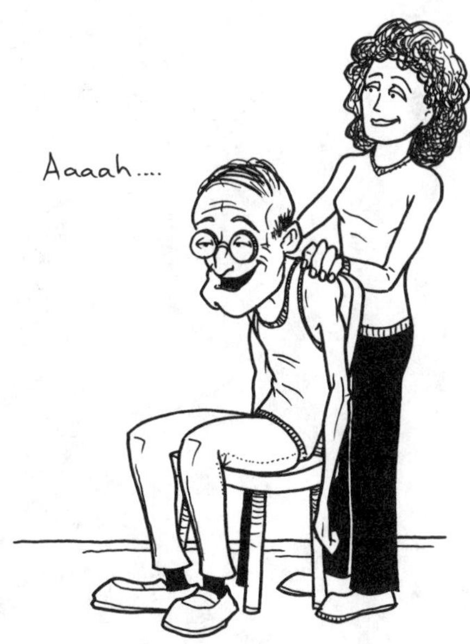

Chapter 21

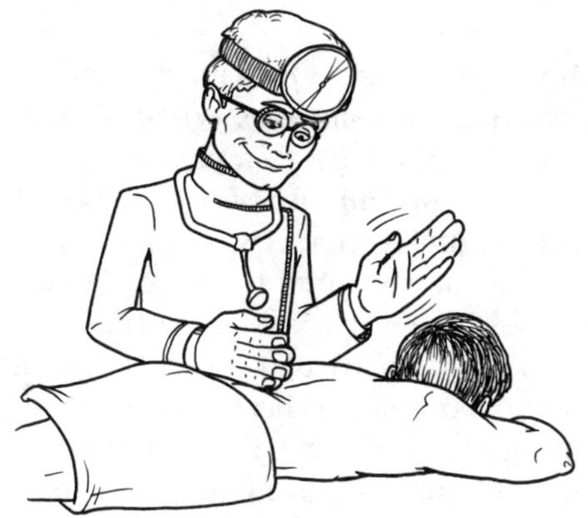

Rx: Massage

In This Chapter

- Massage is relaxing, but can it also cure you?
- What massage can do for nagging complaints, such as back pain, fatigue, insomnia, and indigestion
- What massage can do for more serious health problems
- Should your doctor know if you are using massage as a therapy for your physical problems?

We've focused a lot on all you stressed-out folks out there and how massage can relax you, energize you, and improve your outlook. But can it do more? Can massage heal what ails you?

Obviously, massage does something in the way of healing. After all, many doctors prescribe it and some insurance companies cover it under their health plans. What it does, exactly, depends largely on who you ask and what kind of massage you get.

Some will say massage releases endorphins to dull the pain of symptoms, without actually healing conditions. Some will argue that because massage facilitates circulation, waste product removal, and nutrient delivery, it does help to heal a variety of physical problems. Some will say that massage helps your body to help itself. But few will suggest that massage does nothing for pain, disease, and other maladies. In this chapter, we'll briefly discuss a number of common health problems, from the mild to the severe, and how massage can help.

What Makes You Sick?

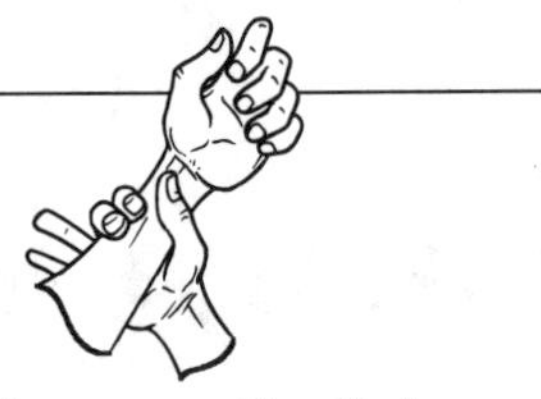

Your Finger on the Pulse

A clear intention is important for massage to be healing. If you gently place your hands on someone and fill your mind, heart, and hands with healing, loving energy, you might be amazed at the response: a slow (sometimes sudden) release of tension. We are more than our bodies—we are energy fields with the ability to communicate on an energetic level.

Just what causes illness or disease? One clue is in the breakdown of the word disease: dis-ease. When the body becomes dis-eased, whether because of a physical or psychological trauma, a slow-build-up of non-healthful habits, or even from too much stress, its systems don't work as efficiently. The body is out of the state of ease, or in a state of dis-ease. Some theories suggest that energy becomes blocked in a particular organ or system; others say certain organs or systems become overtaxed, undernourished, or otherwise out of balance. Genetics surely plays a part, as do our environments, our diets, our activity levels, our states of mind, our points of view, and our degrees of happiness and satisfaction with life.

The truth about the nature of disease is too complicated to paraphrase in a few sentences, but when you are suffering from a physical problem such as chronic pain, your primary concern is most likely getting rid of it. Research has proven that massage therapy can relieve symptoms—and, in many cases, promote cures. Diseases, conditions, and injuries can be eased, corrected, or reversed by supporting the body's natural curative powers.

Is Massage Pampering, Prevention, or Cure?

All of the above, of course! We've told you how massage can pamper you, relieve symptoms, and even how it can often support the curative process. It is also excellent preventive medicine because it keeps your body running at peak efficiency. A relaxed, happy, stress-free, optimistic, and supple body with great circulation is far less likely to get sick than an uptight, anxiety-ridden, tension-filled, pessimistic, tight body with poor circulation. Massage helps to promote the former state of existence and banish the latter.

That doesn't mean healthy, happy people won't get sick, of course. You've heard of the marathon runner who drops dead from a heart attack and the vegetarian who dies of cancer. Disease and death are still mysterious, and factors exist that we can't always anticipate. But we do know that exercising, eating well, and practicing stress-management techniques will lower your risk for getting sick.

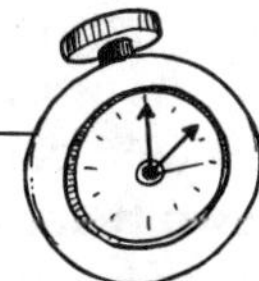

A Massage Minute

According to published studies by the Touch Research Institute, massage therapy clearly reduces various types of stress. Among children who survived Hurricane Andrew, massage therapy decreased levels of anxiety, depression, and the stress hormone cortisol. Preschool children who received massage fell asleep sooner, exhibited more restful naptime periods, had decreased activity levels, and better behavior ratings.

Grown-ups benefit, too! Hospital nursing and physician staff members who were treated with massage therapy, relaxation therapy, and music therapy showed significantly reduced levels of anxiety, depression, and fatigue, as well as increased energy. Massage therapy has also been demonstrated to decrease diastolic blood pressure, anxiety, and levels of the stress hormone cortisol in adults suffering from hypertension.

Massage for Those Nagging Complaints

Luckily, the little complaints are more common than the really big ones, but even the non-life-threatening stuff can be pretty painful, irritating, even life-altering. In fact, chronic pain can be downright debilitating and is often the cause of depression. Can massage help your nagging complaints? The answer is an enthusiastic "Probably!" Read on to find out more.

Oh, My Aching Back!

One of the more common pain-related complaints is back pain. Ever since we humans insisted on standing upright, we've had trouble with our spines. Most back pain is probably caused by muscle strain. Despite the large number of muscles supporting the spine, each muscle still has quite a job and can easily stretch and tear, especially when we abuse our bodies by overextending ourselves or practicing non-healthful posture and movement habits.

Often, it's difficult to get a clear-cut diagnosis for back-pain. You may be prescribed pain medication and sent on your merry (achy) way after a bevy of X-rays and other tests that reveal nothing, but you know it isn't nothing. You know it hurts!

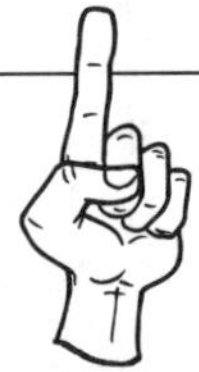

Touch Talk

In between each of the vertebrae in your spine are softer, semi-cartilaginous disks that cushion the vertebrae. These disks tend to wear out as we age. A **ruptured disk** occurs when part of the disk herniates or pushes through the surrounding ligaments of the spine. This condition is extremely painful and may require surgery if pain is extreme and function lost. Sometimes, bed rest is sufficient if the disk isn't fully protruded.

After your doctor has ruled out serious problems such as arthritis or a *ruptured disk*, consider massage therapy to treat your pain. A Touch Research Institute study has shown that massage therapy is effective in relieving lower back pain, but you won't need a study to tell you that after a few sessions with a good massage therapist. Your massage therapist may also counsel you on ways to adjust your posture and other movement habits. Or seek out a bodyworker specializing in movement re-education (see Chapter 12, "More Kinds of Massage"). If you give a massage to someone with back pain, concentrate on the muscles that support the spine (see Chapter 6, "The Body Made Easy," for a reminder of where these muscles are).

Oh, My Aching Jaw! TMJ Syndrome

Temporo-mandibular joint syndrome, or TMJ syndrome, is a surprisingly common and painful condition characterized by dysfunction of the temporo-mandibular joint, which is the joint where the lower jaw joins the skull, just in front of each ear. If you place a finger in front of each ear and open and close your mouth, you can feel the joint working. If you have TMJ syndrome, such a simple movement can be painful.

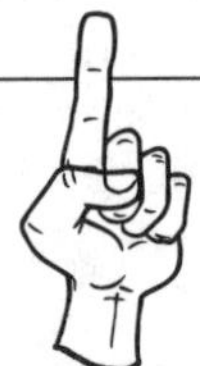

Touch Talk

Tinnitus is the fancy name for ear noise, such as ringing, buzzing, humming, or roaring. A distracting and sometimes extremely aggravating condition, tinnitus can be a symptom of many physical problems, including TMJ syndrome.

Any number of things can cause TMJ syndrome: bad jaw habits such as jaw clenching and teeth grinding, too much gum chewing, uneven food-chewing habits, a jaw or head injury, extensive dental work, or just being born with a jaw that doesn't quite fit together the right way. Eventually, because you use this joint so much, the cartilage that cushions the joint wears away. Nerve endings are exposed and, you guessed it, ouch! Pain may be limited to the jaw or may cause muscle spasms throughout the entire head (including cheeks, teeth, and ears) and even the neck and back. Other symptoms can be clicking or grinding sounds when opening the jaw wide or ringing in the ears (*tinnitus*).

How can massage help sufferers of TMJ syndrome? Deep tissue or trigger point therapy can provide excellent relief and might be covered by your insurance company. Other types of bodywork that claim to relieve symptoms of TMJ syndrome are the Alexander technique, the Feldenkrais method, the Trager method, acupressure, shiatsu, Reiki (see Chapter 12 for descriptions of these types of bodywork), craniosacral therapy, and myotherapy (see Chapter 11, "Welcome to the World of Massage").

Oh, My Aching...Everything! FMS

Fibromyalgia syndrome (FMS) is a painful condition that is often misdiagnosed. FMS sufferers often experience pain in 18 specific tender spots throughout the body (pain in 11 or more can constitute FMS). Other symptoms include muscle spasms, weakness, and stiffness; light, sound, touch, cold, and heat sensitivity; dry eyes and mouth; bloating; depression; migraine headaches; joint swelling and numbness; bladder and bowel irritability; a chronic runny nose and post-nasal drip; dizziness; and disrupted sleep patterns, including extreme fatigue and insomnia.

Massage is one of the best treatments for FMS. Touch Institute studies show that FMS sufferers demonstrated improved sleep patterns and decreased pain, fatigue, anxiety, and depression after massage. Sufferers are typically riddled with painful trigger points, so trigger point work is often an effective treatment for FMS pain. Posture and movement work and massage that improves circulation are also helpful. Acupuncture, acupressure, and shiatsu can help, and many claim that bodywork techniques geared towards balancing energy are also effective. Because craniosacral therapy helps to release restricted energy in the body's fascia—that web of connective tissue throughout the body that constricts and tightens in FMS sufferers, probably causing much of the pain—it can also be effective in relieving some symptoms of FMS. Deep breathing techniques can also be beneficial.

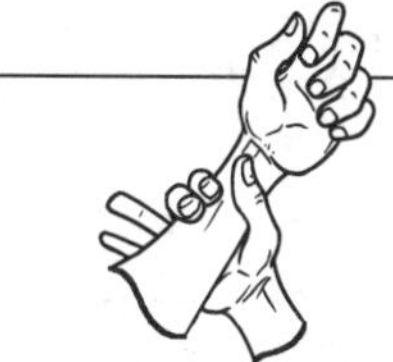

Your Finger on the Pulse

Your jaw is full of trigger points, so massaging gently with your fingers for sensitive areas can quickly reveal where you can press to relieve jaw pain. Try the spot right over the TMJ joint in front of both ears, the spot about one inch above the tops of your ears just in front of your hairline, and the two indentations at the base of your skull just under the ridge on either side of the neck.

The most effective techniques are gentle effleurage, cross-fiber friction, strokes that lengthen shortened muscles, passive stretches, and, in some cases, oscillating vibration. (See Part 4, "Different Strokes for Different Folks," for descriptions of these techniques.) Avoid deep work and any massage over an hour, which is often too much stimulation for the FMS sufferer. Shorter, more frequent sessions are the most effective. Gentle movement such as those employed in Trager or Feldenkrais can be effective for particularly sensitive people who can't handle any degree of Swedish massage.

Many FMS sufferers and physicians stress the importance of a positive attitude, regular and healthy habits, and most importantly, avoidance of high stress, which seems to aggravate FMS symptoms. In general, massage can help FMS sufferers by relaxing them and releasing the stress that is so aggravating to this condition, as well as supporting them emotionally because FMS often has a strong emotional factor and is common in cases of physical and psychological abuse.

Why Am I So Tired?

We all get tired. The days just aren't long enough! Sleep deprivation has become an epidemic. According to the National Sleep Foundation, nearly half of all Americans suffer from insomnia and other sleep-related disorders, and a recent Gallup survey reports that 56 percent of the adult population experiences problems with daytime drowsiness. For some of us, fatigue is a chronic condition caused by Chronic Fatigue Syndrome (CFS). (For more information on sleep disorders, see *The Complete Idiot's Guide to Getting a Good Night's Sleep*.)

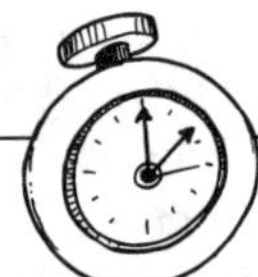

A Massage Minute

More than 30 percent of American drivers admit to having fallen asleep at the wheel at least once in their lifetime, and the National Sleep Foundation estimates that at least 100,000 accidents and 1,500 fatalities per year are due to falling asleep at the wheel.

The best thing you can do for fatigue is to get more sleep! Your body needs sleep to repair and rejuvenate, both physically and psychologically. Regular Swedish massage is excellent for fatigue. However, in cases of Chronic Fatigue Syndrome, the exhausted body's excretory systems may be sluggish, and circulation is probably impaired. Tell your massage therapist if you suffer from Chronic Fatigue Syndrome, and he or she will probably begin with gentle, superficial massage so as not to overtax your circulatory and excretory systems. Massage on a regular basis will eventually bring the body back up to speed and can then become more vigorous (as you become more vigorous!).

Also try acupressure treatments. For you do-it-yourselfers who would like some instant rejuvenation, try massaging 1) the center of your palm, 2) the area behind the tops of your ears, 3) the midline abdominal segment two to four inches below your belly button, and 4) the soles of your feet. And why not take a hint from many other cultures? If you can possibly find the time, sneak an afternoon nap. Just 20 minutes of sleep can be profoundly revitalizing.

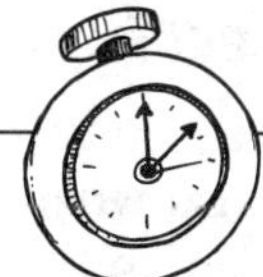

A Massage Minute

In a Touch Research Institute study, people suffering from Chronic Fatigue Syndrome showed immediate improvement in mood, lower anxiety levels, and reduced levels of the stress hormone cortisol after massage. After 10 days of regular massage, emotional stress, depression, insomnia, pain, and feelings of fatigue were all reduced.

Why Can't I Sleep?

Are you miffed on a nightly basis that there isn't anything good on television at 3:00 A.M.? Then you may be one of those insomniacs out there who has time to sleep but can't. Insomnia is characterized by difficulty falling asleep, waking up frequently during the night, waking up too early, or just feeling unrefreshed from sleep. Insomniacs are often tired, irritable, and low on energy. Nonetheless, sleep doesn't come, or doesn't come well.

Insomnia is more frequent in women, in people over age 60, and in people suffering from depression. It may be caused by stress, worry, alcohol, caffeine, nicotine, a medical condition, medication, a change in routine, a too-stimulating sleeping environment, or more mysterious causes. You can take a sleeping pill, which may or may not help. But why not try massage if you just can't relax enough to catch those desperately needed zzzs?

You may find that you can fall asleep on the massage table far more easily than you can fall asleep at home. Hey, grab that sleep while you can get it! Regular Swedish massage may help to balance your body's energies, making sleep less of a challenge. Craniosacral therapy also claims to be an effective treatment for insomnia, as does acupressure.

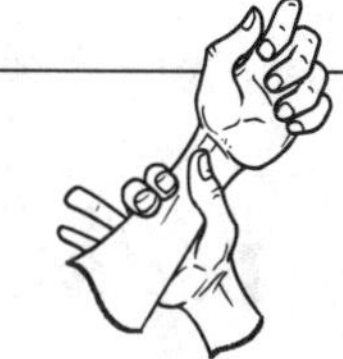

Your Finger on the Pulse

Find the spot directly beneath your little finger in the first wrist crease on the inside of your left hand. Press it three times, for 7 to 15 seconds each press, on this spot to relieve insomnia.

What's Up With My Digestion?

Have you noticed how many television commercials emphasize that if you only take this or that digestive aid, you can eat whatever you want to and not suffer? We think you'd be better off eating healthy, high-fiber, unfried, whole food to keep your digestive system running smoothly. However, some people's digestive systems need a little more help, whether due to chronic indigestion, heartburn, constipation, or something more serious such as *ulcers*.

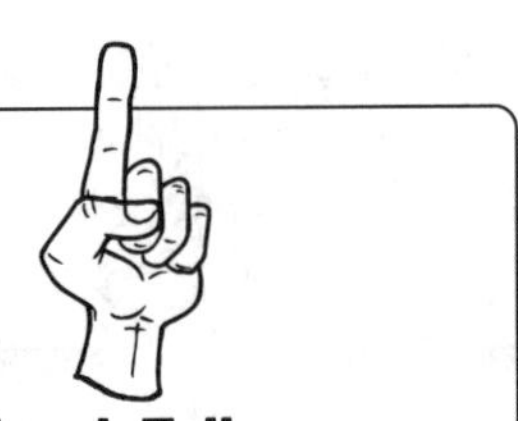

Touch Talk

Ulcers are sores, or localized areas of mucous membrane disintegration. Stomach ulcers are characterized by burning stomach pain when the stomach is empty and are sometimes accompanied by vomiting or bleeding. Soft, bland foods and milk products may reduce symptoms, but the latest research has revealed that dietary habits do not cause stomach ulcers.

Yes, massage can even help your digestive system to run more smoothly. Massage relaxes the muscles of digestion while stimulating the liver and kidneys to promote effective elimination. It can improve the muscle tone of, and increase circulation to, the digestive tract and relieve constipation by stimulating all systems to move. For those digestive problems caused by nervous tension and stress, massage is certainly a good option for treatment. Polarity therapy also claims to address digestive disorders (see Chapter 12).

To help your own digestion, lie on your back, raise your knees, relax your stomach, and gently but firmly press and massage the entire abdomen. Or find the pressure points about an inch or two on either side of your belly button and press for about 10 seconds. And of course, eat fresh, healthy foods, minimally processed, low in fat, with plenty of fiber. And don't forget lots of clear, pure water.

When It's More Serious

Sometimes health problems become more than an inconvenience or a discomfort, and massage can help these serious conditions by making your experience with these diseases easier and less painful. Bodywork also supports your body's efforts to cure itself, so it can certainly contribute to the healing process. However, always check with your doctor before receiving massage therapy or any other bodywork treatment if you suffer from a serious medical condition.

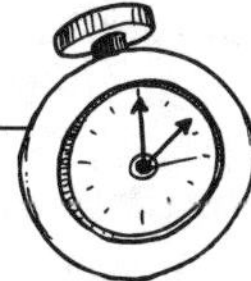

A Massage Minute

Massage is great for many conditions, but should be avoided or limited in some cases: in the presence of fever (over 99 degrees); in the presence of any infectious disease or condition (including severe colds and flu); or on any area of inflammation (skin, veins, organs, tissues), lesions, tissue damage, pus pockets, bruises, varicose veins; and in the presence of any contagious skin condition.

Also, avoid deep massage in cases of swelling caused by kidney or liver problems or increased capillary permeability; high blood pressure that isn't under control; intoxication; a suspected blood clot anywhere; psychosis; osteoporosis (brittle bones due to aging); or scoliosis (crooked spine) unless under a doctor's supervision.

Pre- and Post-Surgical Pain Relief

Before surgery, you may be nervous, agitated, and tense. A pre-surgery massage can relax and calm you and will prime your body to best handle the trauma of the surgical process. (Of course, check with your doctor to be sure massage isn't contraindicated for your condition.)

After surgery, massage is a great way to help your body heal itself. However, you have to be careful. Make sure your massage therapist knows about your surgery. Unless your massage therapist is thoroughly knowledgeable about your surgery and is working with your physician, massage should never be practiced directly on an incision site or over the area where the surgery took place. Your body needs pampering and healing now more than ever, and expert massage can provide it.

Cancer Care

Massage is tricky when it comes to people with cancer. Cancer patients need to be touched because touch helps the body to heal and the whole person to feel more positive and supported. On the other hand, cancer has a nasty habit of spreading, particularly through the lymphatic system, and many types of massage stimulate this system by increasing lymph flow.

That doesn't mean massage must be avoided at all costs in cancer patients, however. The trick is to limit massage to noncirculatory techniques, such as the following:

- Range of motion massage
- Simple laying on of hands
- Energy work, such as Reiki (see Chapter 12), in which the hands stay above the body and manipulate energy without touching
- Gentle reflexology, which reduces stress and boosts the immune system by working on reflex points to various organs

Physical affection is also important. A held hand, a long hug, or an attentive arm around the shoulders can make a big difference to cancer patients who may feel isolated and are probably suffering from the effects of treatments such as chemotherapy.

Immune System Boosting for AIDS

AIDS patients need to be touched, too, and their immune systems certainly need a boost, because the HIV virus that causes AIDS attacks the immune system. One study sponsored by the Touch Research Institute examined the effects of massage therapy on anxiety and depression levels and on immune function in people infected with the HIV virus. Subjects received a 45-minute massage five times weekly for one month. Preliminary findings included significant reductions in anxiety, stress, and stress hormone levels and an increase in the level and activity of the immune cells that attack infection in the body.

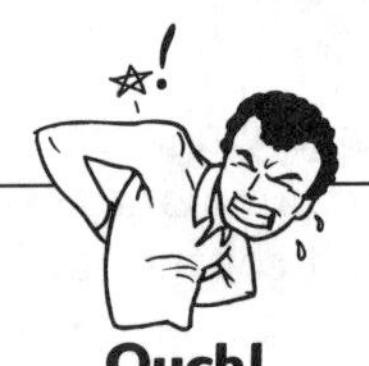

Ouch!

Simply touching someone with HIV can't give you the virus, which must get into your body through the exchange of bodily fluids. Massage can be of great benefit to AIDS patients, but because they are so vulnerable to infection, massage therapists (or anyone) should wash hands thoroughly before giving a massage to someone infected with the HIV virus. Skin lesions should never be massaged on anyone, whether they have AIDS or not.

Massage that relieves stress and is relaxing to the client will benefit the immune system, although circulatory massage may be contraindicated for those with HIV (check with your physician). If circulatory massage is not contraindicated, Swedish massage can boost whole-body functioning and offers the benefit of caring and nurturing human touch, which holistic healers believe is a crucial factor in fighting disease. Energy work, such as Reiki (see Chapter 12), may also be helpful to the immune system, and even movement re-education can help the AIDS patient feel more in control of his or her body and mind.

M-A-S-S-A-G-E Spells Arthritis Relief

As you learned in Chapter 17, "Goin' Round and Round: Increasing Range of Motion," arthritis is a condition in which joints become painfully inflamed. Although many different types of arthritis can occur, the most common types are osteoarthritis and rheumatoid arthritis.

Scientists have yet to develop an arthritis cure, but massage can help to prolong joint mobility. In cases of mild arthritis, Swedish massage, Rolfing, craniosacral therapy, the Alexander technique, and energy manipulation techniques such as Reiki can all be beneficial. Working the muscles that support arthritic joints (without working on the inflamed or arthritic joints themselves) can go a long way towards reducing pain.

However, massage should never be attempted over an arthritic joint and shouldn't be attempted at all in cases of acute rheumatoid arthritis. Also, in cases of a severe flare-up in one joint, massage shouldn't be attempted because an infection may be present, and massage could prompt the spreading of the infection though the body.

Banishing Depression

At least one in six people will experience a major depressive disorder during his or her lifetime, and these numbers appear to be increasing, according to the Harvard Mahoney Neuroscience Institute. More and more people are developing depression at a younger age, and some estimates put the depression rate in young women as high as 50 percent. Depression is characterized by two weeks or more of a depressed mood state including feelings of guilt, fatigue, loss of concentration, decreased energy, loss of appetite and sex drive, and a general loss of interest in everything that once was a source of interest and pleasure.

Depression is highly treatable both through counseling and drug therapy. Another good way to treat mild depression is through touch (in cases of severe depression, check with a therapist or counselor before giving massage). Touch Research Institute studies have demonstrated that depressed teenage mothers who received massage therapy versus those who received relaxation therapy were less depressed and anxious, their stress hormone levels were lower, and their *serotonin* levels were higher. Child and adolescent psychiatric patients had lower levels of depression, anxiety, and stress hormone levels; better sleep patterns; and improved clinical progress after a series of five daily 30-minute massages.

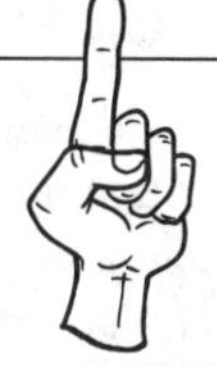

Touch Talk

Serotonin is a chemical neurotransmitter that occurs naturally in the body and is involved in numerous functions including appetite control, sleep, memory and learning, mood, behavior, and depression

Mild depression may be aggravated by the lack of touch experienced by many sufferers, who tend to isolate themselves and avoid touch. Massage's stress-reducing and mood-boosting benefits and the fact that massage may increase your body's production of serotonin just may be a prescription for happiness. The most studied type of massage for depression is Swedish massage, but energy therapies such as Reiki and psychophysical therapies such as Trager, Aston-Patterning, and Feldenkrais may help as well.

Helping to Manage Diabetes

Diabetes is a disease in which the body can't make enough insulin to burn and store carbohydrates, sugars, and starches for energy. In many cases, the disease is inherited. It can also occur during pregnancy and later in life, especially in those who have practiced nonhealthful habits for years and are overweight. Management of the diet is crucial for diabetics.

But massage may be beneficial, too, especially because poor circulation is such a problem in diabetics. A Touch Research Institute study showed that in diabetic children who received massage from their parents, the children's glucose levels decreased to a normal range after one month. Massage that stimulates the circulation may be beneficial and reduce stress, anxiety, and depression, which are common conditions for all disease-sufferers.

Priming the Heart Pump

Massage is a wonderful preventive for heart disease, the number one killer in America. When used in conjunction with healthy dietary and exercise habits, massage can maintain a healthy lifestyle and increase your chances of avoiding or surviving a heart attack.

Even when heart disease is already present, massage may be beneficial for its circulation-enhancing and stress-reducing effects. Because massage, especially Swedish massage, has such an effect on circulation, it must be practiced on heart patients with some caution and under a doctor's supervision. However, human touch can be so healing and emotionally supportive that massage may be extremely beneficial, even if it only involves gently placing hands on the patient and holding them there. Because heart disease is a serious condition, massage should never be attempted without a physician's go-ahead.

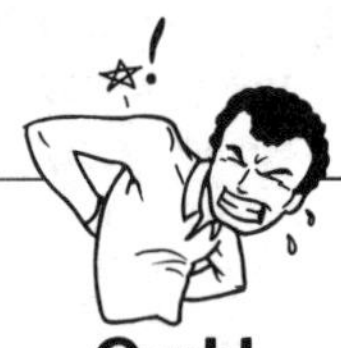

Ouch!

If you are giving a massage and you have any doubts about whether to perform a massage on someone with heart disease (or anyone with a serious medical condition), don't do the massage. Better to be careful. Plus, you could transfer your doubts and anxieties to the person you are massaging, possibly aggravating their condition on an energetic level!

Breathing Easier: Asthma, Allergies, and Respiratory Problems

Breathing problems can result from a huge number of situations: allergic reactions to airborne or ingested substances, *asthma*, pollution, advanced pregnancy (during which lung space is limited), stress or panic attacks, even heart problems. In non-life-threatening situations, massage is a great way to facilitate easier breathing. It can help to open the chest area, relax muscles that may tighten and constrict breathing, and boost immune function, which helps to fight allergic reactions. A Touch Research Institute study showed that when parents massaged their asthmatic children, the children demonstrated increased air flow when breathing, improved lung function, less anxiety, and reduced levels of the stress hormone cortisol.

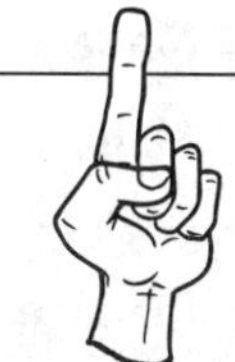

Touch Talk

Asthma is a disease characterized by shortness of breath, wheezing, bronchial spasms, and a persistent cough. Attacks can be brought on by allergies, excessive physical activity, ingestion of certain foods, anxiety, or for no apparent reason. Attacks are frightening and, in rare cases, fatal. If asthma is managed with proper medication and healthy habits, most asthmatics can live normal lives.

Many bodywork techniques can facilitate breathing and address asthma, allergies, and other respiratory problems. The most effective include the Alexander technique, Trager, reflexology, Reiki, and various types of breathwork that can increase lung capacity and function, including breathwork associated with yoga.

Ask Your Doctor About Massage Therapy

No matter what your physical condition, some form of massage can probably help to make it better and help your body to help itself. But when your condition is serious or chronic, always talk to your doctor before receiving massage or bodywork treatment. Every situation is different, and only you and your doctor know your individual symptoms, progression, and reaction to a particular health problem. If your doctor advises against massage therapy, please heed his or her advice.

Chances are, however, that you'll get an enthusiastic go-ahead, as physicians are becoming increasingly aware of the many ways in which massage and touch can augment traditional medical treatment and learning of the many massage techniques and modalities available. We sincerely hope you will be feeling better soon!

The Least You Need to Know

- Massage can help put the body into a state that is more disease-resistant.
- Massage can be helpful for relieving nagging health complaints such as back pain, jaw pain, fibromyalgia, fatigue, insomnia, and digestive disorders.
- Massage can also be helpful for symptom relief and supporting the body's efforts to heal after surgery and in cases of cancer, AIDS, arthritis, depression, diabetes, heart disease, asthma, and allergies.
- Always talk to your doctor first before using massage as a therapy for any health problem.

Chapter 22

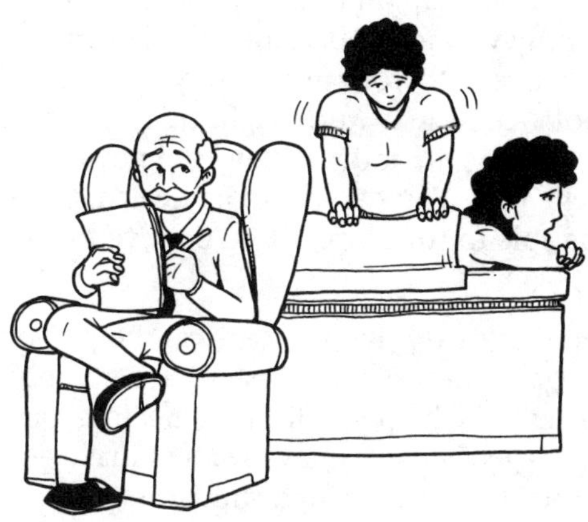

Exploring the Past

In This Chapter

- What if you have a problem with touch?
- Massage for survivors of abuse and trauma
- Finding a massage therapist who understands
- Combining massage therapy and psychotherapy

You know you could benefit from the healing power of massage. Perhaps you even crave supportive, healing touch. But because of something in your past, something that happened to you but that no one should have to experience, you can't quite get yourself to let anyone touch you, especially in a manner as drastic as massage. You're afraid or repulsed. Or the idea just makes you angry. Or maybe your problem isn't with touch, exactly; maybe it's that you aren't willing to make yourself vulnerable ever again.

We want you to know that 1) you're not alone; and 2) what you are feeling is completely natural. Our bodies are programmed both to protect us and to learn from experience. If you've been harmed in the past, either physically, emotionally, or both, your body doesn't want to take a risk like that again, and that powerful instinct probably overrides any rational thoughts you might have about massage being perfectly safe, even helpful. Our instincts are for survival.

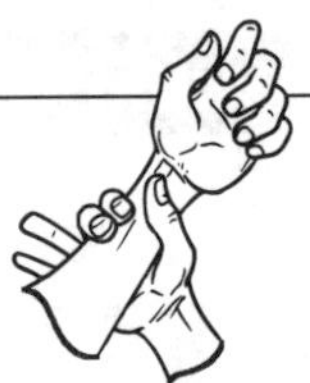

Your Finger on the Pulse

Sometimes fears we aren't even aware of manifest themselves in our dreams. Try keeping a dream journal. Every morning before you get out of bed, immediately write down what you remember about your dreams. Eventually, you may see some patterns emerging. Your own interpretations of your dreams are just as valuable as the dreams themselves—you dreamed those images, and only you know what they mean.

So what do you do? Give up on the idea of ever being touched in a healthy way again because it's just too difficult? Learn to live with your fear, with your guard up? Of course not! Your life is worth fighting for, even if you don't always believe it, and you have the power to reclaim it from the past. You deserve to be healed, to be happy, and to be able to trust again. You deserve to feel safe.

We're not saying that's easy. But massage can help you, and lots of massage therapists know exactly what you've been through. They may help you find the healing path. In fact, many massage therapists have studied massage as a healing journey to work through similar issues in their own lives.

If Touch Has Been Used Against You

Letting someone help you may be your biggest challenge. If someone you were supposed to be able to trust has betrayed you in the past, used touch against you, hurt you, how can you convince yourself it won't happen again? You probably can't, because even if you've got all the proof in the world—say, credentials and testimonials galore about the merits of a particular therapist—deep in your gut, in your fascia, in your very cells, you won't believe it.

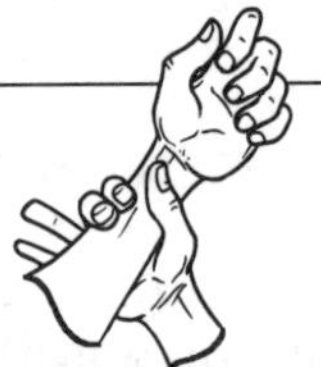

Your Finger on the Pulse

If any touch is too much for you to handle, consider starting your process of self-discovery through meditation, yoga, or prayer. Each can help reintroduce you to your inner self, helping put past traumas in perspective: they are events; they are not definitions of you. Eventually, you may find that you are ready for the next step. The point is to keep working on yourself, forging ahead in your personal journey.

When your body has been abused, it can cause a rift between body and mind. Your mind knows certain things: it wasn't your fault; you should forgive and forget; the new people in your life probably won't hurt you; it's over now. But your body doesn't listen because it has taken over and begun to think for itself in a sense. Maybe part of you stops working. Maybe you experience inexplicable and undiagnosable pain.

One woman we know, as she neared the date of what would have been a horrible marriage, suddenly lost all comprehension of human speech. People talked, and it sounded like gibberish to her. Written words looked like hieroglyphics. In desperation and confusion, she broke off the engagement. She was cured.

If a cure isn't so simple, however, you may need to do a little more work. Work is good—it is the opposite of denial. You have the power to help yourself, the power to move on from your past and into a future owned by you, not by someone else or by the memory of something hurtful.

The first step is to do some learning and networking. Are you depressed, or suffering from anxiety attacks? Are you incapacitated by anger and resentment, or obsessed with your past experience, or so completely removed from it that you feel numb inside and unable to feel any emotion at all? So are many others. Find a therapy group or individual counseling to address these issues.

Do your physical symptoms have an emotional component? For example, many suffers of Fibromyalgia Syndrome, or FMS (see Chapter 21, "Rx: Massage"), have a history of emotional and/or physical abuse. Some theories hold that the pain from FMS is largely caused by a tightening, hardening, and constricting of the body's fascia, the web that runs throughout the body, enclosing and connecting muscles and internal organs. If, as many believe, emotional and psychological experience is stored not only in the brain but also in the body's fascia, such trauma would be recorded here, with dysfunction and then pain as the inevitable result. Precisely because your body is holding all this history, bodywork can be the key to letting it go.

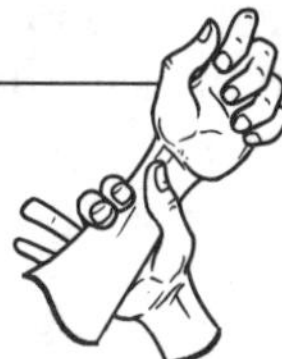

Your Finger on the Pulse

Post-traumatic stress disorder is a condition seen in people who have experienced or witnessed a traumatic event in which intense fear, helplessness, or horror was experienced. People with post-traumatic stress disorder often re-experience the traumatic event through memory, dreams, flashbacks, or intense distress when exposed to cues that resemble the event. Victims may also experience insomnia, fatigue, uncontrolled rage, irritability, nervousness, and difficulty concentrating. The condition usually lasts for more than one month and can be treated with psychotherapy. Different types of bodywork in conjunction with therapy may be even more effective, though the technique must match the client.

When Disaster Has Struck

Maybe you weren't physically or emotionally abused by a person, but your life is still filled with fear. Traumatic events aren't all caused by people. Surviving a natural disaster, such as an earthquake, hurricane, tornado, or flood, can traumatize the body and mind profoundly. Surviving a war, or a plane crash, or a bad car accident can leave physical and emotional scars—often both. From paralyzing, irrational fears to *post-traumatic stress disorder*, experiencing a disaster can be completely debilitating.

Even if your trauma hasn't made you exactly touch-phobic, you may still be saddled with extreme fear. Maybe your fear is limited to never wanting to board another airplane, but maybe it is so severe that you are afraid to leave your home or form close relationships.

Massage can help you, too, by releasing your stored trauma from your body. Massage can reduce your anxiety as it calms your muscles and relieve your stress as it gently reminds your body of how it feels to be normal again. Massage can help you immediately after a disaster or years later, when the effects are still lingering.

Massaging Painful Memories

Letting go of repressed memories of trauma and abuse is scary. That's why for you, the typical massage approach can be, and should be, modified. We've mentioned before in this book that sometimes people on the massage table break into tears or have flashbacks from the past. Don't let this fact scare you away from a potentially healing experience.

A good massage therapist experienced in treating victims of abuse knows how to progress at a rate you are comfortable with. The first session might just involve talking. Your massage therapist will want to know who you are and what you need. Don't be afraid to reveal that you have a problem with touch. You don't need to go into detail if you aren't comfortable with that. But if your massage therapist knows touch is a problem for you, it can give her or him a better idea of how to proceed. Bodywork (and also psychotherapy) can help clarify past from present, slowly diffusing the power of negative memories.

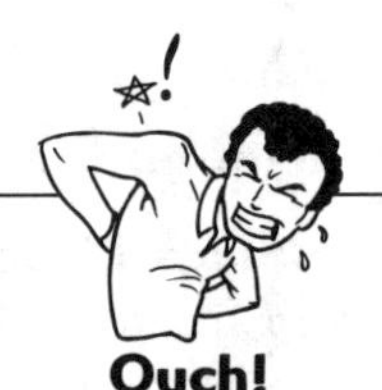

Ouch!

You have to feel safe in the massage space before you can relax enough to be touched, and if the space doesn't feel safe, let your massage therapist know. Together, you may be able to figure out how to change the space. Or maybe there are other places you could go. Don't go along with any aspect of a massage if it doesn't feel right or makes you nervous. Remember, it is *your* massage.

Lying down on the massage table might be difficult, too. If lying down makes you feel vulnerable, your massage therapist should be happy to begin work while you sit or stand. Even then, the massage work may involve little touching. It may involve talking, or visualization, or suggestions for personal exploration of your feelings.

It may take a while to get beyond a gentle laying on of hands, something many massage therapists specializing in abuse and trauma survivors use for a beginning. Even such a simple, still sort of touch can be incredibly healing. Your therapist might start with energy work, which doesn't involve actual touch, instead. If this approach sounds safer to you, let your therapist know. Remember, the more you communicate with the person trying to help you, the better she or he will be able to help.

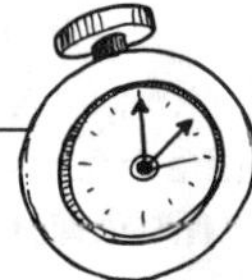

A Massage Minute

According to a Touch Research Institute study, victims of rape and spouse abuse experienced a reduced aversion to touch and decreased anxiety and depression after massage. Similarly, after the Oklahoma City bombing, volunteers gave massages to rescue workers, survivors, and the overworked pathologists on-site, according to a 1997 article in *Life* magazine. The state medical examiner officially noted that massage therapy was working faster than the psychological counseling many were receiving. Hurricane Andrew survivors also showed decreased anxiety and depression levels after massage, and massage is frequently used as a treatment for other disaster survivors, as well.

You Are Still in Control

Of course, communication can make you vulnerable, too. Maybe you aren't comfortable sharing certain information. Then don't! The most important thing to remember about the massage therapy experience is that you are in control, not the massage therapist, not the technique applied to you, and not the conventions of how a massage is supposed to work. You govern the session, and you decide what information to share and what to withhold and for how long. You say what is comfortable and what isn't. Any massage therapist who doesn't understand this is not the massage therapist for you, and you have no reason to stay (even through a single session) if you start to feel anxious or fearful.

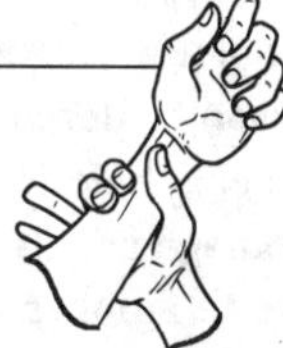

Your Finger on the Pulse

Your massage therapist is morally bound to keep all information you reveal during a massage session in the strictest confidence. Don't be afraid to emphasize this to your massage therapist, however, if it is especially important to you.

Finding a Massage Therapist Who Understands

Finding someone whom you can work with isn't always easy. Sometimes you'll fall in with the right person immediately, but sometimes you may need to do some searching. You can make your search easier, of course, by doing a little research first. Some massage therapists are specifically trained to work with survivors of torture, trauma, abuse, or people who suffer from depression, anxiety, and other psychological or emotional problems.

How do you find such a person? Look in the phone book under massage therapists, psychiatrists, psychologists, counselors, crisis centers, battered women shelters, or your local YMCA or YWCA. Some might advertise their specialties, or call a few of these places and ask if they know someone with this specialty. You don't have to reveal who you are over the phone.

Also try calling other local holistic healers, such as acupuncturists, chiropractors, homeopaths, herbalists, or even midwives. Tapping into this network can be helpful because many have connections with others working in sympathetic disciplines. Remember, you don't have to reveal anything other than the fact that you are looking for someone who specializes in massage for abuse or trauma survivors or people with psychological challenges. They don't know who you are, and for all they know, you are inquiring on behalf of a loved one.

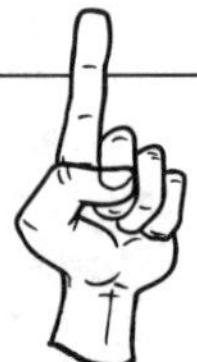

Touch Talk

Phoenix Rising Yoga Therapy is a form of body therapy that uses assisted yoga movements and basic dialogue techniques to guide clients into a body scan to determine where tensions are being held in the body. Sessions encourage clients to work through these tensions (physically, verbally, emotionally) and eventually release them.

Don't be discouraged if someone can't help you. You are helping yourself by searching, and the right person will come along eventually, perhaps only when you are ready. Another option is to consider some of the psychophysical movement re-education techniques. Relearning control over and gaining an understanding of your body and its movements can be supremely empowering. It is your body, after all. Isn't it time you took it back? Techniques such as the Alexander technique, Feldenkrais, Trager, Aston-Patterning, Hellerwork (see Chapter 12, "More Kinds of Massage,"), and *Phoenix Rising Yoga Therapy*, which combine movement education and psychological techniques, might be just for you.

Overcoming Your Fears

The very fact that you are reading this chapter is significant to your healing journey. You are beginning to discover that you are not alone. We understand about fear, about how safe you feel when you keep everything under control. We know that dealing with certain aspects of your past may be the last thing you want to do. We certainly won't presume to tell you that you have to deal with anything.

No one can be an advocate for your happiness like you can, and no one can understand the pace of your personal journey as you do. Maybe people have tried to take your life away from you in the past, but it is yours. Taking control of your own life is certainly a large task, but it is a task you control, a risk you take on at your own speed, and an adventure that is certainly worth the final result.

Therapy Can Help

Speaking of support groups, massage therapy isn't the only therapy you might find helpful. Psychotherapy and other forms of psychiatric or psychological counseling can be a great adjunct to massage therapy. In fact, the roots of bodywork are closely tied to psychoanalysis.

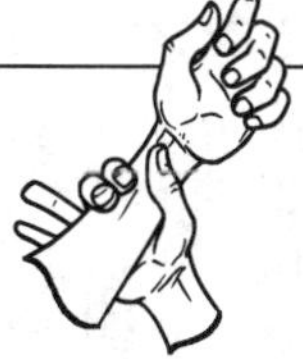

Your Finger on the Pulse

As you travel down your own road to healing and self-discovery, don't forget to cultivate a support system. No matter what has happened to you, there are others with similar experiences. Seek out support groups, look for books and magazine articles about relevant subjects, and scan the Internet. Talk to friends and family members you trust. Unfortunately, abuse, trauma, and psychological pain are all-too-common these days, but that also means you aren't alone.

If, as many believe, psychological and emotional experiences are recorded in the body, then releasing them through massage could be productively practiced in conjunction with psychotherapy or other counseling. As the memories come up, you might not know what to do with them. Some massage therapists are trained to some extent in helping you with this aspect of your therapy, but they are primarily trained in bodywork techniques and not as counselors.

If you decide to begin with bodywork and find yourself confronting emotions that you aren't fully able to process or face, please seek out additional help. Your massage therapist may be able to recommend someone, or ask someone you trust if they know of anyone helpful. Don't feel as though you have to figure it all out on your own. You (probably) aren't trained for that, and someone objective who has experience with situations like yours can guide you toward the answers and understanding you require.

A Massage Minute

Marion Rosen (born 1914) was a Jewish refugee who came to the United States after working with psychoanalysts and physical therapists in Germany. She developed the Rosen Method, which is specifically helpful for survivors of physical and emotional abuse and those recovering from addiction.

The Rosen Method combines gentle touch therapy with verbal support from the massage therapist to help release memories stored in the body that have been prohibiting a client from self-actualization. Rosen Method therapists facilitate and support a client's individual efforts toward release and self-discovery through bodywork. For people in emotional crisis or suffering from mental illness, practitioners recommend that the Rosen Method be used concurrently with psychotherapy.

Embrace the Future

Perhaps the best thing about making the conscious choice to regain control of your life and help yourself through massage or bodywork is that it signals the first step towards a future which you control. When you take the reins of your life and move towards the future you desire, you'll see that happiness is in reach.

Massage therapy and any other therapy you use in conjunction can help you reach out for those reins when you are ready. Yes, you'll still remember your past. It is your past, after all, and worth remembering and learning from, even if it was hurtful or traumatic. But it doesn't have to keep hurting, and it doesn't have to hold you back any more because you have chosen to live!

The Least You Need to Know

- Massage can be of great benefit to abuse and trauma survivors.
- Because traumatic experiences are stored in the body's tissue, massage can release painful memories and purge them from your life, allowing you to move on.
- Psychotherapy or other forms of psychiatric or psychological counseling are a good adjunct to massage therapy.
- You can take control of your life again and find happiness.

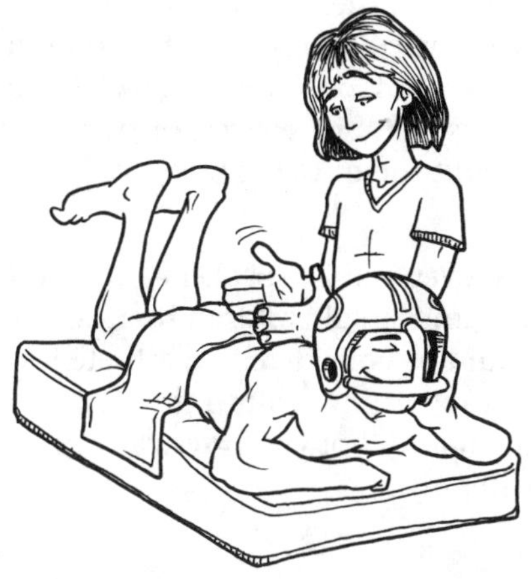

Chapter 23

The Wide, Wide World of Sports Massage

In This Chapter

- You're not a professional athlete—can sports massage help you anyway?
- When to get a sports massage
- How sports massage enhances athletic performance
- How sports massage can help heal sports injuries
- How sports massage can give you a psychological edge

If you're an athlete, any type of athlete, this chapter is for you. Whether you've made sports your career, your favorite hobby, or something you do with the kids when you have the time, your body can benefit from sports massage. Sports massage is based on the techniques of Swedish massage, but it's tailor-made for the needs of the athlete, which include enhanced circulation, supple and strong muscles, and endurance for when it counts: out there on the field, the diamond, the court, the rink, the pool, or even the backyard.

Everyone Who Moves Can Use Sports Massage

But what is an athlete, exactly? Your dictionary might say something like, "One trained in acts of physical strength, skill, endurance, and agility," and that's a pretty broad definition! Just because you don't have a contract with an athletic shoe company or your picture isn't on a cereal box doesn't mean you aren't an athlete.

Weekend athletes who sit at a desk all day and then push their bodies above and beyond their limits just once every week or two are particularly susceptible to injury. If you play in weekend games of football, softball, basketball, or tennis; lift weights or swim laps; or take long bike trips, hikes, dance classes, aerobics classes, or swimming lessons on the weekends, you probably know all about the muscle soreness of an athlete.

Performers of all kinds—dancers, actors, musicians, even public speakers—are athletes, too. Parents of small children are certainly athletes, and small children themselves often behave a lot like athletes-in-training. You could be considered an athlete if your job involves manual labor, such as construction, heavy lifting, painting, cleaning, waitressing, farming, day care, even delivering the mail. All of you physically oriented types can benefit from sports massage's targeted therapy.

A Massage Minute

Sports massage was widely practiced and refined in the Soviet Union before it became popular in the United States. To give their athletes an edge, Soviet trainers began experimenting with ways to help athletes recover more quickly from intense training sessions and found sports massage to be incredibly effective in boosting performance and speeding up healing. In fact, the strength coach for the New York Giants traveled to the Soviet Union to learn about sports massage. The year he returned and started a sports massage program for his team was the year the Giants won the Super Bowl.

When to Get a Sports Massage

Sports massage has several modes, all with different purposes. Ideally, you should get a sports massage before and after an athletic event, as well as on those rest days between performances when your massage therapist can spend some serious time getting your body into peak condition and repairing those recurring problems or new injuries. Many sports teams are now providing their athletes with regular sports massage, but if you are an amateur, you may not have the time, or the finances, for that kind of attention. Read on to determine which type of sports massage will best meet your needs at any particular time.

Massage as Warm-Up

Imagine being suddenly awakened at 4:00 A.M. and being made to step straight from your bed to the starting line of a triathlon. Even the most athletic among us wouldn't be able to start out in top form. It takes a while, especially after a long period of inactivity, to get the body moving. (For some of us, even getting up after sitting at a desk for several hours is a tense experience.) Whether you feel a little stiff or a little sore, you certainly aren't at your personal, physical best if you haven't given your body a sufficient warm-up.

Think of sports massage as a deluxe warm-up. Think how much better you can run or dance or swim after you've been moving around for awhile, doing some stretching exercises, and getting mentally prepared. Then take that difference in performance and multiply times—oh, some huge number. That's what sports massage can do for you. It adds to your warm-up by doing things simple movement and stretching can't do.

The point of the pre-event sports massage is to get your muscles, and your mind, primed for competition. Sports massage gets into the belly of your muscles; draws in vital oxygen; pushes out waste materials that may hinder movement; and stretches muscle fibers, connective tissue, ligaments, and tendons. It warms up joints, pushes out tension, and even helps you to prepare mentally. After all, you're lying there thinking about how your body is getting primed, which primes your mind, too.

Pre-event massage can loosen muscles contracted from too much training so that they are more flexible and ready for competition. It can relax the overly nervous athlete, helping concentration and adding that psychological edge. It can also flush tissues with oxygen and other nutrients just like a physical warm-up while you relax on the table.

Depending on your needs, a pre-event massage might be best up to four hours before competition or just several minutes before. Pre-event sports massage is usually short, about 10 or 15 minutes.

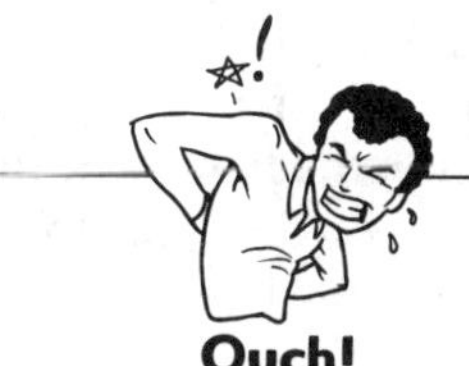

Ouch!

Many sports injuries are due to insufficient warm-up. If your muscles are contracted, they don't work as well and are more susceptible to swelling, pulls, and tears. Tight connective tissue is equally vulnerable. Before vigorous activity, always warm up with 5 to 10 minutes of easy activity that boosts your heart rate and some simple stretches. Of course, a sports massage prior to activity is the ultimate warm-up.

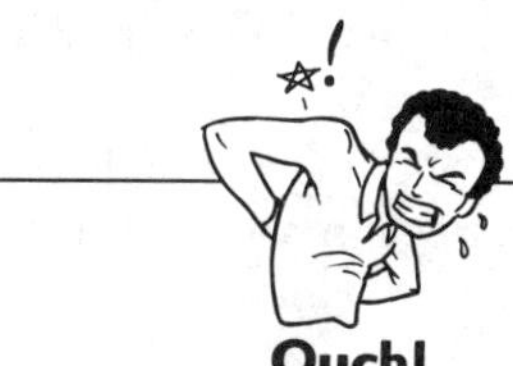

Ouch!

Some athletes don't care for pre-event sports massage, claiming it takes away their nervous edge. You may find you don't jump off that starting line as quickly as you might have if you are too relaxed from a massage. For other athletes, however, pre-event work can enhance performance and take off a nervous edge that might prove debilitating. It depends on who you are and how you compete. For this reason, you may not want to try massage for the first time before an important competition or event, in case you are one of the few whose performance may be jeopardized.

The result of all this work is that when you get out there to perform your sport, your body is prepared. Your muscles are loose, nutrient-filled, and ready for action. Your entire body feels flexible, agile, and alert. Not only will you be less likely to get injured, but you'll be able to push yourself further. Your body will be more likely to do what you ask. You'll be one step closer to fulfilling your athletic potential. Hear 'em cheering?

Massage as Cool-Down

Post-event massage is crucial when you've pushed yourself too hard. Chances are, if you've performed to your limit in the heat of competition, your body will feel the strain. Intensive use causes muscle fibers to contract and to swell slightly. In extreme cases, muscles or tendons and ligaments may tear.

Post-event sports massage combats all these processes by loosening and stretching contracted muscles back to their natural state, encouraging the body's natural repair processes, and mentally calming the athlete after an intense physical and mental performance. Post-event sports massage can be just 15 minutes or over an hour in length.

Massage as Muscle Maintenance

Sports massage on rest days may be the most effective of all types. Maintenance massage involves a longer, more complex process at a clinic or somewhere other than the sidelines or the locker room. Sometimes, post-event or even mid-event sports massage involves quick fixes: deep compression into a muscle spasm or cross-fiber friction to relieve soreness or cramping, for example. But a maintenance massage is the place to scan the entire body, looking for and working on problems, anticipating needs, and generally nurturing the body that is the athlete's tool, perhaps even his or her livelihood.

Maintenance sports massage is like giving your car a regular tune-up. It can locate small problems and resolve them before they become big, or chronic, problems. It keeps everything in good working order and may save the athlete from a major physical breakdown, or injury, in the future.

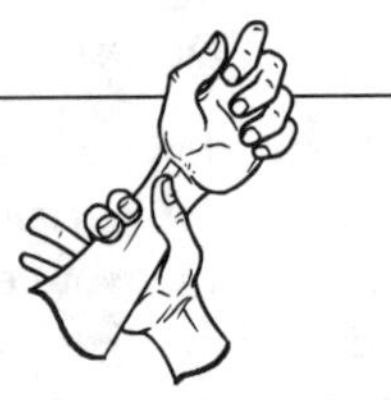

Your Finger on the Pulse

To get the most from your sports massage, take a hot shower, soak in a whirlpool, take a steam bath, or sit in a sauna before your sports massage. When muscles are relaxed and warmed-up by heat, sports massage can work more deeply more quickly, addressing individual problems more thoroughly in the allotted time because the heat has already done some of the work.

Massage for Performance Enhancement

No matter which type(s) of sports massage you use, however, one goal remains constant: performance enhancement. Sports massage in general can bring out the athlete you never knew was there—the athlete who can jump higher, run faster, throw farther, or swim more swiftly than you ever dreamed possible. In a competitive world, performance enhancement is on everyone's mind, so although sports massage is certainly health care, it may also provide the athlete with that extra leverage that makes it possible to win the game, break a record, or attain that personal best.

Different Strokes for Athletic Folks

But how does sports massage do it? How is it different than a regular massage, in terms of the needs of the athlete? Although based on Swedish massage, sports massage concentrates on a few of the strokes and is less concerned with others.

Effleurage and petrissage (see Chapter 13, "Go with the Flow: Effleurage," and Chapter 14, "Oh, How We Knead You: Petrissage"), for example, are used mainly for relaxing the body in preparation for more intense muscle work. The main strokes sports massage utilizes are compression strokes (see Chapter 15, "Groovin' to the Massage Beat: Compression and Percussion"), including direct pressure on trigger points (see Chapter 11, "Welcome to the World of Massage"), and friction strokes, particularly cross-fiber friction (see Chapter 16, " Heat It Up and Shake It Out: Friction and Vibration"). Percussion strokes (see Chapter 15) are good for breaking up congestion in the body after an event and serve to loosen the body while simultaneously waking it up, which is perfect for pre-event sports massage.

These strokes can get deep into muscle tissue, helping to release stubbornly contracted muscles, reduce swelling, and facilitate the removal of toxic waste products in muscle tissue. These strokes also help to loosen connective tissue, making it more flexible and warming it up, in a sense. Because connective tissue isn't blood-filled, it can't be warmed up by the increased circulation resulting from physical activity, the way muscles can be. Stretching and pressing it via massage, however, can break up adhesions and loosen tissue, allowing for more flexibility and decreasing the likelihood of injury.

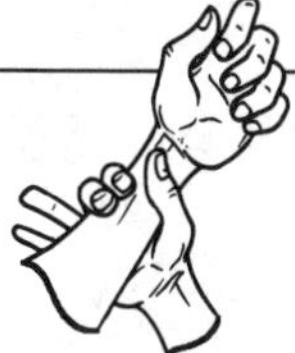

Your Finger on the Pulse

Sports massage is interactive and your massage therapist is also your personal trainer, not in how to perform your sport, but in how to maintain your equipment (your body). Whether suggesting certain stretching exercises, pointing out trigger points, or demonstrating other self-massage techniques, your massage therapist can help you extend the benefits of your sports massage by teaching you what you can do for yourself.

Passive stretching may also be an important component of your sports massage. Flexibility is key to improving performance and preventing injury, so your massage therapist may move you through a series of stretches designed to combat the contractions your overworked muscles may be holding. Range of motion work (see Chapter 17, "Goin' Round and Round: Increasing Range of Motion") and vibration (see Chapter 16) may also be helpful for contracted and stiff muscles.

Sports Massage and Treating Injuries

Your muscles need TLC, but muscles also need to be stressed, or overloaded, to gain strength. The problem occurs when we put too much stress on our muscles for too long. A smart training program involves overloading your muscles a little at a time, and then allowing them to rest long enough to heal. As they heal, they become stronger. But going too far, too fast causes too much injury. That's when the process becomes counterproductive.

When you do overdo it, as you probably will, and your muscles are torn or bruised or just plain sore, sports massage can step up the removal of stagnant waste products, reduce swelling, loosen contractions, dissolve spasms, and generally assuage pain. Pulled muscles that might have taken weeks to heal may feel better in just a few days or less. You'll rebound faster, both on and off the court. And that feels good!

To some extent, sports and injury go hand in hand. When you consistently push your body to the limit, you can't help but exceed that limit now and then. However, you can hardly reach your potential if you are sidelined with injuries every other game. Sports massage is big on injury prevention, and preventing injury should be a concern for any athlete.

As we've explained, sports massage makes your body less susceptible to injury by increasing tissue flexibility and promoting the circulatory process. But when injury has already occurred, sports massage acts like an organic steroid by encouraging more efficient healing. In other words, you'll feel better faster, minor injuries will be less likely to result in chronic pain, and you'll be back in the race.

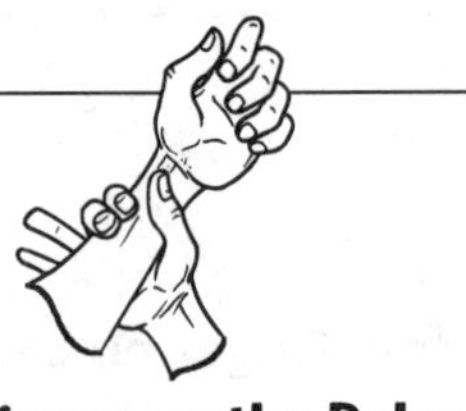

Your Finger on the Pulse

If you experience a strain or sprain, you should know about RICE, an acronym for strain/sprain first aid: Rest (don't use the area), Ice (pack it with ice or cold packs), Compression (wrap it in a bandage or something similar), and Elevation (keep the area elevated above your heart). Practicing RICE immediately and for up to two days after an injury will make a big difference in recovery time.

Sprains, Strains, and Automobiles

Sprains (stretched or torn ligaments) and strains (torn muscle tissue or tendons) are two common sports injuries that massage is particularly able to address. Known as soft tissue injuries, sprains and strains should only be massaged by a trained therapist. Massage can promote healing and drastically reduce recovery time.

When left to heal on their own, strains and sprains can turn into chronic problems, so they should be addressed immediately, unless you want weeks, months, or even years of painful reminders in the form of *shin splints, tennis elbow, Achilles tendonitis, runner's knee, tendonitis of the patella,* or some similar chronic condition.

But you're anxious to get back into action. We understand that. Sports massage can make it happen more quickly. To heal, strains and sprains need good circulation in order to eliminate waste and provide nutritional support to the healing area. Also, any scar tissue that forms can become thick, stiff, and immobile unless it is activated and kept pliable, but sports massage should never be given directly on the injured area while it is still swollen and inflamed, or if there is any indication of infection.

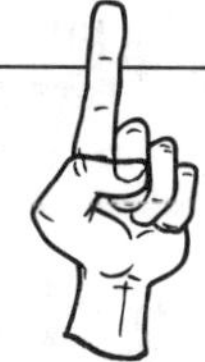

Touch Talk

Some chronic problems resulting from the neglect of minor injuries include **shin splints**, an inflammation of the tendons and muscles on the front of the calf; **tennis elbow**, an inflammation of the tendons and muscles in the elbow; **Achilles tendonitis**, an inflammation of the Achilles tendon (in the heel); **runner's knee**, a softening of the kneecap cartilage; and **tendonitis of the patella**, an inflammation of the tendons around the kneecap.

Relieving Muscle Soreness

Sometimes your muscles hurt, even if they aren't pulled or torn. That's because overuse of muscles forces your body to switch from a state of *aerobic respiration* to a state of *anaerobic respiration.* Anaerobic respiration is a less efficient process for providing the body with energy and results in waste products that must then be flushed out of muscle tissue into the kidneys by the blood.

One of these waste products is lactic acid which, if not flushed from muscle tissue quickly enough (often the case when your body can't keep up with your demands), will cause pain. Sports massage helps flush out lactic acid from overused muscle tissue more quickly than your body can eliminate it on its own.

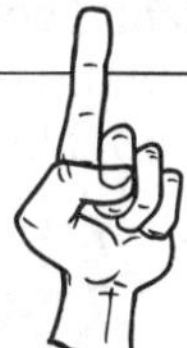

Touch Talk

Muscles require energy to contract, and this energy is provided by oxygen in a process called **aerobic respiration**. However, during strenuous activity, muscles may require more oxygen than is available, forcing the body into **anaerobic respiration**, during which glucose is utilized in the absence of oxygen. Lactic acid is a by-product of this process. If lactic acid builds up in muscles more quickly than the body can eliminate it, muscle pain results.

Addressing Chronic Pain

When minor injuries aren't resolved, they could become chronic. If you continue to use an injured area, it can develop tiny tears, which lead to inflammation, spasms, decreased circulation, pain, and finally loss of use. In other words, when you don't pay attention to your injury, your body will eventually just shut down the whole area.

Sports massage can help nip chronic pain in the bud, but it can also promote the healing process when chronic pain is already a problem. Although serious chronic conditions should be under the care of a physician, sports massage can be used in conjunction with proper rest and medical care to maintain circulation to the injured area and foster the production of healthy healing tissue.

Finding the Zone

You've seen it happen. Your favorite sports team is having an awesome night. They can't miss. They can do no wrong. Every member of the team seems to be a part of a single, perfect, unified plan. The other team, on the other hand, is performing well below their standards: there are dropped balls, people tripping and falling, bungles, bloopers, and blow-outs between team members. Now, you know your team isn't always that good, even if you'd like to believe they are. And the competition? They certainly aren't always that bad, even if you'd like to proclaim they are. What's up?

Although there are different theories on the subject, many believe that there exists in sports (and in life, for that matter) a psychological place called The Zone. When you are in The Zone, suddenly, what once was hard is effortless. Everything you try works. You are infused with confidence, grace, and skill beyond what you thought you possessed. Whether slipping into The Zone while playing basketball at the park, shooting pool at a local tavern, or performing your well-practiced gymnastics routine at the summer Olympics, most of us have experienced this strange and wonderful state of mind at one time or another.

Most of us have been in that other place, too—the Anti-Zone, you might call it. Suddenly, your confidence slips away. You become clumsy. You can't quite think fast enough to keep up, and you make one mistake after another, even trying things you can normally do with your eyes closed. (And have you ever noticed that you are more likely to slip into the Anti-Zone when your competition just happens to be in The Zone?)

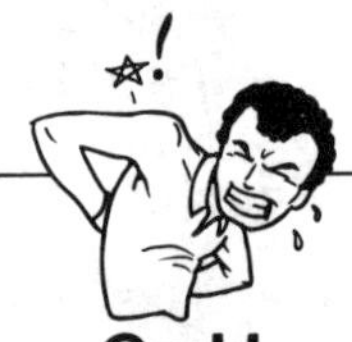

Ouch!

Great athletes know how to push themselves to achieve their goals, but overtraining can result in injury, loss of interest, a higher resting heart rate, insomnia, mood changes, and loss of appetite. If you think you might be overtraining, cut back gradually until you feel good about your athletic performance again.

If only we could get into The Zone whenever we wanted, wouldn't life be a breeze? Many of us might just choose to live there! But although we can't usually invoke The Zone, we can certainly increase our chances of landing there, and one of the best ways for athletes to do so is to get a regular sports massage.

Sports massage has a psychological component, too, and it's no small bonus. Sports massage helps you to use all the tools at your disposal, and that includes your mind. By increasing your body awareness, encouraging your mind to expand its limits in terms of what you can do, and helping to fuse your body and mind in your practice of your sport, sports massage can make The Zone a very familiar place.

Peak Performance Through Body Awareness

The non-athletic among us might only consider our bodies once in awhile: when we want to be sure we look good in a new outfit, when we hope our bodies will carry us through some emergency situation, or when they break down and cause us pain and inconvenience. For an athlete (and remember our expanded definition of that word at the beginning of this chapter), the body is more central in consciousness than it is for those who tend to live primarily in their heads.

But athletes can become even more body-aware through sports massage. If you are a runner, for example, you might notice when your heel suddenly starts to hurt or your left knee acts up yet again. You probably also notice when you are lacking in energy or feeling particularly good, but sports massage can get you even more tuned in. As you lie on the massage table having your body worked on in such an attentive and specific way, you have the time to pay attention to the details of your pains or strengths. What happens to your energy when that trigger point is activated? Where is that shooting pain coming from? Why isn't your right elbow bending like your left elbow?

Both by careful observation and by maintaining a dialogue with your massage therapist ("What is that muscle?" "What hurts right there?" "Does that feel tight to you, too?"), you'll find that your body becomes more intimate friend than useful machine. The result? Your body knows what you want, and you know what it wants. In the spirit of friendship, when the pressure is on and your goal is peak performance, your body will oblige.

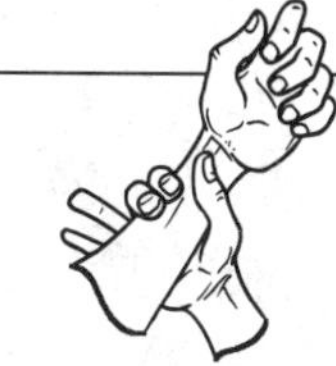

Your Finger on the Pulse

Got pain? Have a ball! Press a softball into a muscle spasm or trigger point, such as in a biceps, shoulder muscle, or hip, and roll it around. Or for hard to reach areas such as your back or buttocks, put a tennis ball on a firm surface, and then lie gently on the ball so it can move over the painful spot. Don't practice this technique over areas of inflammation or injury.

From Ordinary to Extraordinary

Sometimes, your body will even oblige beyond your wildest dreams. When you're in The Zone, you may accomplish feats of athletic genius. "Where did that come from?" you may wonder in amazement. You may even have a sort of out of body experience where you watch yourself performing like a superstar, almost as if it wasn't you at all.

Evidence of this kind of achievement is everywhere. You've heard the stories, and you've probably seen it happen, too: the blow-out Super Bowl that was supposed to be neck-and-neck, the kid who hits five home runs at his first Little League game, the ballet dancer who moves an audience to tears, Michael Jordan most of the time. (Do you think Michael Jordan receives sports massages? We'd bet on it!) We might be tempted to say these feats of extraordinary achievement are a matter of luck, but what is luck? It surely has to do with many factors, some so variable as the weather or location or time of day, but most of it is probably to do with a sudden inner confidence, tapping into previously untapped potential, and an abrupt, momentary, profoundly effective fusion of mind and body.

The Ultimate Mind/Body Experience

Being in The Zone is the ultimate mind/body experience. It isn't just about physical performance at all, and anyone who has been there knows that's true. Your mind rides high in The Zone, and you know before you even try that you'll make that shot, that hit, that record, that quadruple lutz.

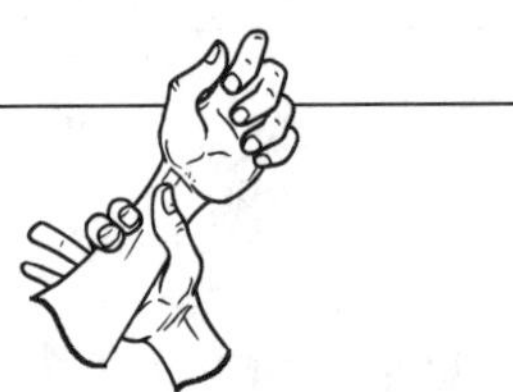

Your Finger on the Pulse

Other types of bodywork can benefit the athlete in addition to sports massage. Movement reeducation techniques such as the Alexander technique (see Chapter 12, "More Kinds of Massage") can teach the athlete to use his or her body in a more effective, graceful, and efficient way. Weightlifting or walking, swimming or skiing, dancing or horseback riding can be enhanced when the body is used more consciously.

When you are in The Zone, your mind and your body work together—something we all wish could happen all the time, but which most of us haven't quite mastered. This mind-body fusion could be a clue to what we are capable of as humans, a brief glimpse into our evolutionary potential. Maybe someday, The Zone will be The Norm for the human race.

Anything that helps to integrate your body and mind can help you to have more frequent access to The Zone, and sports massage is one of the many possibilities. The body has a consciousness all its own: Memories and knowledge stored in its tissues, an awareness of pain and of particular strengths, the intricate network of messages being sent from one place to another through the system of nerve cells. In sports massage, as in regular massage, the body's knowledge is stimulated, almost as if the massage therapist is asking the body, through touch, "Will you tell us what you know?" Through massage, the body can communicate its secrets to the conscious mind and begin the mind-body dialogue, introducing you to a more complete and accomplished participation in your favorite physical activity.

Thinking and Acting Like a Champion

For those of you who need just a little more convincing, remember the theory behind creative visualization? When you envision yourself accomplishing something, you help your body move towards the actual accomplishment. It's just one more type of mind-body dialogue, but this time the mind starts the conversation.

So if you think and act and see yourself as a champion—in control of your body, excelling at your sport, experiencing joy from the very act of participation—your body will know what to do. If you're also receiving regular massage, your body will be more able to fulfill your mind's desire.

The Least You Need to Know

- If you use your body, your body can use sports massage.
- Sports massage can warm up muscles before a sports event, help relax and repair them after an event, and keep them in top condition on rest days.
- Sports massage can enhance your athletic performance.
- Sports massage can help sports injuries such as sprains, strains, muscle soreness, and chronic pain to heal more quickly.
- Sports massage gives you a psychological edge as well as a physical edge because it helps to integrate mind and body into a unified force.
- If you think, act, and see yourself as a champion, your body will do its part to make you a champion.

Chapter 24

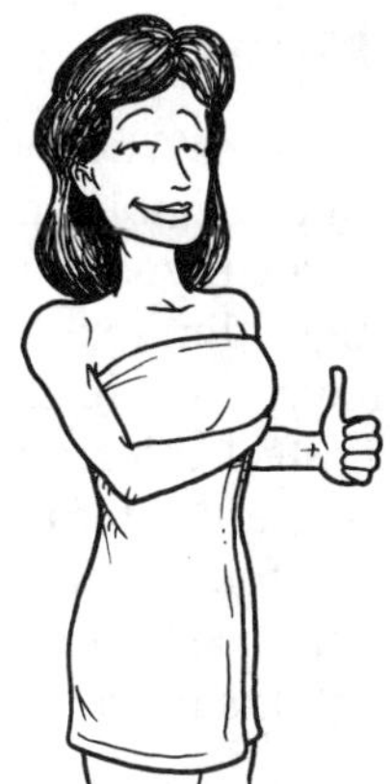

For Women Only

In This Chapter

- Massage and the fertility cycle
- How massage can make that time of the month a little more bearable
- Is massage beneficial during pregnancy?
- What's so important about postpartum massage?
- Massage and menopause

You are woman, and even though we can't hear you roar from here, we know you could do it if you wanted to. Maybe you roar often, but chances are it isn't always because you're feeling your female power. Being a woman is wonderful, but it isn't easy. We have to contend with our own biological processes, cultural expectations, and the inner pull of wanting to be both nurturers and achievers in our own right.

With all that pressure, we're quite sure you could use a massage, and massage can help women in many female-specific ways, from the many discomforts associated with our fertility cycle (PMS to menopause) to our self-esteem. Self-esteem is an important part of female existence (or any existence) and can easily get a little shaky in this complicated society that expects us to be all things to all people while still appearing eternally fresh-faced and ready for aerobics class.

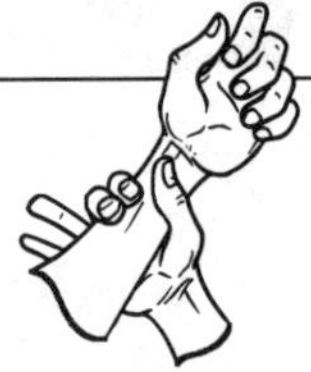

Your Finger on the Pulse

Creative visualization can be a good adjunct to massage when you aren't feeling your best. Close your eyes before, during, or after a massage and visualize the ideal you—not necessarily thinner or curvier or with better hair, but happier, more energetic, doing the things that, to you, mean really being alive. Keeping this picture of yourself in your mind will help to make it a reality.

The Truth About Beauty

It isn't easy to feel beautiful these days. When you look in the mirror and your face doesn't resemble any supermodel you've seen on this planet, you might feel distinctly unbeautiful. If your thighs don't look like the thighs on your daughter's bouncy young preschool teacher, and your hair is sporting steel-colored strands, beauty may seem like something reserved for the young, the dewy-complected, the taut and toned. But none of that superficial stuff has to do with true beauty, because the truth is, beauty isn't skin deep. It's much deeper.

This isn't always easy to remember (the media certainly doesn't help remind us), but beauty begins in your soul, in the you that is far beneath the layers of skin, fascia, muscle, and bone that make up your physical self—no matter how much that skin, fascia, muscle, and bone does or doesn't resemble the skin, fascia, muscle, and bone on that supermodel in *Vogue* (or whomever embodies your idea of the ultimate beauty).

The best way to bring this beauty to the surface is not by working on the surface, but by working beneath it. For example, do something good for yourself, such as a self-massage of the hands, feet, or face. Hold a positive picture of yourself in your mind as you do this act of kindness for yourself. The next time something negative happens in your life, come back to this feeling, thought, and physical action.

Bodywork in its many forms is a far more effective beauty ritual than a slew of cosmetics, wrinkle creams, hair dyes, cellulite busters, crash diets, expensive clothing, or fine jewelry. Massage relaxes your exterior self, making it, in a sense, more malleable and permeable so that the inner you can shine through. Even if the inner you is buried way down deep and you haven't seen her in a long, long time, bodywork can help her to surface by integrating your physical, emotional, and spiritual selves into a beautiful whole. When that inner beauty emerges, you'll know it, because beauty is a lot more about how you feel than how you look to someone else in some objective sense.

When you feel healthy, strong, centered, aligned with gravity, awake, alive, and full of energetic joy, you can't help but be irresistibly beautiful. Everyone will notice, but you probably won't even care because you'll know that beauty means embracing life, and you're far too busy enjoying yourself and feeling great to waste time worrying about what that guy over there thinks about the size of your thighs.

Kiss PMS Good-Bye

You probably feel less beautiful when suffering from *PMS* than you do at any other time (except maybe when you are nine months pregnant and waddling to the bathroom every three minutes). Not everyone suffers from PMS, but those of us who do don't want to hear about those of you who don't—unless you choose to sympathize by giving us a massage!

Of course, every woman is different, and you may not experience anything more than an intense need for pure and unadulterated chocolate and some uncomfortable bloating in your abdomen, breasts, or thighs. But many experience a range of symptoms including backache, headache, irritability, food cravings, constipation, depression, acne, painful or swollen breasts, absent-mindedness, insomnia, clumsiness, fatigue, and even uncharacteristically violent or suicidal behavior. Those fluctuating female hormones sure do pack a punch!

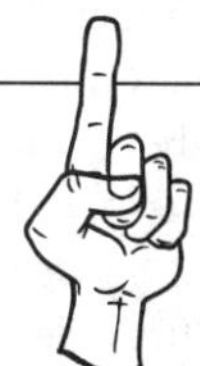

Touch Talk

PMS, or **premenstrual syndrome**, is a condition characterized by a wide range of symptoms and is probably related to the fluctuation in hormones experienced during the menstrual cycle. Some researchers believe that the disorder originates in the brain and may be linked to levels of seratonin, the neurotransmitter linked to depression.

The one consistent symptom among women suffering from PMS is the cyclical nature of symptoms, which typically appear during the week before a woman's period (or when a woman ovulates), begin to subside with the onset of menstruation, and are absent during the week following menstruation. Women should have at least five symptom-free days per month. Most of us have more, thank goodness, but that doesn't make the uncomfortable days any better!

But you don't have to accept your discomfort and hide from society for three-fourths of every month. One great way to alleviate PMS symptoms is to get a massage. (Exercise helps a lot, too, but we're willing to bet that a massage sounds a lot more appealing when you're feeling big, achy, and bloated.)

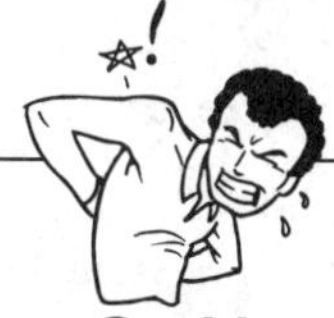

Ouch!

Eating certain foods just before you expect PMS symptoms can aggravate symptoms in many women. Even if you crave them, try to avoid chocolate, anything with caffeine, alcohol, excess salt, red meat, sugar, and overly processed foods.

Massage can help you deal with PMS in a lot of ways. In general, the increased circulation and feeling of well-being you get from a great massage will help you feel pampered and healthy, taking the edge off PMS. If you look around, you can find a wide variety of books diagramming acupressure

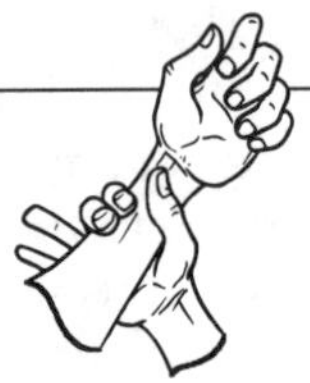

Your Finger on the Pulse

For bloating, irritability, and/or depression, press with your thumb on the spot about four finger-widths below your knee on the inside of your calf, right between the leg bone and calf muscle. Massage in a circular motion for about 10 seconds. Or have someone gently press their palm about two inches below your belly button and hold, for pain relief. A foot massage can relax your whole self, too, and you can give yourself one any time.

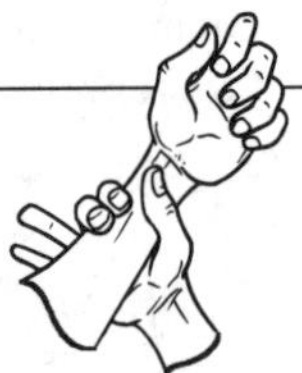

Your Finger on the Pulse

In Eastern thought, femaleness and the moon are yin. Study the moon and perceive its effects on you. How does your menstrual cycle synchronize with the moon's cycle? Observe the beautiful regularity of the moon's waxing and waning, and then carry that reverence over to your own body. Your cycle is similarly splendid, even if it doesn't always feel that way.

and shiatsu pressure points for everything from bloating to irritability. According to some forms of acupressure, PMS means that chi is stagnating in your liver, and disarming the liver through acupressure can cause PMS discomfort to dissolve away.

If you're suffering from PMS, tell your massage therapist, who has probably developed specific methods for alleviating PMS discomfort. If you're giving a massage to someone suffering from PMS, or advising your massage partner on what you need for your own symptoms, focus on effleurage (see Chapter 13, "Go with the Flow: Effleurage") to connect the whole body-mind in a positive way and create the "flow" (pun intended). Deep effleurage also helps to shuttle waste products through the lymphatic system, which is appropriate at a time when your body is cleansing anyway.

Going Full Cycle: Celebrating Menstruation

In our view of a perfect world, the onset of menstruation would be a time of joyous celebration. A big party celebrating fertility and initiation into womanhood would usher a young girl into the ranks with a feeling that something mysterious and wonderful had happened to her. Because menstruation is something mysterious and wonderful!

Unfortunately, however, the onset of menstruation is more often accompanied by embarrassment, confusion, even shame. Remember the little girl in junior high who wouldn't come out of the bathroom stall until someone called her mother? (Maybe it was you.) Our culture still isn't quite comfortable with the mystery of female fertility, making it difficult for us to feel good about that time of the month. (Those pretty, thin, unbloated women on TV chattering about wings and pouring little tubes of blue fluid onto the latest invention in menstrual protection don't help much either.)

If menstruation were more openly celebrated, maybe we wouldn't feel the pain so severely. But even if we did, it would have more meaning, seem more worthwhile. No wonder so many of us experience menstrual pain. All that repressed negativity about menstruation is sure to surface as some sort of physical discomfort.

In any case, worth it or not, menstrual cramps hurt! Can massage help? You bet your box of winged maxi pads it can! Your massage therapist probably has effective techniques for helping with menstrual cramps, but try massaging the liver and small intestine reflexes on the feet (see the figure in the section on Reflexology in Chapter 11) and any other relaxing massage strokes that feel good to you at the moment.

Lower back massage can help ease menstrual cramps, and massaging the abdomen may help, but it may also aggravate the pain, especially if massage in that area makes you tense. Remember deep breathing during painful moments.

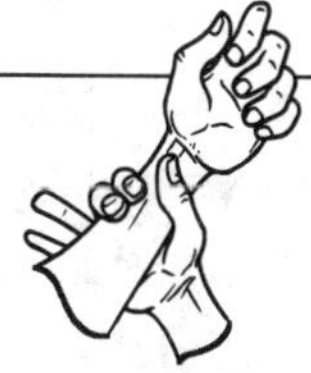

Your Finger on the Pulse

Deep breathing can bring relief from menstrual pain. Also try pressing the point about four finger-widths below your kneecap on the outside of your leg bone. Apply pressure in a circular motion for about 10 seconds. When your flow is very heavy, press the spot about four finger-widths below the navel and massage gently.

So You're Having a Baby!

When you're pregnant, you may find yourself frequently caught up in a state of wonderment at what's happening to your body. You are producing life—wow! You probably dream about what your baby will look like, whether it's a boy or a girl, what kind of mother you'll be, and what your hopes and dreams are for this new little life you've created.

Between reveries, however, you may also notice a few other changes. You may spend a lot more time in the bathroom—either because you're periodically losing your lunch (if you could even stomach any lunch) or because your bladder seems suddenly to have shrunk to the size of a thimble. Where did those huge breasts come from, and why do they hurt so much? Your veins start to pop out and turn blue, your joints get looser, achier, and less coordinated, and a lot more of you is getting thicker and wider than just your abdomen. (Is that really your butt?)

Toward the end, your back really hurts. You've got heartburn like never before. You've lost all physical

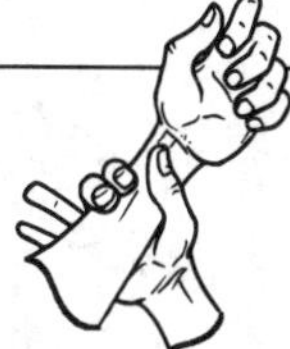

Your Finger on the Pulse

As your baby grows, your lungs, bladder, and stomach all play second fiddle and temporarily lose capacity. Massage and deep breathing exercises in early pregnancy can help to open the chest and ribs, giving you more breathing room in the upper chest. Don't decrease your fluid intake—you can put up with frequent trips to the bathroom for a few more months! Smaller, more frequent meals can reduce heartburn.

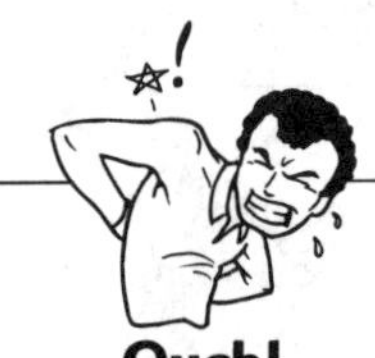

Ouch!

After the 20th week, pregnant women shouldn't lie on their backs for more than a minute or two. The weight of the baby can hinder your blood flow and possibly the baby's, too. You'll also feel like someone dropped a bowling ball on your stomach! Pregnancy massage is typically administered while you lie on your side, well supported by lots of pillows, especially between the knees, under the head, and anywhere else that feels the need for support.

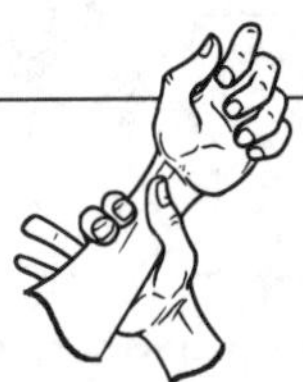

Your Finger on the Pulse

In the third trimester of pregnancy, water retention is common and you may find yourself atop puffy feet and ankles bearing no resemblance to the ones you remember. To minimize water retention, put your feet up as often as possible, especially when sitting for long periods. Cut back on salt intake, and drink lots of purified water (48 to 60 ounces per day is ideal).

and mental coordination, and you finally understand the true meaning of hemorrhoids. (For any guys reading this chapter, you're probably feeling pretty smug right now. We suggest you keep your mouths shut and offer to give us a massage.)

As glad as you are to be pregnant, you probably wouldn't mind a little relief from the less transcendent aspects of your hormone-wracked existence. Massage during pregnancy can be the perfect way to ease your discomfort, but it's important in a few other ways, too.

You're experiencing your body in a new way, and your impending labor may be mysterious and not a little frightening. Many women are very fearful of the pain of labor. We watch darned carefully when those TV programs and movies show women screaming in pain, bathed in sweat, and clenching within what seems to be an inch of their lives. Scary stuff! But part of the reason the process of labor is so scary is because it is unknown, and worse yet, our own bodies are relatively unknown to most of us.

Because massage reacquaints us with our bodies, regular massages by therapists who specialize in pregnancy massage can be a great boon to the pregnant woman. You may have noticed that people seem to think you are, quite suddenly, as fragile as a delicate piece of crystal. People you don't even know rush to help you, opening doors, carrying groceries, even letting you move to the front of lines. What they usually won't do, beyond a cursory belly rub (which you probably didn't ask for) is touch you. What if they broke the baby?

Even massage therapists without much experience with pregnant women may be a little reluctant to touch you beyond very gentle effleurage. But someone who knows the pregnant body can give your body the touch it craves and will also know how to work deep enough to make a difference, relieving muscle and joint pain, helping your body to realign with its shifted gravitational center, facilitating intestinal movement to help with constipation and heartburn, and jump-starting your circulation to relieve fluid retention.

Experienced massage therapists can also work with your body to prepare it for labor, both by helping to educate you about what your muscles, bones, and joints will be doing as you work to give birth to that baby, and by working those muscles, bones, and joints in a manner that will facilitate the birthing process. Your massage therapist may work on certain trigger points to relax clenched or painful areas, range of motion exercises to loosen and relax sore joints, and lots of Swedish massage to enhance circulation and keep blood and nutrients flowing inward, where the work of labor takes place, rather than to your extremities, where it tends to flow when you are nervous, tense, or clenched against pain.

Massage serves different purposes throughout a pregnancy:

- Ideally, massage sessions should begin before you become pregnant, when your massage therapist can work safely on your abdominal area to prepare it for pregnancy.
- Because miscarriage is more common in the first trimester, massage during this time generally focuses on areas of the body other than the abdomen, facilitating circulation as blood volume increases and gently relaxing the body to help minimize first-trimester discomforts such as nausea.
- During the second trimester, pregnancy massage focuses on opening up the chest area to prepare for decreasing lung capacity as the baby grows, keeping those loosening joints strong and aligned, and relieving muscle soreness associated with the body's adjustment to its changing center of gravity.
- Third trimester massage works to relieve the pain of spreading joints and overtaxed back muscles. The abdomen can be gently massaged and rocked, trigger points may be released to unclench the body for labor, and nurturing relaxation strokes may be employed to remind the expectant mother of her important and miraculous role in the birthing process.
- Massage during labor can go a long way toward reducing labor pain and relaxing you. Even though it may seem like an impossible feat to relax the laboring body, massage can make labor much more enjoyable (at least between contractions!) and stress-free. According to some studies, stress may interfere with the labor process, and massage may help speed labor by reducing stress.

Although you may not have considered asking your massage therapist to help you with labor and be present at your baby's birth, chances are, she (or he) would probably be honored. In addition, take a massage class with your labor partner, ask your massage therapist for some tips, or at least read up on the subject so that your labor partner can help you through the process with some knowledge of what techniques are best.

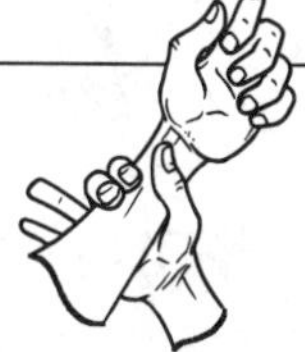

Your Finger on the Pulse

Okay guys, one of the best things you can do for your pregnant partner is to learn some pregnancy and labor massage basics. As her labor coach, you can make a big difference in her pain and anxiety levels during the childbirth process, and you'll also feel more connected (literally, via touch) to the whole process, as well as to her.

Labor massage is like pregnancy massage and should be done with the pregnant woman lying on her side with lots of supportive pillows. Focus on the lower back, which is often an area of pain during labor. Massage the feet, hands, and shoulders to help in relaxation, which can also be done when the laboring woman is sitting. Avoid percussion, vibration, and deep tissue work that is jarring to the system. At some point, a laboring woman may want all touching to cease and desist immediately. You should, of course, obey.

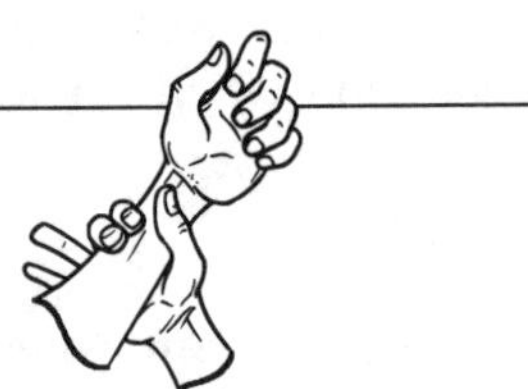

Your Finger on the Pulse

A new mama may be reluctant to entrust her baby to anyone else's care, but it's important for baby to spend time with Daddy. Alternatively, Grandma, Grandpa, or proud aunt and uncle can help baby to learn new faces, and when you return a happy, relaxed mama, you may find your offspring picks up on your mood and becomes a happier, more relaxed baby.

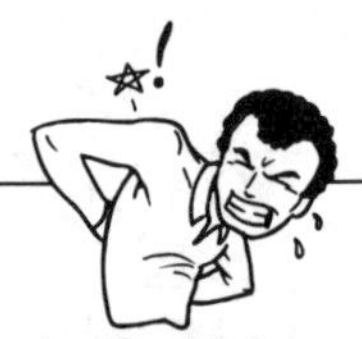

Ouch!

Check with your doctor before receiving your first professional postpartum massage. Depending on what type of birth you had and how you are recovering, you may be able to receive a massage right away, or your doctor may suggest you wait for a certain amount of time. Listen to your doctor, and don't jump back into any activity before your body is ready.

New Mama Massage

Once labor has ended, it's easy to forget about your own needs. Suddenly, you've got this tiny, helpless, completely dependent, absolutely beautiful baby. You created it (with some not-insignificant help from your partner, of course), and now you get to take it home and care for it—for the next 20 years or so (or more!). And talk about need. This little creature needs you more than anybody will ever need you. For the next few years, you'll be completely absorbed in attending to the needs of your child, and at first, before you're used to it, the prospect can be overwhelming.

Add to that hormones raging out of control, no more than an hour or two of sleep at one time, and the stress that comes with a major life change, and you've got one tense mama who could really use a good, thorough, postpartum massage. "Massage?" you might giggle hysterically. "Ha, ha, ha! Who has the time? Who has the energy? Who has the money? And what would I do with the baby?"

Calm down. Sit. Relax. Take a deep breath. It isn't easy to be a good mother when your nerves are so frayed that you can hardly put together a complete sentence. Postpartum massage is important in restoring your body to its pre-pregnancy state. The increased circulation can help your body to heal. The relaxation response can help make breastfeeding a little easier. Many women don't experience backaches until after birth because the sudden shift in their centers of gravity throws the back out of whack; massage can help to ease these aches and pains as well.

Don't forget the emotional side. For nine months or so, you have been lavished with attention. You were

Pregnant Woman and received all the pomp and circumstance deserving of your state. Then, precipitously, you were simply Mom. Where did all that attention go? To your pride and joy, your little bundle, your baby. Not that you mind—when your baby gets lots of attention, it's almost like the attention is going to you, but not quite. Considering that you're also feeling pretty emotional these days, the sudden lack of attention can be disconcerting. Not that you're some spoiled toddler who needs to be the center of attention all the time, but gee whiz, you got so used to it, and now it's all just gone.

Well, what do you think massage is for? Sure, it's for a lot of things, but one of the best parts of postpartum massage is that, for one precious hour, all the attention goes to you. You'll be kneaded, stroked, and nurtured. Your massage therapist will be completely focused on you, your needs, your aches and pains, and your body. Believe us, you need it. In fact, you deserve it!

Keeping your body and mind operating in peak condition is the best way to be a good mother. If you are so stressed out that you don't know which way is up, you'll be less available and present for your infant. (Which spewing end of that baby gets the diaper? You knew yesterday...)

Home massages are great for supporting you postpartum, too, if you can get your partner or a friend to give them to you regularly (explain to your partner how much he will benefit by your improved mood). The best strokes for now? Long, flowing effleurage strokes, gentle petrissage, foot massages, face massages, and anything that gives you that sense of well-being.

Easing Through Menopause

The other end of our fertility cycle certainly isn't the other end of our lives as women. Women live approximately 10 to 14 years before beginning their fertility cycles, but they can live far longer than that after their fertile years. Even though the whole fertility process is sometimes inconvenient, you may feel mourning at its passing. This is natural and normal, like saying good-bye to any other stage of life. Yet it's just one more passage, like the end of childhood, or graduation, or becoming a parent.

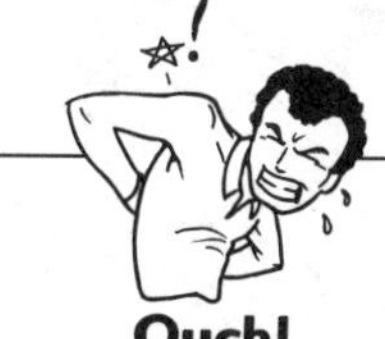

Ouch!

After menopause, many women experience bone loss due to decreased estrogen levels. Be extra careful when massaging over postmenopausal bones, which can break more easily. Concentrate on fleshy areas and work muscles without putting too much pressure on bones.

After menopause, you may feel stronger, more in control of your life, less subject to your body, and more in charge of your spirit. But menopause itself may have its own uncomfortable symptoms—dizziness, depression, heart palpitations, decreased sex drive, shortness of breath, and, of course, the notorious hot flashes, to name a few.

Massage can ease you through menopause in much the same way it eases you through the other hormone-intensive stages of your life. It increases your circulation so your body works better. It gives you increased energy and a more positive outlook. Best of all, it is self-care, and you deserve self-care just as much now as you always did. If you haven't given it to yourself until now, it's high time!

The Least You Need to Know

- Beauty is deeper than the skin, and massage can help to release the inner you so that you radiate beauty.
- Massage can help reduce symptoms of PMS and menstruation.
- Massage can ease pregnancy and prepare the body for labor, as well as facilitate labor itself.
- Postpartum massage helps new mamas regain their pre-pregnancy bodies, energy, and self-esteem.
- Massage can help ease the transition of menopause.

Chapter 25

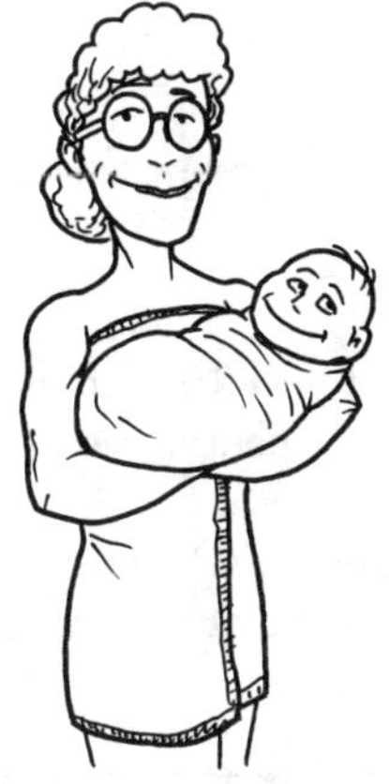

Massage for the Rest of Us

In This Chapter

- Infant massage essentials
- Cool kid massage
- Men and massage
- Massage for seniors

Even though we devoted a whole chapter to women, we don't want the rest of you to think you're somehow less able to benefit from massage. Babies, kids, men, and seniors all have special needs and health concerns that massage can address with finesse, so read on to see what massage can do, specifically, for you.

Oh, Baby!

In the early part of this century, the popular view was that babies should be touched as little as possible, for fear that they might end up spoiled, whining brats who would never understand the concept of not speaking until being spoken to. John Broadas Watson, author of *Psychological Care of Infant and Child*, published in 1928, wrote "Never hug and kiss (your children), never let them sit in your lap. If you must, kiss them once on the forehead when they say good night. Shake hands with them in the morning." Mothers were encouraged not to coddle their children and to work against their natural inclinations to touch their children. An entire generation grew up touch-starved due to the popularization of this attitude.

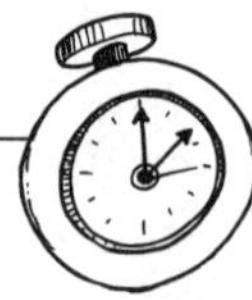

A Massage Minute

Massage is an excellent therapy for babies born prematurely. A famous Touch Research Institute study showed that pre-term infants given regular infant massage gained 47 percent more weight, become more responsive, and were discharged six days earlier from the hospital (saving $15,000 per infant). Eight months later, the massaged babies demonstrated higher weight and better mental and motor development than their peers. Later studies have shown that the massaged infants had an increase in insulin, which enhances the absorption of food.

Then along came the insightful Dr. Benjamin Spock, whose book *Baby and Child Care,* first published in 1945, completely changed the face of parenting. He firmly advocated natural childbirth, rooming-in, holding and touching a baby immediately after birth, breastfeeding, and carrying the baby against the body whenever possible instead of toting the baby around in an infant seat. He was also a strong advocate of parental instinct and encouraged parents to use their own judgment rather than follow expert advice on how to raise their babies. Suddenly, mothers everywhere were being redirected to follow their natural instincts.

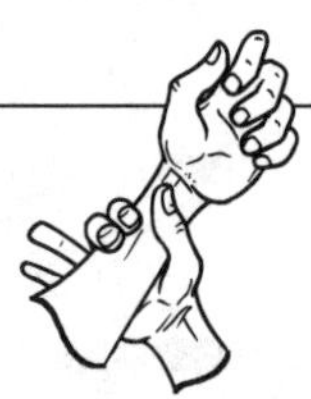

Your Finger on the Pulse

Most people now know breastfeeding is best, but in the first week or two, before mother and baby are breastfeeding pros, breastfeeding can be frustrating even to those committed to the process. Stress can inhibit milk flow, causing many mothers to give up, even though the benefits of breastfeeding are dramatic for baby. A pre-feeding infant massage can relax both mother and baby and get everything flowing more easily.

Although Dr. Spock never mentions massage per se, he recognized and validated the benefits of touch for infants. He noted that in many nonindustrial areas of the world, babies are held against their mothers constantly and breastfed on demand. He cited a study performed by two doctor friends, John Kennel and Marshall Klaus, in which mothers in the United States who were allowed to be with their babies immediately after birth were observed: "They don't just look at (their babies). They spend a lot of time touching their limbs and bodies and faces with their fingers. Months later these mothers have easier relations with their babies, and their babies are more responsive than in the case where mothers don't have these opportunities to touch soon after birth."

Dr. Spock also noted (with distaste) how many ways our society has distanced mothers and babies: Anesthetized childbirth, bottle feeding in the hospital, propping bottles on babies' chests, putting babies to bed on hard mattresses in distant cribs, infant seats, and playpens. Luckily for babies today, the trend is in the opposite direction. Most mothers know it's very difficult to spoil an infant, and that all a baby's needs should be met to ensure a sense of security and confidence later in life. But many mothers may also wonder how they can best meet their babies' touch needs.

Infant massage is a wonderful way to bond with your baby, both physically and emotionally. Most babies love it, it reduces *colic* and stomach distress, and it also helps new mothers to relax and feel more comfortable handling their babies.

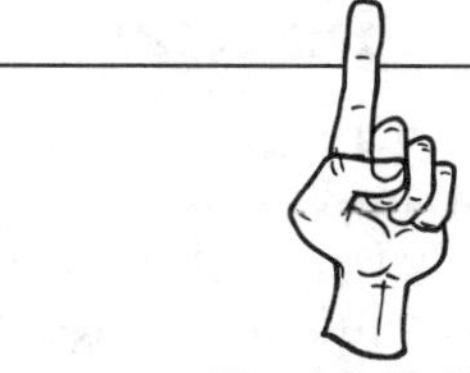

Touch Talk

Colic is characterized by intense, inconsolable crying/screaming sessions lasting three hours or longer. No one knows for sure why some babies experience it and others don't. Some theories hold that colic is related to gastrointestinal distress; others claim it is a matter of overstimulation. No matter what the cause, massage can be extremely effective in calming some colicky babies.

It's Not Easy Being a Baby

Perhaps you envy your baby. "That must be the life," you think. "Nothing to do but sleep, eat, and play." Think again! It's not easy being a baby. Not only are babies unable to clearly communicate their needs (beyond crying and some uncoordinated groping and kicking), but their little systems aren't quite up to par yet. That means tricky digestion, unpredictable muscle control, blurred vision, and the fastest year of growth your baby will ever experience. It also means that when a diaper is wet, or something hurts, or baby is hungry or tired or just plain wants to be somewhere other than where you've put her, her only recourse is to hope you figure it out. Talk about stress!

Infant massage can address several of these problems. It helps to reduce stress, which may in turn reduce colic. It relaxes tiny muscles, promotes circulation to help brand new digestive systems work a little more smoothly, and it feels really, really good. A baby recognizes the mother's smell soon after birth and quickly learns to trust that mom will provide. If mom also touches, strokes, and rubs baby into a calm, relaxed, and happy state, life as a baby may not seem so hard after all!

Of course, Dad can give infant massages, too—a great way to bond with the new baby. Although baby hasn't been inside the father for nine months and the father isn't experiencing lactation or the dramatic maternal hormones that could be tailor-made for baby to recognize, baby will know dad's voice if he's been around a lot and will appreciate the loving touch only daddies can supply. Infant massage is a great way for new fathers to establish a loving touch bond with their newborn sons or daughters.

Tiny Techniques

Infant massage isn't exactly like grown-up massage. A baby's muscles make up only about one-fourth of its total body weight; an adult's muscles make up about one-half of body weight. Babies are not developed enough to have knots of tension, so the primary infant massage stroke should be gentle effleurage (see Chapter 13, "Go with the Flow: Effleurage"), which stimulates circulation and tones internal organs. Strokes should be long, slow, and soothing for baby.

Also, remember two important things: Babies can't ask for a massage when they might like one, but they also can't tell you, in so many words, when they don't want to be touched. Try to be sensitive to your little one's mood and know when it isn't time for a massage. Just as important, you should be relaxed and in the mood before massaging baby. Babies are incredibly sensitive to your energy, and if you are tense and nervous about what you are doing, or grumpy or irritated, your baby will pick up on that and won't enjoy the experience. Fill your body with peace and love before bonding with your baby through a massage.

A few rules to keep in mind when massaging an infant:

- Use a mild, unscented massage oil.
- Use gentle, long flowing strokes and simple range-of-motion movements.
- Always ask baby's permission. Even though baby cannot verbally respond yet, your asking will help make you more sensitive to baby's mood.
- Be gentle.

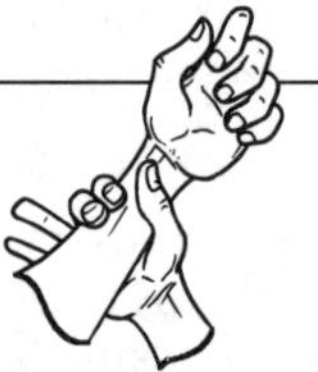

Your Finger on the Pulse

Your baby will probably enjoy some passive stretching exercises, such as bringing his arms out to a *T*, and then back over the chest or spelling the alphabet in the air with his feet.

But just how do you give an infant massage? To get you started, we'll give you some suggestions, but feel free to vary the process according to your baby's likes and dislikes:

- First, relax. Take a few deep breaths. Smile. Show baby your hands, and ask permission to give baby a massage.
- Look into baby's eyes and slowly bend forward. Perhaps wiggle your nose against baby's nose, or give baby a gentle kiss. Hello, baby! I love you! Gently trace your finger around baby's eyes, down the nose, in circles over the cheeks, around the lips, and around the ears. Make tiny circles with your fingers over the jaw joints. Baby is probably already smiling!
- Babies are least vulnerable around their legs and feet, which they use constantly. Your baby will probably welcome attention here, so it's a good way to start and to get baby comfortable with massage. Work your way up and down each leg in a very gentle wringing motion. Progress slowly, with baby's permission.

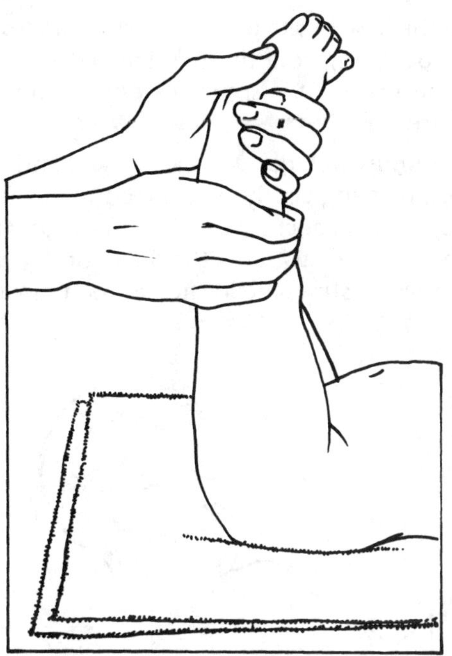

Gently smooth your hands up each of baby's legs all the way to the tops of the toes.

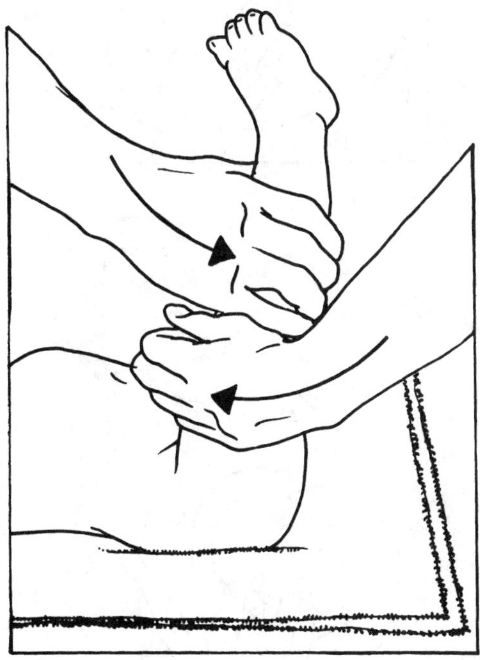

Now, in a gentle wringing motion, slowly work your way up and down each leg. Maintain eye contact with your baby and speak softly and reassuringly as you massage.

- Move your thumbs all around the base of the feet where there are so many nerve endings. Press lightly on each toe. Using your thumbs, stroke the top of each foot toward the ankle, then circle the ankle. If the spirit moves you, sing a little song to baby and massage with the rhythm.
- On to the tummy! Rub baby's tummy in large, circular strokes, and move over baby's tummy with your palms, pressing gently. These techniques are good for relieving gas pain and also may calm a colicky baby. Moving your hand in a clockwise direction helps with digestion, as this is the direction for elimination. Baby's lower left side is where the intestines are located as food moves toward the bowel.

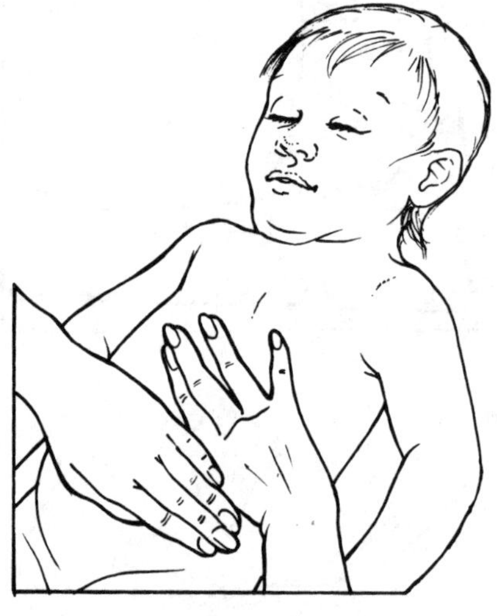

Rub baby's belly with large circular strokes, pressing gently.

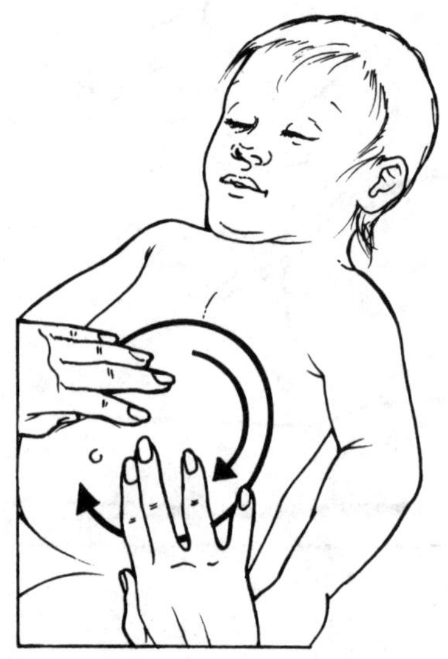

With your fingertips, continue to massage the belly by pressing gently in a clockwise direction, to aid baby's digestion.

- Now, move up to the chest. Massage baby's chest in little circles with your fingers. Say "I love you!" as you place your hand over baby's heart. Always remembering to be gentle, draw one hand across the chest to the right shoulder, and then the other hand across to the left shoulder. Cross my heart, I love you!
- Lift baby's arm and glide your hand in one smooth motion (think of a playground slide) over palm, wrist, inner arm, under the arm, down the side, the hip, the leg, and all the way to the little feet. Wheeee!
- Massage baby's arms and fingers just like you did their legs and toes. Baby might not extend arms out. Let baby hold arms in whatever way is comfortable, and massage them in that position.
- Return to the face and repeat those first facial strokes.
- Now for the back. Most babies (and most grown-ups!) find backrubs very relaxing. Turn baby over and massage baby's back with long effleurage strokes from neck to buttocks. Walk your fingers down each side of baby's spine (don't press directly on the spine). Rub in a circular motion with your fingers gently over baby's entire back. Then, move your hands up and down, back and forth over baby's entire backside, just as you did over baby's legs. You might even try some very light finger tapping on baby's little buttocks muscles.
- End with feather strokes (see Chapter 13) from crown to toe and lots of soothing baby talk. Look deeply into baby's eyes with love. You'll see that love reflected back at you—the ultimate reward for giving a great infant massage!

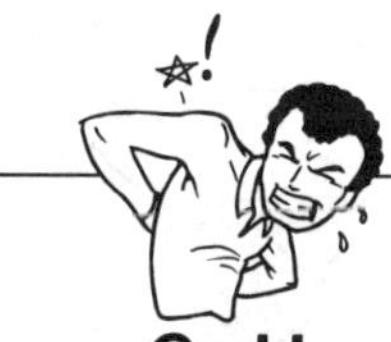

Ouch!

Keep tummy rubs gentle, and wait about an hour after a meal to do a tummy massage. Otherwise, lunch (or breakfast or dinner) will probably end up eliminated out the wrong end and all over you!

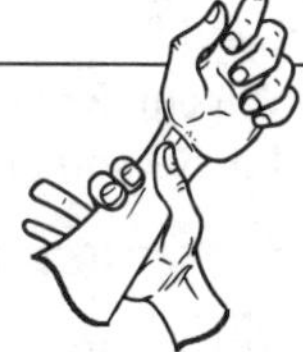

Your Finger on the Pulse

Every baby is an individual. Very young or ultrasensitive babies may be catapulted into hysterics or withdrawal by too much stimulation. For them, slow, gentle effleurage is best. A few babies, however, especially those over six months old, enjoy a lot more stimulation and can be massaged briskly, playfully, and actively (although still gently). Vary your technique according to your baby's personality.

Cool Kid Touch

Sometimes it's easy to go for days without touching your kids in a meaningful way, especially when toddler tantrums, excessive extra-curricular activities, pre-teen blowouts, or general kid rebellion suddenly dominates family life. Kids do love massage though, if you can get them to sit still long enough. As resilient and unbreakable as

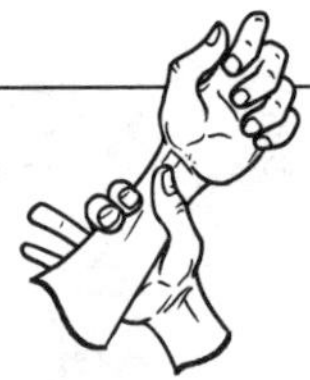

Your Finger on the Pulse

Kids and water go together like peanut butter and jelly. Try some basic yoga, range-of-motion, or massage techniques when playing with your kids in the pool, where they may be more willing to participate. You'll have to make it a game: "Let's all be dolphins!" "You be the boat and I'll sail you." "I'll bet you can't completely relax in my arms while I move you around!"

kids may seem, they can strain muscles and experience stress just like grown-ups. When your kids get older and start school, you may not find yourself in close physical contact with them as often as you were when they were babies, and massage can bring you back together on this level, too.

Let's Play

But how do you get that little ball of toddler energy to agree to a massage? How do you convince your third-grader to turn off the television and relax with you or your seventh-grader that massage is cool? How do you let your teen know that massage is great for combatting anxiety and depression?

The trick is to turn massage into play. Kids understand the language of play, and you have to speak their language if you want to communicate at all. For toddlers, massages will last about as long as their attention spans—five minutes max. But a cheerful, "Let's play the massage game!" may be all it takes to get things started. Let your toddler reciprocate after you've given him or her a massage by giving one to you (toddlers are great imitators—you might actually get a good one!).

With grade-schoolers, you could play massage therapist or set up a play spa to which your child can pay a visit, perhaps as a rich and famous movie star or a world-renowned athlete. (What grade-schooler wouldn't like to pretend to be Michael Jordan getting a massage?)

With pre-teens and teenagers, massage can be a great way to connect. Kids this age sometimes find it difficult to talk to their parents, but if you set up a weekly massage appointment (or call it something more teen-friendly, such as "spa visit" or "one-on-one time"), your child may find it easier to open up. Cherish this time and try not to spoil the massage by judging or condemning what your child tells you. Just listen, and help her or him to relax.

Chances are, your pre-teen or teen is under a lot of stress, even if you don't think he or she has any reason to be. Peer pressure, school, struggles with authority and achievement, and the simple need to define oneself and be an individual while still being accepted by the group are all tough challenges. Remember? Being a teenager isn't any piece of cake. Give your teen the gift of touch in a no-strings-attached (talking isn't required), stress-free oasis.

A Massage Minute

Massage may be more of a survival technique than a luxury for teens, who frequently experience high levels of anxiety, depression, and stress, and low self-image. According to the American Academy of Child and Adolescent Psychiatry, thousands of teenagers commit suicide in the United States each year. Suicide is the third leading cause of death for 15- to 24-year-olds and the sixth leading cause of death for 5- to 14-year-olds. Studies show that massage can reduce depression and anxiety levels in adolescents. Tune in to your teen and suggest regular massage, either by a professional massage therapist or by you, before you sense that life is becoming overwhelming for your teen.

The Lessons Massage Teaches Kids

The family that is comfortable with affection and touch has a more solid, lasting bond. Kids who learn that touch is a healthy, positive way to show affection are likely to form better relationships and be more self-confident than children who were rarely touched, whose parents were awkward with physical affection, or who were touched in an unhealthy or violent way. Raising a child in an environment where touch is a way of life and massage is a natural and frequently employed stress-relieving, healing, and health-maintenance technique means raising a child who cares about others and isn't afraid to show it and a child who cares about his or her own body, health, and spirit.

Mucho Macho

If you are a man, you may be perfectly willing to get a massage—if someone wants to give you one for free, if you could ever find the time, if your partner suggests it and you suspect it will lead to more intimate kinds of touch, or if you need to relieve your stress. You might even accept a massage from a male massage therapist—as long as none of the guys found out about it!

But guys are notoriously unwilling to really care for themselves in the way massage cares for the body/mind. You guys have no problems indulging yourselves in some ways. You like to buy stuff (especially electronic stuff!), and you like to have a nice evening out now and then. Maybe you like to buy gifts or take vacations, and you'll probably spend months shopping for a new car. But a massage? Isn't that kind of wimpy?

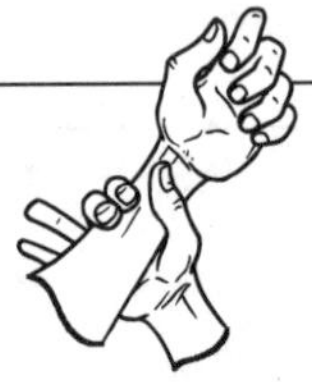

Your Finger on the Pulse

For all you athletes out there, whether professional or weekend, consider the benefits of sports massage, which prepares your body for competition and helps you heal more quickly afterwards (see Chapter 23, "The Wide, Wide World of Sports Massage"). Fast becoming an integral part of professional sports training, sports massage can benefit anyone with an active lifestyle. Massage wouldn't hurt you armchair athletes, either. It might even inspire you to get moving!

We'll let you in on a little secret: Real men get massages, and give them, too. Men have long known that swapping massages with their partners in the bedroom can lead to a fun evening for all. An increasing number of star and amateur athletes are making sports massage part of their fitness regimens. Top executives are discovering that massage can relieve stress and make them more productive. Even your regular guy on the street is becoming more open to the idea of massage as an effective way to relieve stress, even if it takes a gift certificate from a loved one to get him there.

But massage is about more than stress-relief and muscle repair. Massage is about touch—nonsexual, supportive, caring touch—and how it can improve your health, your life, and your relationships. Think about your touch comfort level, and then think about your relationships. Are they comfortable, affectionate, loving, and fun? The more comfortable you are with touch, the better your relationships will be. Massage is a great way to help you become more comfortable with the kind of touch that is health-enhancing but doesn't have an ultimate goal (you know the goal we mean).

What about giving a massage? Plenty of you are really good about giving your partners massages, and believe us, your partners are appreciative. But a lot of men we know admit that they don't give their partners massages more often because they are lazy. "I'd rather get one than give one!" they admit. Or they only think of it as a nice form of foreplay.

But giving a massage is more than just a prelude to getting one. Giving a massage can be a therapeutic touch experience in itself. You are still in physical contact, sharing loving energy. Giving a massage can grant you more intimate knowledge of your partner's physical, emotional, even spiritual self. Learn your partner's body without thinking ahead to where the whole thing might lead. Live in the moment of the massage, and you might be surprised at what you will learn. Your relationship may well become deeper and more meaningful, and that can only benefit you both.

Vulnerability Equals Strength

But back to the professional massage: lying there on a massage table, all unclothed, practically yelling out that your body needs some care—how manly is that? At home, do you want to admit to your partner that you need a massage, not sex? That, emotionally, you need to be touched? Here's another little secret, guys: Vulnerability equals strength. By opening yourself up to regular, non-goal-oriented massages, you are helping yourself open up to being helped, and that can be quite comforting, even empowering. The man who allows himself to be nurtured, who pays attention to his mental and physical health needs, and who can open himself up emotionally will get help, will be mentally and physically healthier, and will be more ready for successful and fulfilling personal relationships, especially as he becomes older and more vulnerable. What's stronger than that?

A Massage Minute

Contrary to the stereotype, getting older is not easier for men than women. Sometimes it's a lot harder. Women are traditionally conditioned to be more open in sharing emotions and are thus better able to communicate their attitudes and feelings about aging. Men don't traditionally learn to be as open about emotional issues and may feel less able to express their feelings about the aging process.

But you know the stereotype: The woman who wants a commitment, the man who runs the other way at the very mention of the *c* word for fear it will emasculate him in one fell swoop. Our society tends to raise boys to believe that autonomy and strength are the most important characteristics for men, while a nurturing instinct and the desire for family are what women want.

We say, baloney! Apart from the stereotypes and locker room talk and which planet each of us is from, humans are social animals, and they need each other. They need to be touched, held, needed, supported, and loved. Fulfilling those needs makes for strong relationships, strong individuals, and a stronger, more vital society.

Intimacy Equals Knowledge

Studies show that from birth, boys are handled, held, and caressed less often and for shorter periods of time than girls. According to the Hite Report on Male Sexuality, men wish they could receive more non-sex-related touching from women. But something holds many men back from asking for more nonsexual touch. What is it?

Just as men are often loathe to appear weak, they also don't want to appear interested in intimacy. Sure, sexual intimacy is great, but emotional intimacy? Yikes! We certainly don't mean to offend the enlightened among you who have already discovered the power of intimacy, but the fact is, lots of you—through no fault of your own—just aren't comfortable with the concept.

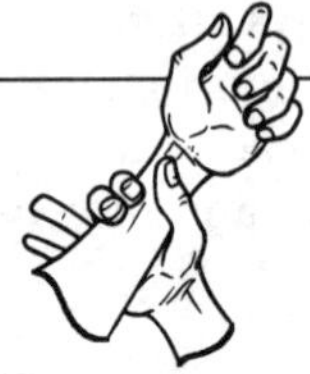

Your Finger on the Pulse

You may not always have the time to get or give a full-blown massage, but don't let that stop you from physical communication. A loving shoulder rub after dinner, a foot massage, a quick scalp massage, or a really long hug are all intimate ways for couples to stay in touch when they only have a few spare moments together.

Intimacy is a personal, passionate exploration of a relationship and may be highly couple-specific in approach. But intimacy will almost always reveal things about your partner and about yourself you never realized were there. It can open up a whole new dimension to a relationship. And it can make you feel secure, strong, and virile knowing you've bared your inner self to someone else who still loves you—maybe even more than before.

But what does all this have to do with massage? Getting regular massages, even if just to improve your athletic performance, address some health problem, or relieve your stress, is a big step towards acknowledging your need for touch. Why did that hour of Swedish massage feels so incredibly good? Because it relaxed and primed your body, yes, but also because it fulfilled a basic and undeniable human need for human contact. Regular reciprocal massage with your partner can strengthen the infrastructure of your relationship because you will be communicating on a body-mind level through the power of touch, which is pretty intimate and pretty darned manly.

Senior Touch

Aging brings with it certain trials as well as rewards. You seniors are older than you once were, but you are also wiser. Your minds and bodies have experienced more and understand more than those who haven't lived as long. But all that experience can be a little rough on the human body, and certain systems in your body may not work like they used to. Of course, even these changes have their positive side:

- ➤ Your digestion gets a little touchy, so watching your weight becomes easier!
- ➤ You lose muscle tissue and bone mass, yet another form of en-LIGHT-enment.
- ➤ Your skin thins and, along with other tissues including blood vessels, loses elasticity, giving your face even more character!
- ➤ Your nerves don't conduct signals as quickly, so you gain patience.
- ➤ You may not sleep as well or have the same appetite you used to have, so you have more time for reading, painting, listening, and creating.
- ➤ Your senses aren't quite as sharp, making meditation easier.
- ➤ Your immune system doesn't work quite as efficiently, making you more sensitive and in tune to the changing environment around you.

Staying active (both physically and mentally); eating a low-fat, high-fiber diet; managing stress; and receiving regular massage or other forms of touch can continue to broaden your ever-expanding horizons.

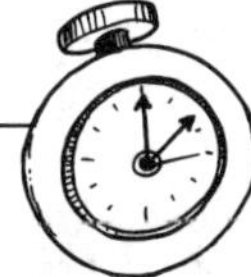

A Massage Minute

Research published in the May 1998 issue of *Alternative Therapies Journal* on the effects of various alternative health therapies for seniors has demonstrated (primarily through anecdotal evidence) the effectiveness of the following for combating cardiovascular disease: a sense of hope; faith and a personal spirituality; a social network; regular attendance at religious services; the ability to practice forgiveness; use of imagery as a relaxation technique or for healing; meditation; music therapy (the use of music to encourage healing); hypnosis; energy or spiritual healing; yoga (see Chapter 12, "More Kinds of Massage"); T'ai Chi (a traditional martial arts form involving relaxed breathing and slow, graceful motions to balance body and mind); qigong (see Chapter 12); and Aikido (another martial arts form).

Time Is on Your Side

Aging has a lot of perks. You are wiser, you have a greater and more objective perspective on life, and you have lots of experiences to draw from and memories to enjoy. Your kids are grown, and you can make yourself a priority again. You've still got an undetermined amount of future ahead of you to learn more and do more.

Having seen your share of history, you may also have developed a more open mind, a broader concept of living, and a more tolerant perspective. After all, you've seen things happen in your lifetime you never would have believed possible when you were in your teens or twenties. Perhaps you have a sense of the limitlessness of human endeavor, or the mutable nature of what society deems acceptable, or the importance of recognizing life's spiritual side.

You've also probably figured out, over the course of your life, that touch is important to your well-being. Yet as many people age, experience the loss of friends and family members, and suffer from an increasing number of health problems (whether major or minor), frustration and stress can set in. The result? Many seniors find it easier to withdraw

Your Finger on the Pulse

You know exercise is important, but you may not feel comfortable jogging or even walking around the block on that hard sidewalk. Try water aerobics, water yoga, or water walking, either in a class or on your own. Just as water massage is less stressful to your body, so is water exercise. Plus, exercising in the pool is just plain fun.

and don't seek out the relationships and touch they need—especially those who have lost a spouse and whose children have moved far away.

But this isn't the time to be alone and untouched. Seniors need touch just as much as anyone. Therapeutic massage is a great way to receive the health-enhancing benefits of touch because it is specifically formulated to increase circulation to the skin and internal organs, boost energy and mood, and improve the functioning of all your internal systems that may be slowing down just a bit. Massage can make your body feel years younger, and that's a great feeling, especially if, like many seniors say, your mind still feels decades younger than your driver's license claims!

AquaMassage: Use It or Lose It

If you've already begun to experience some of the symptoms of aging, such as loss of bone and muscle mass and thinned, drying skin, you may find that some traditional massage techniques aren't particularly comfortable. Massage therapists are trained to tune in to individual bodies and exert just the right amount of pressure and friction, but some seniors are particularly sensitive to, say, a too-vigorous Swedish massage.

AquaMassage to the rescue! AquaMassage is a general term for any massage or bodywork performed in the water. Different from hydrotherapy, in which you are treated with water in the form of saunas, whirlpools, showers, and so on (see Chapter 11, "Welcome to the World of Massage"), AquaMassage includes, for example, water shiatsu (or Watsu, see Chapter 11) and water yoga. Water not only cushions your bones and joints, but it also gives your entire body a lightness and buoyancy that reduces stress and makes the bodywork process more relaxed and enjoyable.

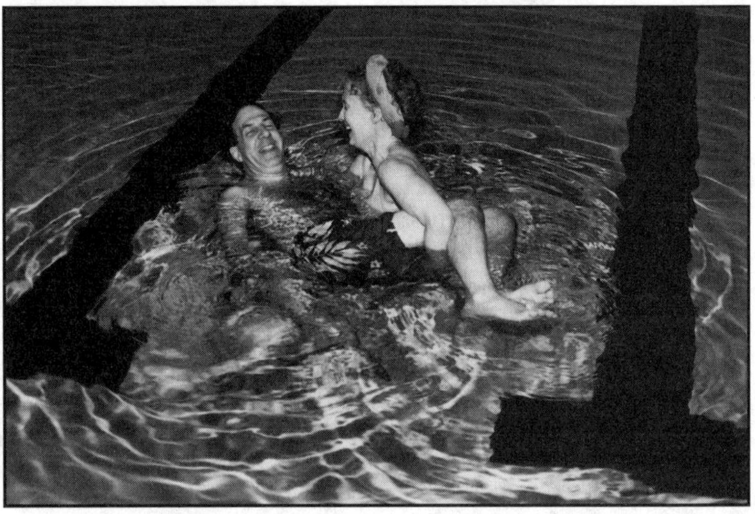

Laughing together is a great way to get started.

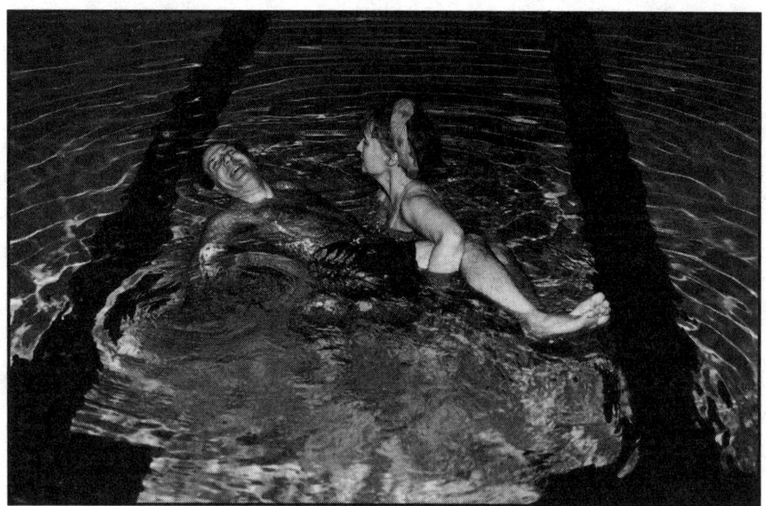

Bob's body slowly opens into a spinal twist as Joan supports his flat back with one arm, and her other arm holds his knees over to one side.

For some, water massage and exercise are the only comfortable forms, and both are important to maintain a general relaxed mental state and flexible body. If you don't use that body, you'll keep losing function, so if you find that life on dry land is a little too jarring, get into that pool! You'll probably be hooked for life.

No Pain, Supreme Gain

Despite what you may have been brought up to believe, exercise, massage, and life in general don't have to hurt to be effective. In fact, they shouldn't hurt! Make it a habit to tune in regularly to your body, as though it were your favorite radio station. Lots of static today? Maybe you are being too hard on yourself. Can't get a good signal? Maybe you aren't engaging in enough physical or mental activity. Coming in clear? Now you've got it!

You can reduce stress to your body and your mind in many ways, during exercise, during massage, and even during your everyday living. Here are a few feel-good hints (you younger folks take note, too—these tips can benefit anyone):

- Stay active. Exercise your body and your mind every day. Take a walk in the fresh air, ride a bicycle, go to an exercise class, do a crossword puzzle, read a challenging book on a new subject, and discuss current events with friends.
- Exercise with really good shoes. Spend a little extra to get the cushioning and support you need. Your feet shouldn't hurt after a walk.

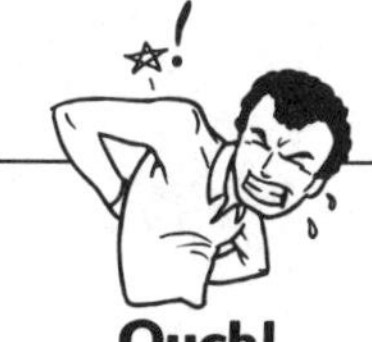

Ouch!

If you suffer from *osteoporosis*, a condition in which aging bones lose mass, become more porous, and are more easily broken, let your massage therapist know. She or he will be able to adjust the pressure of strokes accordingly to circumvent injury.

- Maintain at least a few really close relationships. Talk to someone else every day, even if for just a few minutes on the phone. Isolation, loneliness, and depression can all compromise your health.
- If you aren't comfortable lying on a massage table, ask your massage therapist about seated massage. No aspect of the massage experience should be painful, and if it is, speak up.

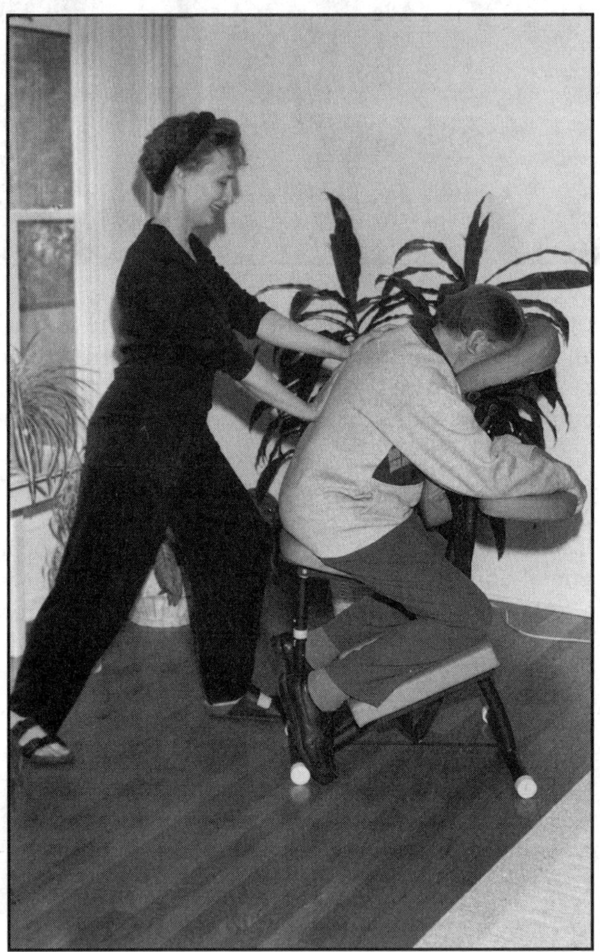

John enjoys total relaxation in this chair massage. His knees are comfortably supported and Joan is able to massage his back, neck, and arms fully.

- If an hour of massage is too much, try a shorter session. Fifteen- to 30-minute sessions can have all the benefits of a longer session.
- Eat a healthy diet, but remember to enjoy yourself, too. If you really love that morning cup of coffee or that glass of wine with dinner, it probably does more good to your psychological state than harm to your physical state. (But don't overdo it, of course. A pot of coffee or a whole liter of wine per day will eventually compromise just about anyone's health.)

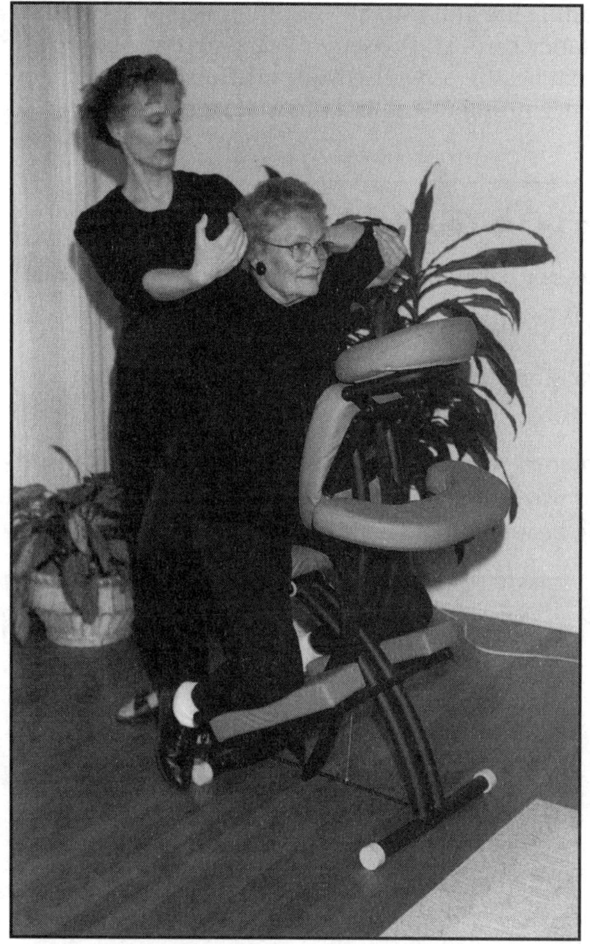

Joan assists Leona in a slight backbend during her seated massage.

- Cultivate a positive attitude. You've earned the right to be happy and enjoy life. You've also earned the right to relish and embrace this stage of your life, taking full advantage of your experiences and understanding. Dwelling on past mistakes, regrets, tragedies, even how young you once were, won't do you any good. Be forthright. Repair damaged relationships if you can, but if you can't, move on. Look ahead, and seek out joy in the life you have now, with all its richness and complexity.
- Have goals. What do you want to accomplish today? This week? This year? Can you help someone else with their goals? Your listening skills are so appreciated in a fast-paced world filled with busy signals. Help the world grow through your wisdom. Keep making plans with those around you and looking forward to the future. The future will then embrace all of us with open arms.

Bringing massage into your family life and into all your life stages will bring an added richness to your life. From infancy through the senior years, massage improves your physical, mental, and emotional health, as well as your relationships to others. A life filled with loving touch from beginning to end is a life well worth living!

The Least You Need to Know

- Infant massage can help your baby and you to relax, bond, and feel great.
- Massage is great for kids, especially when disguised as play.
- Men can benefit physically and emotionally from therapeutic, non-goal-oriented touch.
- Massage, especially combined with exercise and other healthy mental and physical habits, is a good way for seniors to appreciate the aging process and rejoice in the everlasting beauty of the changing seasons of life.

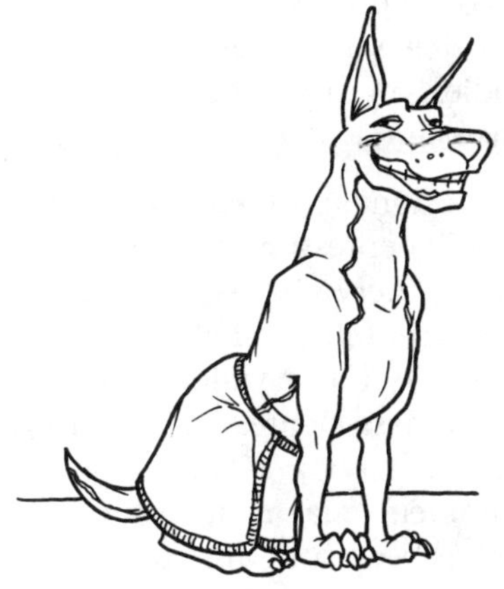

Chapter 26

Massage for Pets

In This Chapter

- Why your pet needs a massage
- Does pet massage have similar benefits to human massage?
- Do people actually make a living at pet massage?
- How do I massage my pet?

You might look at this chapter title, then glance over at your dog or cat stretched out in a square of sun on your couch, snoozing soundly, and think we're crazy. How could an animal get more relaxed than that? And what does any creature obviously so accomplished in the art of relaxation need with a massage?

Actually, much of this book could be rewritten in reference to pets only. Many of the benefits of massage, types of massage, and positive effects of massage apply, and have been applied, to our fellow creatures in the animal kingdom. Animals need touch just like humans, and newborn animals die without touch, just like we do. Animals are prone to stress and tension just like humans, and your stress level is one of the major causes of stress in your pet, because pets are sensitive to their owners.

For animal athletes or working animals, such as show dogs and horses, farm and herding dogs, police dogs, and guide dogs, massage can relieve the aches, pains, and strains of overworked bodies, promote healing, prevent future injury, and enhance performance.

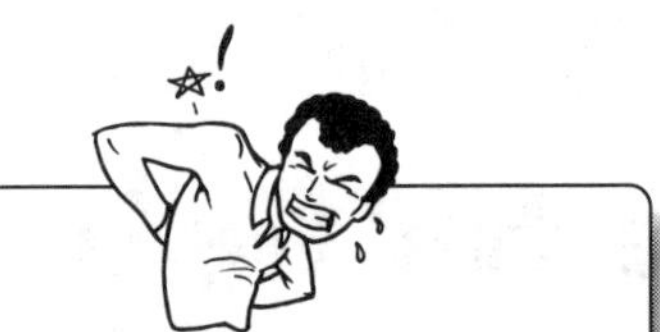

Ouch!

Never use pet massage as a substitute for regular veterinary care. If your pet is sick, in pain, or seems anxious or depressed, see your vet first. Then, in conjunction with professional care, you can treat your pet with massage.

Pets have their share of emotional problems, which massage can address, as well: depression, anxiety (including *separation anxiety*), nervousness, insecurity, and fear. Because our pets can't tell us what's wrong, untreated pain can manifest itself in a variety of behavioral problems, such as nippiness, depression, lethargy, irritability, even destructive behavior. Massage that seems to cure behavior problems may really just be relieving pain an animal has been suffering from for a long time.

People's attitudes about their pets have changed dramatically in the last few decades. Dogs who used to be relegated to backyard doghouses have been brought inside and made official family members. Fewer people let their cats roam the streets, keeping them inside and making them family members, too.

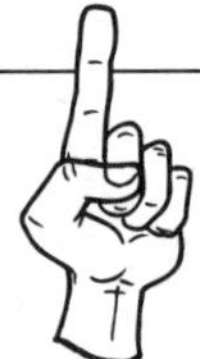

Touch Talk

Separation anxiety is a condition in pets (especially dogs) brought on by your absence. This condition is common in puppies who have been with their owners constantly for several months and are suddenly left alone all day, sick dogs, and dogs with overly dependent emotional relationships with their owners. Symptoms include destructive behavior (eating your sofa, digging, shredding garbage), depression, chronic barking, nervousness, and disintegrating health.

Perhaps as people become more physically disconnected due to the advances of communication technology (how many e-mail pals do you have?), they are seeking the touch they require and the unconditional love they desire from their pets. People spend more time with their animal companions. (Even the term *pet owner* has become politically incorrect in favor of *pet companion*—who's to say we have the right to own our pets, anyway?)

They also spend a whole lot more money on pet health care, high-quality pet food, grooming, and pet products than ever before. Have you seen the pet supply catalogues these days? You can buy fancy wooden sleigh beds and other pet-sized fine furnishings; gourmet treats made from the finest of ingredients; pet seat belts; battery-powered canine oral hygiene machines; fancy creme rinse conditioners, perfumes, and a bevy of natural coat and skin care products; cooling and heating pads; puppy-carrier backpacks; and supplements too numerous to mention, from all-natural arthritis remedies to multivitamins and whole-food concentrates.

Silly as some of these luxuries may sound, our pets not only require but deserve our love and attention. That doesn't mean we have to spend a fortune on a bedroom set for Snooky, however. All pets really need are some basics: food, water, shelter, health care, and love. More than anything, they want your attention and your touch. What better way to provide it than through regular pet massage?

Massage and Mother Nature

Massaging your pet certainly isn't unnatural. Equivalents to massage or other forms of touch can be found everywhere in nature. Primates engage in touch all the time, from grooming each other to carrying and nursing their babies for several years. Birds preen each other, fish swim in close-knit schools, horses nuzzle, and lizards frequently choose to bask in the sun while sitting on a fellow lizard's back. Cats (tame or wild) and dogs (tame or wild) love to curl up together to sleep, sometimes so inextricably that you can't distinguish which limbs and tails belong to which animal. Virtually all animal mothers lick, paw, and otherwise physically manipulate their young. And where would your dog or cat rather sit: Out there alone in the kitchen or on your lap, on your feet, or spread over every inch of pillow not taken up by your head? So to say that animals need touch, seek out contact, and can benefit from massage isn't so far-out after all.

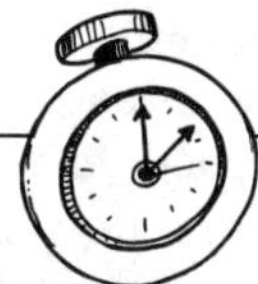

A Massage Minute

An increasing number of veterinarians practice aromatherapy. Aromatherapy remedies have been shown to decrease respiratory problems in cats housed in animal shelters, calm and relax anxious pets, and alleviate symptoms of depression, lethargy, and separation anxiety. When used in a diffuser, essential oils can benefit both pet and owner. Some essential oils can be irritating to sensitive pets, however, so only use remedies and concentrations recommended or approved by your veterinarian.

Some pet product suppliers have aromatherapy kits for pets. Or you can create your own combinations. For example, essential oils that help to relax an anxious pet are lavender, sweet marjoram, neroli, basil, verbena, and pine.

Pets Have Muscles, Too

A lot of people tend to *anthropomorphize* their pets. We feel their pain. When they look embarrassed, we imagine they are feeling embarrassment the way we do. When they are sick or injured, we apply our own feelings about being sick to our pets.

Different people have different theories about how accurate such projection is. If we all evolved from the same place, originally, it makes sense that many of our mental processes would be similar. On the other hand, a pet's perspective is also so different from ours and the influence of culture, not really a factor for pets, is so pronounced in us, that surely their perceptions are vastly different. When an animal is sick or in pain, for example, it probably understands the discomfort differently than we do—but that doesn't mean the experience is any less intense.

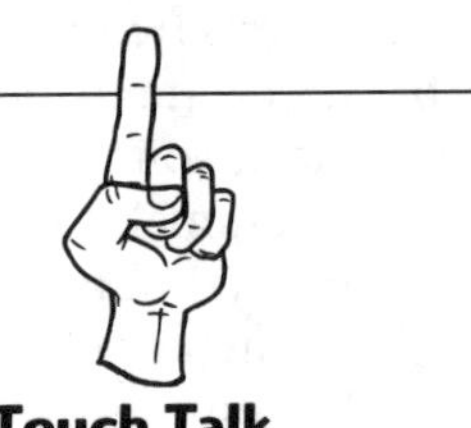

Touch Talk

To **anthropomorphize** is to assign human characteristics to a non-human, such as an animal. Although some controversy exists as far as what is and isn't anthropomorphism (for example, if you say your dog is jealous, is that accurate?), many pet owners admit that they probably anthropomorphize their pets frequently.

But no one can argue that humans and pets have one important feature in common: muscles! Because pets have muscles, they can experience all the same muscle symptoms, pains, and injuries that humans can.

Pet massage has become an important industry for very active pets who use their muscles frequently. Testimonials abound of show dogs whose performance skyrocketed after massage relieved their pain and put their bodies back in order, or horses who were lame and were miraculously cured by acupressure, or injured working dogs who were given their lives back through chiropractic manipulations. Even if your pet is just a regular house pet who exercises moderately and spends lots of time lying on your lap, it has muscles that can occasionally get strained and that would certainly benefit, even when they aren't injured, from the relaxing touch of massage.

Don't You Have Enough to Do?

"Oh, c'mon," you might be protesting. "I can barely find time to get a massage myself—and I should take more of my precious time to get my pet massaged?" Think of it this way. What is your pet to you? An alarm system or a best friend? A beautiful addition to your finely decorated home or a beloved family member? A status symbol or a loyal companion? Is a simple massage too much to ask for the creature who is always there for you, who can sense your moods and knows when you need comfort or a snuggle or a friendly lick on the nose?

Pet massage isn't time-consuming if you do it yourself. You can incorporate it into your regular grooming routine or when you would be petting your pet anyway, while watching television in the evenings or as you enjoy your morning cup of tea with your pet at your side. If you hire a professional, it's usually less expensive than a massage for a human (and well worth the benefits). Visiting a professional pet massage therapist might not be something you want to do weekly, but such a visit could be a special birthday treat or an occasional, out-of-the-blue, thanks-for-being-there reward for your pet.

Visiting a Pet Massage Professional

Depending on where you live, it may not be so easy to find a pet massage therapist. But their numbers are increasing, and if you live in or near a relatively large city, you'll surely be near several.

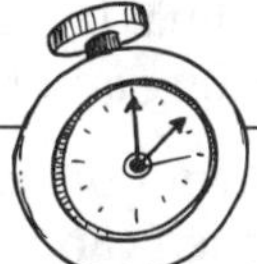

A Massage Minute

Pet massage therapists practice a variety of techniques. Some were trained in massage therapy schools and then extended their practices to include pets. Some continue to practice on humans as well as their pets. Others are more specialized, focusing on, for example, acupressure, acupuncture, pet reflexology, or even energy therapy. Pet chiropractors are also appearing with increasing frequency, and some veterinarians practice chiropractic care in conjunction with regular health care. Other pet massage therapists may specialize in horses, or dogs, or cats, or small animals, or performance animals only.

How do you find all these forward-thinking pet practitioners? If your vet tends toward the holistic approach, he or she can probably make a referral. Or look for a holistic vet in the phone book if yours is more traditional and not familiar with pet massage (although by now, most vets have at least heard of it). Homeopathic and naturopathic practitioners may also treat pets and may know of people qualified in different manual therapies for pets. Your human chiropractor may know of someone (or may even be able to work on your pet him- or herself). Ask around. Sometimes the best way to find the perfect person is by finding someone who has helped a friend or a friend of a friend.

Your Pet's Health Is in Your Hands

Pet owners are far more aware of how to take care of their pets these days. Leash laws, vaccination programs, higher quality pet food, and education at veterinary visits have all served to increase the length and quality of our pets' lives. You know that your pet

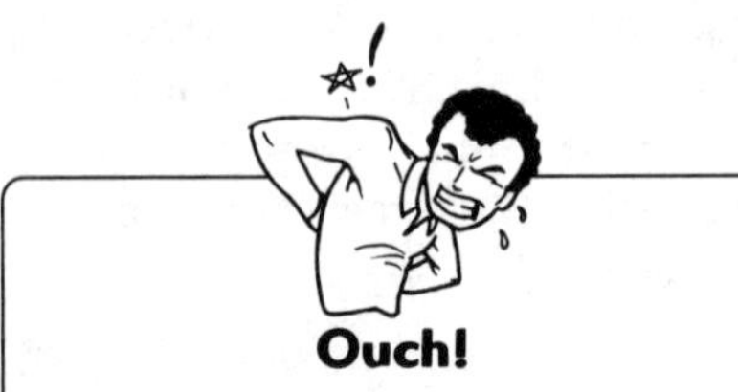

Ouch!

Your pet may not be able to say the word "Ouch!," but it will let you know if you do something that hurts. If, when massaging your pet, something you do elicits a yelp, a nip, a yowl, a scratch, or causes your pet to run away, you've obviously hit a sore spot. Make an appointment with your vet to have the problem checked out and eliminate any serious causes.

will be healthier if you practice good pest control, keep your pet heartworm-free, feed it a good natural diet, and allow it to get plenty of exercise.

If you exert the effort to take care of your pet in all these ways, you probably care a lot about your pet and consequently give it lots of affection. But making a real commitment to touch, stroke, massage, and really communicate with your pet may be one of the most important things you can do. Massage isn't something most veterinarians will include in their list of things you must do to keep your pet healthy, but the physical and psychological benefits of massage and the human-animal bond it solidifies will help your pet to stay strong and healthy.

If your pet is already suffering from a health problem, touch can help your pet's body to heal itself. Read on to find out how to give your particular pet a great massage. (Note: So as to avoid the impersonal *it* pronoun, we will randomly refer to dogs as he and cats as she. We hope all of you with female dogs and male cats won't mind.)

The Canine Caress

Dogs live to please, and when your relationship with your dog is a strong one, there isn't much your dog won't do if he understands what you want. Repay your best friend's loyalty and devotion with lots of pet massages. Here's how to do it:

- Call your dog to you and have him sit (or stand). Gently begin to pet him in the way your normally do. Spend at least a minute or two with gentle, all-over petting. Dogs are creatures of habit, and if you suddenly start doing something different, your dog may get nervous. Plus, this petting gets your dog's body ready for deeper touch.
- Work up to your dog's face. Gently hold him underneath his jaw and look into his eyes. (Try not to come down with your hand from above. Dogs are more comfortable if you approach them from below their heads.)
- Ask your dog if he would like a nice, relaxing massage. Feel your own intention—to calm, relax, and soothe your pet—so that your positive energy is transmitted to your dog.
- With one hand still under his muzzle, gently stroke the top of your dog's head with your other hand. Extend each stroke over the ears. Dogs' ears are filled with nerve endings, and stroking the ears is a great relaxer. Don't pull the ears, but stroke them firmly and thoroughly with long effleurage strokes. Pick up each ear and apply some gentle, slow friction strokes. Then stroke your dog's cheeks and muzzle, very gently.

- Work your way down to the back of the neck. Now you can really get into the muscles. With your fingers, feel your dog's muscles beneath the skin. Dog muscles are smaller than human ones, of course, but you should be able to feel them. Work the back and sides of the neck area, and don't press on the windpipe (at the center front of your dog's neck). Dogs tend to hold a lot of tension in the neck, and releasing this area by kneading the muscles can relieve pain, stress, and anxiety in many dogs.

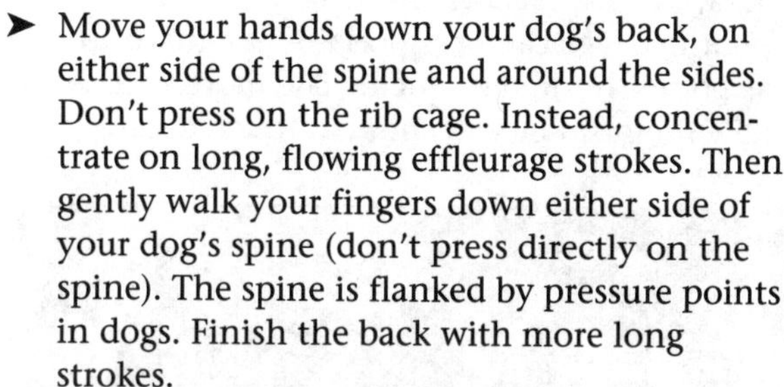

- Move your hands down your dog's back, on either side of the spine and around the sides. Don't press on the rib cage. Instead, concentrate on long, flowing effleurage strokes. Then gently walk your fingers down either side of your dog's spine (don't press directly on the spine). The spine is flanked by pressure points in dogs. Finish the back with more long strokes.
- Now, have your dog lie on its side. Very gently stroke down each leg several times, and then squeeze and hold each leg muscle for about 10 seconds. Apply gentle cross-fiber friction across the leg tendons, and then gently rub on and in between the paw pads and nails with your finger. Move each digit in tiny circles, and then flex and extend each leg joint. If your dog suffers from *hip dysplasia*, moving the back legs at the hip joint will probably be painful, so avoid any hip range-of-motion exercises in dogs suffering from this painful condition.
- Have your dog lie on the other side and repeat the leg strokes with the remaining two legs.
- Finish your dog's massage with head-to-toe, super-gentle effleurage strokes. If your dog is asleep by now, great! But chances are, he's probably just basking in that relaxed feeling. Leave quietly or remain at your dog's side and allow him to get up at his own pace. For some dogs, it may take awhile. Other dogs may jump right up, ready for a rousing game of catch. That doesn't mean your massage didn't work—it just means your dog is feeling great, which was your goal!

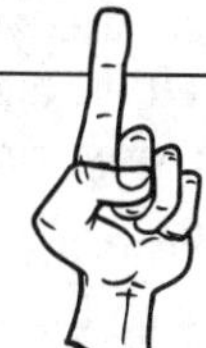

Touch Talk

Hip dysplasia is a congenital defect more common in large dogs. An abnormal hip joint results in pain, limping, hopping, and difficulty getting up and down from sitting or lying positions. Arthritis frequently develops in the hip joint. Hip dysplasia is commonly treated with weight and exercise control, pain relievers, or surgery in severe cases. Dogs with hip dysplasia should be under the care of a veterinarian.

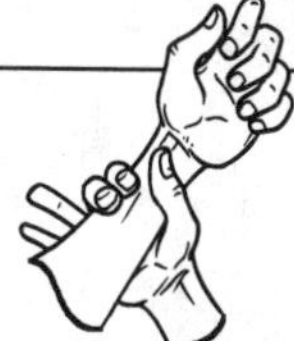

Your Finger on the Pulse

One of the perks of regular pet massage is that your pet will become more comfortable with being touched. This can be a lifesaver when you take your pet to the veterinarian. Some pets are particularly sensitive to touch, but pet massage can desensitize them, to some extent, so that being touched is relaxing and calming rather than traumatic.

Fortunate Felines

What's more luxurious than a stretching, purring cat? Not much! Cats love luxury, so chances are, your feline friend will relish massage. You probably already pet your cat with effleurage strokes, without even realizing it! Who can resist petting a cat with those long, firm, flowing strokes?

Some cats are touch-magnets, even pressing their bodies against your hands when you're trying to work at the computer or pay bills or even sleep. Other cats, however, are very touch-sensitive and shy away from human touch. Have you ever tried to pet a cat whose body seemed to cave in and draw back wherever you tried to touch it? Both types of cats can enjoy massage, but massage can be especially helpful for the touch-shy cat, teaching it to trust and even relish human touch. (The more kittens are held when young, the more comfortable they will be with human touch as adults.)

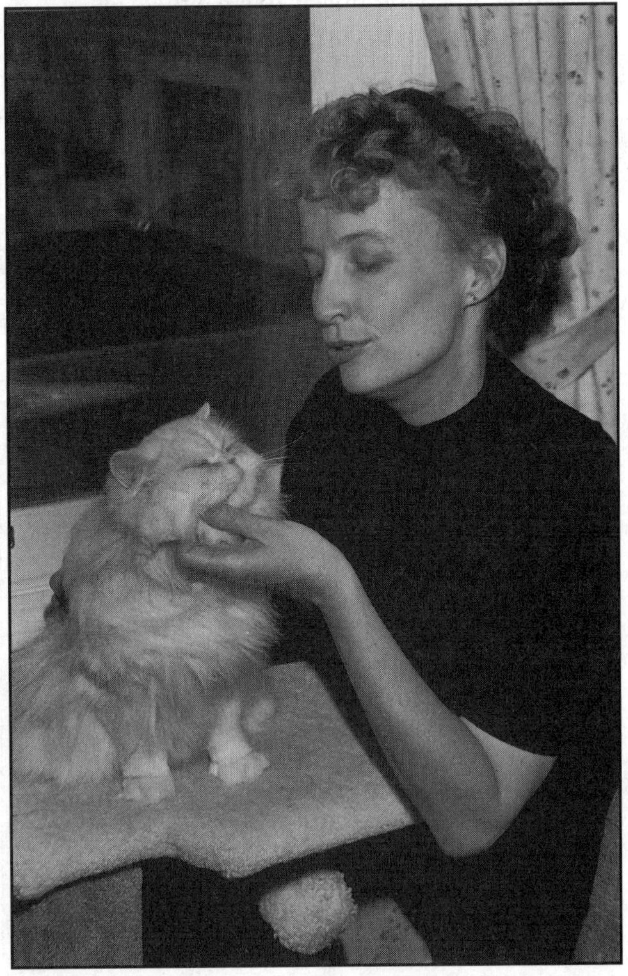

Joan purrrrs with her cat, Mufasa. As she strokes his chin, she's gradually massaging her other hand around his shoulder girdle. Cats keep lots of tension there from all their jumping around!

Massage can also help to relax anxious cats and may solve behavioral problems. We once knew a cat who would hide in the hall over the stairs of a split-level home. Whenever anyone descended the stairs, this cat, with claws extended, would pounce on the unsuspecting human's head, take a few swipes, and then disappear instantly. Who knows how this cat might have relaxed with a few weeks of daily massage? We suspect she'd be much better behaved. (We also suspect that every person leaving that house could use a good massage!)

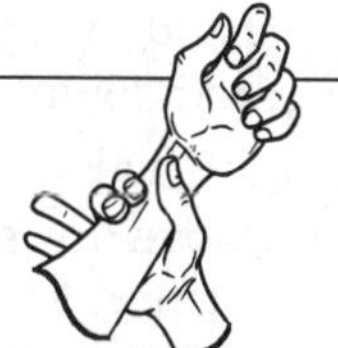

Your Finger on the Pulse

When massaging your pet, be particularly aware of trigger points. Cool, depressed areas or warm, raised areas are probably more sensitive. Gently pressing on these areas may relieve pain, but if your pet reacts in pain to any pressure or massage technique, stop immediately and return to gentle, reassuring strokes.

Here's how to massage your cat:

- Find your cat. (Sometimes this is the hardest part, unless your cat is the type who lives on your lap.)
- Depending on your cat's personality, you may have to progress slowly. Some cats take to massage immediately. Others need a few days, or even weeks, of introductory, practice stroking. In either case, begin with long, soothing strokes along your cat's back. Pet your cat the way you usually do. Anything sudden and unusual may scare your cat away. Spend at least two or three minutes with these familiar strokes.
- Talk soothingly to your cat. If she acts nervous or pulls away from you, try again later. You don't want your cat to remember the massage experience negatively. When your cat seems really comfortable (that rumbling purr is a sure sign!), proceed.
- If your cat lies down, great. If not, don't force her into any particular position. You can work around her preferences. Begin with very soft, gentle strokes around the face and ears. Talk to your cat and ask if you may massage her. She may not be sure, but may let you proceed with caution. With your fingers, lightly stroke her cheeks, nose, and chin. She probably won't mind some scratching, either. Gently rub her ears and stroke the back of her neck.
- As with dogs, many cats hold tension in their necks, so this is a good place to begin the serious business. Concentrate the stroking around the back of the neck, feeling with your fingers for the muscles beneath the skin. Press gently into the muscles to release tension. Remember to stay in tune with your cat. You should be able to tell what she likes and doesn't like.
- Your cat carries lots of tension in her shoulders, too. After all, cats love to perch up high, and these joints and muscles are jolted every time your cat jumps back down to a chair or the floor. Gently knead your cat's shoulder muscles.
- Work your way down your cat's back. Rub with your thumbs down each side of the spine (don't press directly on the spine), while spreading the rest of your

hand over your cat's flanks. Move your thumbs in a circular motion. Move up and down your cat's back a few times, massaging the entire back with small, circular movements. Be careful not to press on the delicate ribcage.

- Move down your cat's back legs, kneading the muscles and applying cross-fiber friction across the tendons. Some cats are extremely sensitive when it comes to touching their feet, but if your cat will allow it, press into the paw pads and massage between them. (Your cat may resist at first but be willing to let you try this after a few weeks of regular massage. Don't push it.) Flex and extend each joint in your cat's legs. Some cats are also sensitive about their hip joints, so be careful with these, too.
- Work back up to the front legs and massage them in the same way, kneading muscle, applying friction to tendons, massaging paw pads, and flexing and extending joints.
- Lightly stroke your cat's chin, the underside of her neck, and her chest. Your cat's underside is probably more sensitive than her back, so use a lighter touch, but try to cover the entire area.
- End the massage with more long, firm strokes from nose to tail. Your cat should be purring loudly or be sound asleep. Either way, you've done your job! She'll soon be back for more—if she'll even let you stop. You may have to go through the whole procedure again!

A Massage Minute

Pet massage is as good for you as it is for your pet! Many studies have demonstrated that owning a pet, from a puppy to a tank of tropical fish, is relaxing and a great way to reduce stress. More recent studies suggest that giving your pet a regular massage has a further relaxing effect and may even reduce blood pressure in people suffering from hypertension. So give your own health a boost while you express your love and affection to your pet. (But we suggest you refrain from trying to give your tropical fish a massage. They probably wouldn't enjoy it.)

Happy Horses

Massaging a horse is a little bit more of an undertaking—horses have a lot more surface area than a dog or a cat! But horses can derive great benefit from massage. Just as in humans, equine massage increases circulation, speeds up the elimination of waste materials, relaxes muscles, and can even calm and reassure anxious or nervous horses. In fact, equine massage is often credited for solving behavioral problems in horses.

Equine sports massage is big these days for increasing performance and speeding up the healing of injuries in performance, race, and hunting horses. The techniques used in human sports massage are only slightly modified and applied to horse athletes. Acupressure and acupuncture have also been used quite successfully on horses, even curing lameness with nothing more than work on one ear (thought to correspond to the entire body). Lots of pet massage professionals are experts at working on horses; classes on equine massage, sports massage, and acupressure abound, and if your horse is in the show circuit, you may already have seen equine massage therapists at work.

As far as what you can do at home, massaging your horse isn't like massaging your cat. Horses are large and frequently try to nip the hand that massages them. If you aren't very comfortable with horses and knowledgeable about horse anatomy, your horse will pick up on that. The whole experience might make your horse more nervous than before, and you could even get hurt. On the other hand, someone comfortable with horses and well-trained can make a huge difference in a horse's health, performance, and behavior. If you still want to try to do it yourself, check out some of the equine massage and equine acupressure workbooks available (see Appendix B for some suggestions), but also consider taking a course in equine massage.

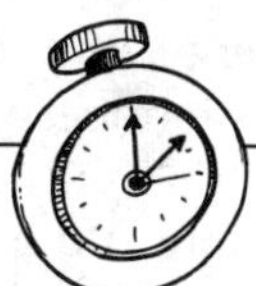

A Massage Minute

A horse's primary activities will determine where it is most likely to experience soreness. Younger horses who haven't yet been ridden tend to experience shoulder stress from bucking and playing. Horses who are ridden frequently tend to experience back stress. Dressage (a type of performance event that involves intricate movements on the ground and no jumping) horses tend to experience neck and hind-end muscle stress. Jumpers and racehorses tend to have leg problems. Because all horses have such thin legs and poor leg circulation, equine massage can be extremely helpful for maintaining and healing legs.

Horses love to be stroked, brushed, rubbed, and reassured of your commitment to them. Simple touch, through which you can transmit your loving, healing energy, will help your horse to heal and strengthen the animal-human bond.

Smaller Animal Massage

Maybe a horse is too big of a commitment for your life right now, and you've even held off on getting a dog or a cat, but you did buy Junior that hamster or gerbil, guinea pig or white rat, rabbit or ferret. Can these smaller creatures benefit from massage, too? They certainly can.

Sometimes nervous by nature, ferrets can benefit from the calming effects of massage. However, they also might be less likely to stay still through a long massage than a dog or a cat. If you've got a ferret, follow the steps for a cat massage, but don't force your pet to enjoy the massage. If your ferret scampers away or acts nervous, stick to gentle stroking, and then try again another time.

Hamsters, gerbils, and guinea pigs have skin, and muscles, and nervous systems, too. They are certainly prone to stress, especially if they get lots of unwelcome handling from younger children (which you shouldn't allow if you own one of these animals, anyway—they are living beings, not educational toys, and no one should keep them unless they are old enough to handle them sensitively).

Regarding technique, you must treat very small mammals delicately. They have tiny muscles and tiny bones. Soft, slow, gentle stroking over the entire body is all you need to, or should, do. You may see quick results, however. Your tiny pet may become calmer, less nervous, and healthier. You may notice a healthy weight gain, increased appetite, sounder sleep, more energy, and even a shinier coat. Again, though, be sensitive to your pet. If your hamster doesn't want to be held, don't force it. Stick to very short periods of daily stroking. Eventually, your pet will become more accustomed to the routine and will enjoy it more and more.

Exotic Pet Massage

If your tastes run more along exotic lines, you may have a pet snake, or lizard, or tarantula. You may keep saltwater fish. Or maybe you prefer our feathered friends, and your best friend is a Greater Sulfur-Crested Cockatoo, a Macaw, a Yellow-Naped Amazon Parrot, or on the less pricey side, a parakeet or a cockatiel. Can your pet benefit from massage, too?

That depends. Some exotic pets don't require and may even suffer from human touch, such as certain tarantulas. Aggressive or venomous pets should, of course, be left alone. Other exotic pets (certain docile tarantulas, lizards, snakes) could care less one way or the other, although you might enjoy touching them.

As far as reptiles are concerned, few people claim that these scaly creatures need human touch. Snakes tend to curl up together, and lizards tend to climb over each other or bask in a stack of two or three, and this may serve some beneficial purpose. But everyone who keeps reptiles knows that the more you handle your pet, the tamer it will be. A 12-foot Burmese python who hasn't been touched in years is going to be a far more dangerous pet than one who is taken out, stroked, and allowed to slither around its owner's arms every day.

Birds are another story. Parrots of all kinds, from tiny blue parakeets to huge macaws, love to be stroked, scratched, and pet. If you raise a parrot from a baby, you can accustom it to human touch right from the start, and you'll have a tame and affectionate pet. If you adopt an older bird, you may have to start gradually. Eventually, most parrots (there are exceptions) will learn to relish your touch.

To give your parrot a good rub, start with whatever area seems to make your bird the least nervous. Some parrots will shove the tops of their heads into your hand in an attempt to get you started. Scratch your bird's head, rub its neck, stroke its face, and massage lightly with your fingers around the place where the wings join the back. Some birds even like a gentle tummy rub. The key is to figure out what your bird likes best. Spend some time petting and stroking your parrot every day, and your bird will probably be noticeably calmer, happier, and healthier.

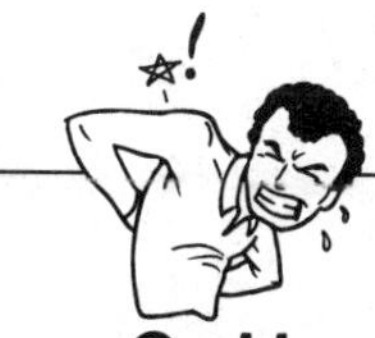

Ouch!

Reptiles are unpredictable. Large reptiles should be handled with caution, and never by people who are inexperienced. If you own a reptile, whether a boa constrictor or a tiny turtle, begin to handle it gradually, always wash your hands before and after touching it (you can infect your pet with germs, and some reptiles may carry salmonella, which can make you sick), and never be rough or make sudden movements.

The Least You Need to Know

- Pets can benefit from massage in all the ways that humans benefit.
- In the wild, animals frequently touch each other.
- Your pet deserves a massage.
- You can do pet massage at home or find a pet massage professional.
- You can massage your dog, cat, horse, smaller mammals, and even some exotic pets on your own with a few simple techniques.

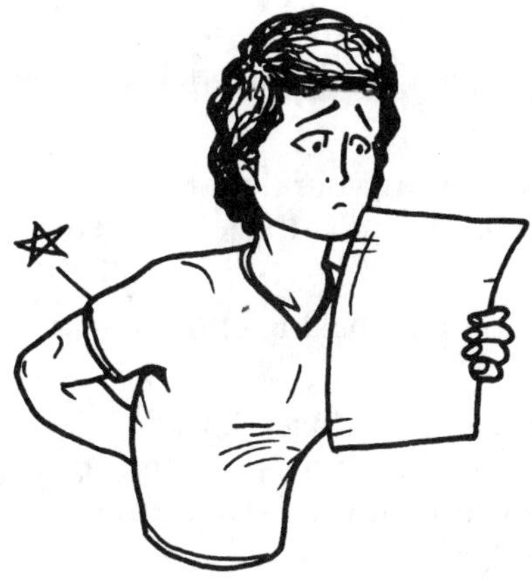

Appendix A

The Right Touch: Personalized Massage Sessions

Whether it's a relaxing five-minute break or a full, luxuriously invigorating hour, massage may be just what you need to melt away tension. The therapeutic effects of even a brief daily massage on your overall health and well-being make it definitely worth your while to incorporate a little healing touch into your busy schedule. Here are some great ideas for massage sessions to start with. You can mix and match, or use our suggestions to create your own massage sessions. But, whatever you do, keep in touch!

5-Minute Self-Massages

You can try these quick and easy self-massages at home, at school, in your car, or at your desk in the office. In short, anywhere you need some fast tension relief!

Get A-Head

After this refresher massage, you'll be "a-head" of the game!

- With the tips of your fingers (not your fingernails), massage your scalp from nape to crown as if you're giving yourself a thorough shampoo.
- Work the imaginary lather all around your head. Be sure to get the back, sides, and front of the scalp. Take your time.
- Next, finger-tap with light, percussive movements all around your face. Tap around the sinuses, over the forehead, and over the cheeks.
- Continue this light tapping for a minute or so to encourage circulation to the head.

Palm Calm

It's all in the hands, especially in reflexology! Let's take a quick break to work the whole body through your palms.

- Begin with your left palm. Pull gently on each finger (using your right hand to work your left), one at a time, then rotate each finger around at the joint where the finger enters the palm.
- Now push all around the left palm with your right thumb, making little circular movements.
- Move to the back of the hand and trace down between each finger. Use your breath…on the exhale, trace down between one finger. Inhale deeply, come to the top of the next finger, then slowly exhale as you trace down between the next finger. Follow between each of the fingers in this way.
- Let your slow, deep breath help guide your rhythm.
- Switch hands and repeat. Your entire body will hum with satisfaction.

15-Minute Massages

A 15-minute massage with a partner can work wonders to refresh and focus your day. Make it a habit.

Back-Up a Buddy

How about a back tune-up for a buddy?

- Have your friend sit in a chair with full back facing you.
- Place your palms on both sides of the back and walk your hands up and down along each side of the spine. Slow down your own breath and movements, and you'll find your friend will follow suit.
- Now, take your thumbs and walk them up and down either side of the spine, concentrating more minutely on the area while staying off the spine.
- Next, repeat these strokes (first "walking" with the palms, then with the thumbs) down each arm.
- Move up to each shoulder and knead the shoulder muscle. Slow down—no need to hurry.
- Now, concentrate on the neck. Work your thumbs along either side of the neck vertebrae.
- End with a gentle scalp massage, as if you were giving your friend a thorough but gentle shampoo.
- Break the dreaded news: Massage is over!

Clear the Air

Is your friend feeling blocked, stagnant, and in need of an energy clearing? You can do one in 15 clarifying minutes.

- Without touching your partner, ask him or her to sit in a chair, eyes closed.
- Slowly move your palms over the surface of your partner's body *without touching*. Stay about an inch or two above the skin. Begin at the crown of the head and work down the face, scalp, neck, shoulder, arms, back, etc., until you've reached the feet. Then move back over the body, wherever energy feels "heavy."
- Try closing your eyes after you've moved over the body a time or two, and notice different heat intensities over different parts of the body. Move around the body, concentrating on the areas that feel hotter or more stagnant. Imagine you are smoothing the energy so that it flows evenly over the body.
- Think of smoothing the energy, cooling the hot spots by stirring them up and encouraging flow. Or, imagine you are calming turbulent waters so the energy is like a calm, gently flowing body of water over the body.
- Tell your partner what you are doing and feeling as you go so your partner can tune into his or her energy fields as you clear them.

30-Minute Massages

A 30-minute massage is a great way to relax at the end of the day, and to spend quality time by staying in touch with the people you love. You can find 30 minutes, can't you? Turn off that TV!

Musical Massage Interlude

Massage and a little soft music is a great way to wind down at the end of the day—smoothing away the day's tensions and preparing your body for tomorrow.

- Put on your partner's favorite slow, relaxing music.
- Ask your partner to lie face down on the floor. For comfort, first put down a folded blanket or quilt.
- Begin with hand-over-hand compression strokes (see Chapter 15) over your partner's entire back and backs of legs. Continue for five minutes.
- Now focus on just one side of the back and choose two of the effleurage strokes from Chapter 13 (Hand over hand, Loose fists, Forearm, Fanning, and Feather). Continue for five minutes, working to perfect your strokes.
- Then move to the other side of the back and repeat your effleurage strokes for five more minutes.
- Next, concentrate on the back of one leg alternating any two effleurage strokes of your choice for five minutes.

- Repeat on the other leg for five minutes.
- End your musical massage interlude with five minutes of compression strokes up and down the entire back side, from neck to toes.

Foot Fancy

Give a foot massage to a friend. For this 30-minute massage, spend fifteen minutes on each foot. It feels great to help someone put his or her best foot forward!

- Begin with the toes. One at a time, move each toe in little circles, first one way, then the other.
- Next, walk your thumbs up, down, and around the ball of the foot. Take your time.
- Make your hand into a fist and roll it up and down the arch of the foot.
- Circle your thumbs around the heel. Massage gently around the back of the heel where the Achilles tendon lies.
- Now, massage the calf with effleurage and petrissage strokes (see Chapters 13 and 14).
- Repeat the above sequence on the other foot. Then do it all again, if you like (or if your partner begs you!).

One Full Glorious Hour of Massage

A full hour of massage is a wonderful gift for someone you love. Make the offer. Arrange a trade. You'll be glad you did. (Is it better to give than to receive? Well, we think both are good!)

- Begin with your partner lying face up on the floor or on a massage table. Ask your partner to close his or her eyes.
- Begin your massage on the face. Very slowly and gently move all around the face making little circles with your fingers. Movements on the face may seem faster than they actually feel to the one receiving the massage, so slow down! Spend 10 languid minutes on the face.
- Next, move to the sensitive neck area. Place your hands on either side of the spine, palms up, and roll your fingers up the back of the neck (imagine your hand doing a forward somersault, fingers first) in a wavelike motion. Watch the chin bob up and down.
- Extend out to the shoulders and continue to the rolling motion. Slowly build into a petrissage (kneading) of the shoulders (see Chapter 14). Continue working the shoulders for 10 minutes.
- Work down one arm at a time, first with long, flowing effleurage strokes (see Chapter 13) that move from shoulder to fingertips. Vary the stroke technique (try

different strokes described in Chapter 13, such as Hand over Hand, Thumb over Thumb, Loose Fists, Forearm, and Feather).

- Follow with petrissage strokes to the arms. Vary the strokes (try different strokes described in Chapter 14, such as Kneading, Wringing, Pulling, Skin-Roll, Pac-Man). Spend five minutes on each arm, for both effleurage and petrissage strokes.

Now, take a short transition break. Place your hands on your partner's stomach and hold for a few minutes.

- On to the legs. First, cover each leg with a series of effleurage strokes, then into petrissage strokes, as with the arms. Spend five minutes on each leg.
- Ask your partner to turn over, to lie face down. Now, work your way back up.
- First, one leg at a time, effleurage and petrissage your way up the backs of the legs, spending five minutes on each leg.
- And now the GRAND BACK FINALE! Spend 10 minutes on the back. Begin with long, flowing effleurage strokes and follow with kneading petrissage strokes. Cover the entire back area. Spend the last minute or so with light, effleurage feather strokes.
- When you are finished, simply place your hands on the center of your partner's back and rest there. Feel the beautiful energy you have just shared. Let this energy settle and rest within both of you. Listen to the soft music of your breaths.
- Slowly remove your hands. Leave quietly and allow your partner to get up in his or her own time.

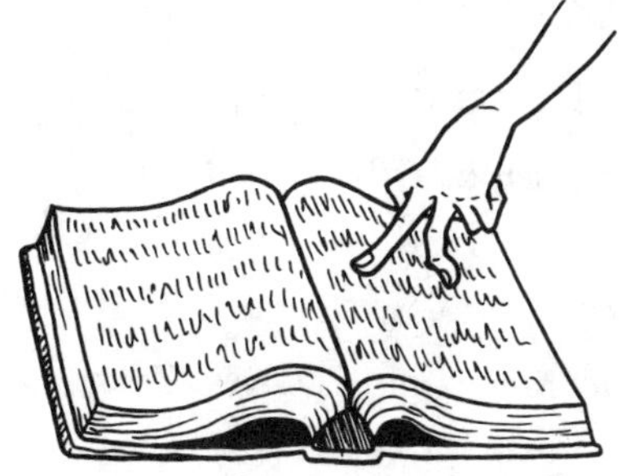

Let Your Fingers Do the Walking: Suggested Reading

Beck, Mark F. *Milady's Theory and Practice of Therapeutic Massage*, second edition. Albany, NY: Milady Publishing Co., 1994.

Berry, Carmen Renee. *Is Your Body Trying to Tell You Something*? Berkeley, CA: PageMill Press, 1997.

The Boston Women's Health Collective. *Our Bodies, Ourselves, A Book By and For Women*. New York: Simon & Schuster, 1979.

Bone, Breath & Gesture: Practices of Embodiment, edited by Don Hanlon Johnson. Berkeley, CA: North Atlantic Books, 1995.

Budilovsky, Joan, and Eve Adamson. *The Complete Idiot's Guide to Yoga*. New York: Alpha Books, 1998.

Byers, Dwight C. *Better Health with Foot Reflexology*. Saint Petersburg, FL: Ingham Publishing, Inc., 1996.

Calais-Germain, Blandine. *Anatomy of Movement*. Seattle: Eastland Press, Inc., 1993.

Calais-Germain, Blandine and Andree Lamotte. *Anatomy of Movement Exercises*. Seattle: Eastland Press, Inc., 1996.

Chaitow, Leon. *Fibromyalgia & Muscle Pain*. San Francisco: Thorsons, 1995.

Chateau, Leon. ND, DO. *Soft-Tissue Manipulation*. Rochester, VT: Healing Arts Press, 1988.

Chopra, Deepak, M.D. *Perfect Health: The Complete Mind/Body Guide*. New York: Harmony Books, 1991.

Claire, Thomas. *Bodywork: What Type of Massage to Get—and How to Make the Most of It*. New York: William Morrow, 1995.

Damian, Peter and Kate Damian. *Aromatherapy: Scent and Psyche*. Rochester, VT: Healing Arts Press, 1995.

Davis, Laura. *The Courage to Heal Workbook*. New York: Harper & Row Publishers, 1990.

Dodd, Barbara, ND, R.D. *Full-Body Reflexology: An Illustrated Guide*. Pleasant Grove, UT: Woodland Publishing, 1996.

Downing, George. *The Massage Book*. New York: Random House, 1972.

Fischer-Rizzi, Susanne. *Complete Aromatherapy Handbook: Essential Oils For Radiant Health*. New York: Sterling, 1990.

Fromm, Eric. *The Art of Loving*. New York: Harper & Row, 1956.

Goleman, Daniel. *Emotional Intelligence: Why It Can Matter More Than I.Q.* New York: Bantam Books, 1995.

Hands-On Healing, edited by John Feltman and the eds. of Prevention Magazine Health Books. Emmaus, PA: Rodale Press, 1989.

Hanna, Thomas. *Somatics*. Reading, MA: Addison-Wesley Publishing Company, 1988.

Hay, Louise L. *Heal Your Body*. Carson, CA: Hay House, Inc., 1998.

Ingham, Eunice D. *Stories the Feet can Tell Thru Reflexology, Stories the Feet Have Told Thru Reflexology*. Saint Petersburg, FL: Ingham Publishing, Inc., 1984.

Jarmey, Chris and Gabriel Mojay. *Hammersmith*. London: Harper Collins, 1991.

Jora, Jurgen. *Foot Reflexology*. New York: St. Martin's Press, 1991.

Leigh, Michelle Dominique. *Inner Peace, Outer Beauty: Natural Japanese Health and Beauty Secrets Revealed*. New York: Citadel Press, 1995.

Massage & Bodywork magazine, the official publication of the Associated Bodywork and Massage Professionals (ABMP).

Massage Therapy Journal, the official publication of the American Massage Therapy Association (AMTA).

Masson, Jeffrey Moussaieff and Susan McCarthy. *When Elephants Weep: The Emotional Lives of Animals*. New York: Dell Publishing, 1995.

Mattes, Aaron L. *Flexibility Active and Assisted Stretching*. Sarasota, FL: Aaron L. Mattes, 1990.

McClure, Vimala Schneider, *Infant Massage A Handbook for Loving Parents,* New York: Bantam Books, 1989.

Montagu, Ashley. *Touching: The Human Significance of Skin*. New York: Harper & Row, 1986.

Ohashi. *Reading the Body: Ohashi's Book of Oriental Diagnosis*. Middlesex, England: Penguin Books Ltd., 1991.

Palmer, David A. *The Body Entrepreneur*. San Francisco: Thumb Press, 1990.

Pitcairn, Richard H., D.V.M., and Susan Hubble Pitcairn. *Dr. Pitcairn's Complete Guide to Natural Health for Dogs & Cats*. New Edition, Emmaus, PA: Rodale Press, Inc., 1995.

Prudden, Bonnie. *Pain Erasure: The Bonnie Prudden Way*. New York: M. Evans & Company, Inc., 1980.

Ratcliff, J.D. *I Am Joe's Body*. New York: Berkley Books, 1993.

Rush, Anne Kent. *The Modern Book of Massage: Five-Minute Vacations and Sensuous Escapes*. New York: Dell Publishing, 1994.

Sandifer, Jon. *Acupressure for Health, Vitality, and First Aid*. Rockport, MA: Element, Inc., 1997.

Schatz, Mary Pullig, M.D. *Back Care Basics*. Berkeley: Rodnell Press, 1992.

Shaw, Eva, *60-Second Shiatzu*. New York: Henry Holt & Co., 1995.

Siegel, Bernie S., M.D. *Peace, Love & Healing*. New York: Harper & Row, 1989.

Spock, Benjamin, M.D. *Baby and Child Care,* Revised Ed. New York: Hawthorn Books, Inc., 1976.

Stone, Robert J. and Judith A. Stone. *Atlas of the Skeletal Muscles*. Dubuque, IA: Wm C. Brown Publishers, 1990.

Teeguarden, Iona Marsaa, M.A., and Senior Teachers of Jin Shin Do Acupressure. *A Complete Guide to Acupressure*. Tokyo/New York: Japan Publications, Inc., 1996.

Thie, John F., D.C. *Touch for Health*, 4th Revised Ed. Sherman Oaks, CA: T.H. Enterprises, 1994.

Travis, John W., M.D., and Regina Sara Ryan. *Wellness Workbook*. Berkeley, CA: Ten Speed Press, 1988.

Zidonis, Nancy and Marie Soderberg. *Canine Acupressure: A Treatment Workbook*, 1995.

Zidonis, Nancy and Marie Soderberg. *Equine Acupressure: A Treatment Workbook*, 1995.

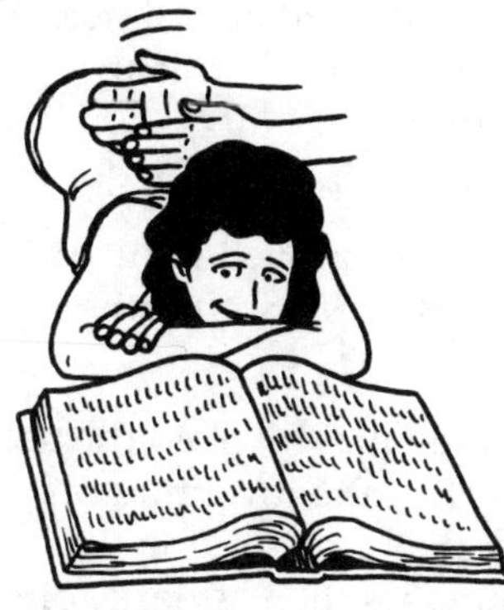

Appendix C

Touch Talk Glossary

Abduction: Any movement that moves a body part away from the body's midline.

Achilles tendonitis: An inflammation of the Achilles tendon (in the heel).

Active ROM movements: Movements of a joint through its range of motion that you make yourself, without assistance, such as circling your arms.

Acupuncture: A method of healing in which needles are inserted into certain areas of the body to free or reactivate stagnant chi, developed centuries ago in China. Originally, needles were made from bone and stone. Later, they were made from steel. Some historians believe an original purpose for acupuncture was to lance infections.

Adduction: Any movement that brings a body part toward the body's midline.

Adhesions: Abnormal connections between tissues, such as muscles stuck together with connective tissue, that are caused by injury, stress, or misuse. Massage can break apart adhesions to restore normal function to muscles and connective tissue.

Aerobic respiration: The process through which muscles derive energy to contract, provided by oxygen.

Amma: An ancient Chinese system of massage. It incorporates centuries of experience gained by Chinese health practitioners on the effects of stimulating certain points on the body in various ways.

Anaerobic respiration: The process through which muscles derive energy to contract, during which glucose is utilized in the absence of oxygen. Lactic acid is a by-product of this process. If lactic acid builds up in muscles faster than the body can eliminate it, muscle pain results.

Anatomy: The study of the structure of the body and the interaction of its parts.

Anthropomorphize: To assign human characteristics to a nonhuman, such as an animal.

Applied kinesiology: A technique that first tests muscles for strength and range of motion, analyzes posture and lifestyle, then prescribes an appropriate treatment program that may include particular massage techniques, acupressure work, craniosacral work, a specific diet, vitamin and herb use, and exercises meant to mobilize joints.

Aromatherapy: The therapeutic use of pure essential oils, either applied to the skin or inhaled through various methods. This term is also used to describe scent-oriented therapies that use plant oils.

Aromatics: Both a practice and a product, the practice of aromatics involves the use of plant fragrances in general, not limited to essential oils. Before the invention of steam distillation, oils were typically infused with a plant's essence by soaking the plant in the oil. These oils are more appropriately called aromatics than essential oils.

Asthma: A disease characterized by shortness of breath, wheezing, bronchial spasms, and a persistent cough. Attacks can be brought on by allergies, excessive physical activity, ingestion of certain foods, anxiety, or for no apparent reason.

Aston-Patterning: Founded by Judith Aston, this technique involves movement re-education that combines the techniques of Dr. Ida Rolf with patterns of movement. It eventually grew to include fitness training and ergonomics.

Axon: The central extension of a nerve cell that carries impulses away from the cell.

Ayurveda (Ayur-Veda): The oldest (over 5,000 years old) system of scientifically based health care. Literally translated as "science of living" or "art of life," Ayurveda combines diet, exercise, meditation, and a regular routine into a philosophical system of energy balancing. Ayurveda has recently enjoyed a surge of popularity in the West because of the writings of Deepak Chopra, M.D.

Bodywork: The systematic manipulation of the body through massage, movement, energy work, or other manual therapies.

Bone marrow: The red type is a soft, spongy, blood-vessel-filled tissue in the center of bones. The yellow type, also at the center of some bones, stores fat. Red bone marrow manufactures the majority of red blood cells, which nourish bones and the rest of the body, and white blood cells, which protect against infection.

Bronchial tubes: A subdivision of the trachea, which is part of the lungs.

Bursae: Fluid-filled sacks that cushion muscle, tendons, and skin from bones in high-impact areas, such as shoulders or knees.

Cartilage: A tough, elastic form of connective tissue, also known as gristle, with the primary function of cushioning and protecting bones and joints.

Cerebrospinal fluid: The fluid that flows through and around the brain and down around the spinal cord. This fluid helps to bring nutrients to and carry waste from the brain and spinal cord, but it mainly serves as a shock absorber to protect these delicate and essential organs.

Chakras: Centers of psychospiritual energy in the body. The seven primary chakras are located at the base of the spine (Saturn), on the spine behind the pelvic area (Jupiter), behind the stomach area (Mars), behind the heart (Venus), in the throat (Mercury), in the middle of the brow (Sun), and at the crown of the skull (Thousand-Petalled Lotus). There are also many subtler chakras.

Chi: Life force energy that flows through and around the body and throughout the universe. In Japan, it is called *ki*, in India *prana*, in Tibet *rlun*, in ancient Greece *pneuma*. Westerners call it a number of things, all along the lines of "life force energy." Many Westerns have also adopted the Eastern terms.

Chiropractors: Doctors who treat disease and other medical problems by manipulation of the musculoskeletal system.

Circadian rhythms: Your internal rhythms of temperature, hormone levels, and energy. Circadian rhythms vary among individuals (especially between morning people and night owls), but most people tend to have high energy in late morning and late afternoon, an energy slump an hour or two after lunchtime (siesta time), and the need for a long period of sleep beginning a few hours before midnight.

Cold pressing: The process of pressing oil from the plant.

Colic: A condition in infants characterized by intense, inconsolable crying/screaming sessions lasting three hours or longer. No one knows for sure why some babies experience it and others don't. Some theories hold that colic is related to gastrointestinal distress; others claim it is a matter of overstimulation.

Collagen: From the Greek word *kola*, meaning glue, collagen is a gelatinous substance found in connective tissue, bones, and tendons.

Compression: A type of friction massage stroke involving a rhythmic pressing motion performed with the hands or fingers.

Connective tissue: A matrix of tough, fibrous material that provides a support system for the entire body and lubrication for joints.

Craniosacral therapy: A technique that involves gentle pressure and manipulation of the craniosacral system, or the bones and soft tissues of the skull, face, vertebrae, and sacrum (the bones at the base of the spine). This technique balances the flow of cerebrospinal fluid, which is thought to balance the entire body. Dr. John Upledger, an osteopath, coined the name.

Creative visualization: A technique for attaining what you desire, such as material possessions, spiritual goals, or certain life situations, by regularly visualizing yourself already in possession of what you desire.

Cytoskeletal structure: Sometimes referred to as the cell's individual nervous system. Connected on a molecular level to the body's entire tissue matrix, the cytoskeletal structure gives the cell its shape. Some researchers believe the cytoskeleton is a storehouse for cellular memory, which can then be communicated to the rest of the body through the tissue matrix.

Decoction: The process of obtaining an extract by boiling plant parts.

Deep tissue massage: A general term referring to several variations of Swedish massage that concentrate on freeing the body's connective tissue through intense physical manipulation.

Dendrite: A threadlike branch of a nerve cell that conducts impulses towards the cell body.

Disk: The soft, semicartilaginous disks that cushion the vertebrae.

Effleurage: From the French verb *effleurer,* meaning "to graze, to skim the surface of, or to touch lightly," this is the term coined by Dr. Johann Mezger (1839–1909) to refer to a long, gliding massage stroke.

Endorphins: Chemicals that work within the brain to relieve pain, affect emotions, and contribute to feelings of euphoria after intense physical activity. Chemically similar to morphine, endorphins are the brain's "homemade" painkillers.

Energy channels: Specific channels that run through the body like rivers, through which life-force energy flows.

Energy meridians: See Energy channels.

Energy therapy: A type of bodywork that manipulates, unblocks, and balances the body's energy field.

Esalan massage: A combination of Swedish massage and sensory awareness techniques, including passive joint movements and deep tissue work in a nurturing and ideally, an aesthetically pleasing environment. The technique is named after the Esalan Institute in Big Sur, California, where Esalan massages are given outside on a cliff overlooking the ocean.

Essential oils: Aromatic oils distilled from organic plant sources, including flowers, leaves, and bark. Only oils produced by steam distillation are technically pure essential oils. Different essential oils are thought to have different, potent effects on body, mind, and spirit.

Extension: Any movement that increases the angle of a joint. The opposite of flexion.

Fascia: The layer of fibrous connective tissue underlying and separating your skin from the organs, bones, and muscles beneath it. Your fascia supports your nerves and blood vessels. When kneaded and manipulated through massage, the fascia is loosened, releasing toxins and stimulating circulation.

Feldenkrais method: Founded by Moshe Feldenkrais, D.Sc., an Israeli physicist from Russia, this system of movement re-education is meant to optimize human function by raising a client's awareness about limiting movement patterns and habits.

Fibrosis: A process in which fibrous tissue forms in the body. When this fibrous tissue develops where it wouldn't normally belong, such as around the site of a muscle injury, it can limit function, causing stiffness or even pain.

Flexion: Any movement that decreases the angle of a joint. The opposite of extension.

Gluteus muscles: The muscles of your buttocks, responsible for extending, abducting, and rotating the thigh. One of the largest muscle groups in your body, they are a common place to hold tension.

Hard end feel: Refers to the limit of a joint's range of motion because of bone prohibiting further movement.

Hedonism: A philosophy that states that pleasure is the principal good and all action should have pleasure as its aim. In psychology, hedonism refers to the idea that all human actions have pleasure as their purpose.

Hellerwork: Founded by a former aerospace engineer and student of Ida Rolf, Joseph Heller, Hellerwork combines movement re-education, massage, and dialogue between client and massage therapist.

Hip dysplasia: A congenital defect more common in large dogs. An abnormal hip joint results in pain, limping, hopping, and difficulty getting up and down from sitting or lying positions. Arthritis frequently develops in the hip joint. Hip dysplasia is commonly treated with weight and exercise control, pain relievers, or surgery in severe cases.

Homeostasis: The tendency of a system (a body, a group, an ecosystem) to maintain an equilibrium or balanced state.

Hydrotherapy: Water therapy that uses the healing power of water in conjunction with massage or movement, or simply for soaking, streaming, spraying, or otherwise applying water, in its various forms and temperatures, to the body.

I.Q.: Intelligence Quotient; a number that signifies a person's mental development. It is obtained by multiplying the person's mental age (determined by a test) by 100 and then dividing the result by chronological age.

Infusion: The process of pouring boiling water over plant parts and steeping them or soaking plants in vegetable oil. Some plants require solvents such as alcohol to release their essences.

Interstitial fluids: The fluids between cells and blood vessels within the body. Through various processes, these fluids are constantly transferred in and out of cells, helping to remove waste products and deliver nutrients.

Keratin: The substance out of which your nails and hair are primarily made; keratization is the process by which living cells (such as those in the hair roots and nail bases) become dead, tough material without nerves or blood vessels.

Ki: See Chi.

Larynx: A box of cartilage at the back of your throat containing your vocal cords; it's your voice box.

Ligaments: Bands of connective tissue that support joints and bind bones to other bones.

Limbic system: The brain's emotional center. A more primitive area of the brain (present in evolution long before higher brain functions evolved), the limbic system reacts to sensory signals and cues the body to act without analysis or interpretation.

Lotus position: A seated yoga pose in which the legs are crossed and each ankle is placed on top of the opposite thigh. Often used for meditation, this position is said to resemble the beauty and symmetry of the lotus flower.

Lungs: The primary organ of respiration in which the exchange of oxygen and carbon dioxide takes place.

Manual lymph drainage: Developed by Dr. Emil Vodder and wife Estrid in the 1930s in Europe, this technique facilitates the lymphatic system's processes by massaging the body with slow, light strokes. Widely practiced in Europe, where it is often used to alleviate post-surgical pain and swelling, manual lymph drainage is more recently becoming popular in the United States.

Massage: The systematic and manual manipulation of the soft tissues of the body.

Metabolic rate: Your "rate of living," referring to the processes within your cells that transform food into energy. Ideally, your metabolism is balanced (or in a state of homeostasis) so that you produce as much energy as you need.

Metatarsals: The five bones that extend from the area of the heel toward the first bones of the toe, almost like pre-toes. They can be likened to the metacarpals in the hands.

Muscle belly: The thicker, middle part of the muscle.

Muscle insertion: The place where the other end of the muscle attaches to the skeleton, a muscle, or deep skin layers and where movement takes place, usually further from the body's center than the origin.

Muscle origin: The place where a muscle attaches to a relatively immovable part of the skeleton, usually closer to the body's center.

Myotherapy: One type of trigger point therapy made popular by Bonnie Prudden.

Neuron: A nerve cell.

Orthobionomy: A bodywork technique developed by Arthur Lincoln Pauls. "Ortho" means "to correct or straighten," and "bionomy" means "study of life processes." According to Dr. Pauls, orthobionomy restores the body's natural understanding of itself by safely and slowly moving the body in the direction of its habitual holding patterns that are blocking energy or causing pain.

Osteopaths: Doctors who typically combine traditional medical treatment with structural manipulations and a holistic perspective.

Passive ROM movements: Movements of a joint through its range of motion made by someone else without your assistance, such as a massage therapist circling your arm for you while you stay relaxed.

Petrissage: A French noun translated as kneading or, figuratively, forming, is the term coined by Dr. Johann Mezger (1839–1909) to refer to a kneading massage stroke.

Phalanges: The toe bones; the word also applies to the finger bones.

Phoenix Rising Yoga Therapy: A form of body therapy that uses assisted yoga movements and basic dialogue techniques to guide clients into a body scan to determine where tensions are being held in the body. Sessions encourage clients to work through these tensions (physically, verbally, emotionally) and eventually release them.

Physiology: The science of vital processes, mechanisms, and functions of organs and organ systems.

Phytotherapy: The use of plants for therapeutic purposes. It includes herbal medicine, which uses whole plants or plant parts in various forms, from tinctures and teas to powders and pills, and aromatherapy. The ancient art of phytotherapy has been practiced since the beginning of humankind in every civilization and on every continent.

PMS: See Premenstrual syndrome.

Pneuma: See Chi.

Polarity therapy: Founded by Dr. Randolph Stone (1890–1981), a doctor of chiropracty, osteopathy, and naturopathy who traveled widely and was well versed in Oriental and East Indian theories of healing. Dr. Stone based his technique on a combination of osteopathy, acupuncture, and Ayurveda to balance the body's energies.

Post-traumatic stress disorder: A condition seen in people who have experienced or witnessed a traumatic event in which intense fear, helplessness, or horror were experienced.

Prana: See Chi.

Pranayama: The Hindu word for yoga breathing exercises designed to help you master control of the breath and, ultimately, your life force.

Premenstrual syndrome: Also known as PMS, a condition characterized by a wide range of symptoms probably related to the fluctuation in hormones experienced during the menstrual cycle. Some researchers believe that the disorder originates in the brain and may be linked to levels of seratonin, the neurotransmitter linked to depression.

Pressure points: Points along energy channels where energy tends to pool or get blocked. Pressing or massaging these points can help to rejuvenate energy flows through the channels.

Psychophysical therapies: Types of bodywork that work with both the body and the mind in terms of how they affect each other, such as how an emotional trauma can cause physical distress to the body. By releasing repressed emotions, for example, physical dysfunction can be corrected.

Qi: See Chi.

Reflexology: A system of massage based on the concept that the stimulation of certain areas of the body (typically the feet, hands, and ears) can affect the health and function of other areas, systems, or organs in the body.

Rlun: See Chi.

Rolfing: Also called the Rolfing Method of Structural Integration, it is a form of structural integration developed by Ida P. Rolf, Ph.D. Its purpose is to restructure the body in response to gravity by deep tissue manipulation, to correct misalignments caused by bad habit and trauma.

Rotation: Any movement that revolves a body part around an axis.

Runner's knee: A softening of the kneecap cartilage.

Ruptured disk: Occurs when part of a disk herniates or pushes through the surrounding ligaments of the spine. This condition is extremely painful and usually requires surgery.

Separation anxiety: A condition in pets (especially dogs) brought on by your absence. This condition is common in puppies that have been with their owners constantly for several months and are suddenly left alone all day, sick dogs, and dogs with overly dependent emotional relationships with their owners. Symptoms include destructive behavior (eating your sofa, digging, shredding garbage), depression, chronic barking, nervousness, and disintegrating health.

Serotonin: A chemical neurotransmitter that occurs naturally in the body and is involved in numerous functions including appetite control, sleep, memory and learning, mood, behavior, and depression. The newest and most effective antidepressant drugs are selective serotonin re-uptake inhibitors (SSRIs) that make serotonin more available in the brain.

Shiatsu: A specific method of massage that uses finger pressure on tsubos to manipulate chi.

Shin splints: An inflammation of the tendons and muscles on the front of the calf.

Soft end feel: Refers to the limit of a joint's range of motion because of soft tissue such as skin and muscle prohibiting further movement.

Somatics: A broad term meaning "of or relating to the body," that can be applied to many types of bodywork in which the student is actively taught techniques for increased self-awareness and self-mastery—to move, feel, and exist with consciousness and forethought.

Sports massage: A variation of Swedish massage specifically tailored for the athlete. Sports massage lessens the chance for injury, decreases recovery time, and optimizes performance.

Springy end feel: Refers to the limit of a joint's range of motion because of tendons, ligaments, or other connective tissue prohibiting further movement.

Steam distillation: Involves passing steam through plants and collecting the vapors and is the only way to extract a plant's pure essential oil.

Structural integration: A general term (originally it referred to what is now known as "Rolfing") for a type of massage that works to integrate the body's structure by reorganizing it through physical manipulation of the body's muscles and connective tissue so it can exist in better harmony with gravity.

Swedish massage: A popular form of massage based on a system developed by Per Henrik Ling (1776–1839) of Sweden. Ling developed a system of movements called Medical Gymnastics based on the then-fledgling science of physiology. The Ling System was also called Swedish Movements or the Movement Cure, and spread through Europe, then the United States. In the United States, the technique was known as The Swedish Movement Cure, and eventually evolved into what we now call Swedish massage.

Tapotement: From the French verb *tapoter,* the word is translated as "to pat, to tap, or to strum" and is the term coined by Dr. Johann Mezger (1839–1909) to refer to the percussion stroke.

Temporomandibular joint syndrome: Also known as TMJ, this condition is a chronic, painful condition usually resulting from jaw trauma, such as a car accident or a major dental procedure. "Temporo" means skull bones, and "mandibular" refers to the jaw bone, or mandible. TMJ can be characterized by clicking or other jaw noises, pain, and dysfunction of any of the jaw muscles.

Tendons: Tough connective tissues connecting muscle to bone.

Tennis elbow: An inflammation of the tendons and muscles in the elbow.

Tinnitus: Ear noise, such as ringing, buzzing, humming, or roaring. A distracting and sometimes extremely aggravating condition, tinnitus can be a symptom of many physical problems, including TMJ syndrome.

TMJ: See Temporomandibular joint syndrome.

Trachea: The passageway between your larynx and your bronchial tubes; it's your windpipe.

Trager method: Founded by Milton Trager, M.D., this technique combines painless touch (called "Psychophysical Integration"), exercises the client performs, and mental/movement exercises (called "Mentastics"), to release blockages in the body as an approach to healing.

Trigger point therapy: A term referring to several types of therapy in which trigger points, or sensitive areas in tight muscles that cause pain in various parts of the body, are pressed firmly until the tension releases.

Tsubos: The Japanese name for the specific points on the body that can be pressed or rubbed to stimulate chi.

Tui na: Literally push-pull, the term for modern Chinese massage.

Ulcers: Sores or localized areas of mucous membrane disintegration. Stomach ulcers are characterized by burning stomach pain when the stomach is empty and are sometimes accompanied by vomiting and/or bleeding.

Vis medicatrix naturae: A term coined by Greek physician Hippocrates (460–377 B.C.), who is considered the "Father of Medicine." This term refers to the body's natural ability to heal itself.

Yang: In Chinese philosophy, the male element and opposite of/complement to yin. Also represents sun, light, heat, spirituality.

Yin: In Chinese philosophy, the female element and opposite of/complement to yang. Also represents moon, dark, cold, earthliness.

Index

A

B

C

H

L

M

N

O

P

Q

R

S

T

U-V

W-Z

YES, send me my copies of Joan's wonderful tapes!

Special Audio Tape Offer:

❏ "Foot Massage, For Body, Mind, and Sole" **$7.95**

Massage Video

❏ "My Swedish Massage with Joan" **$19.95**

Massage Audio

❏ "The Art of Massage Made Simple" **$10.95**

Yoga Audio

❏ "Beginning Yoga with Joan" **$10.00**

❏ "Breathworks!" **$10.00**

❏ "Sun-Salutations with Joan" **$10.00**

❏ "Total Relaxation...with Shavasana" **$10.00**

Yoga Book

❏ *The Little Yogi Water Book* **$8.00**

Shipping/handling charges:

Audio/Book—Add $2.50 for 1–2 items; add $.50 for each additional item. ______

Video—Add $4.50 for first video tape; add $1.00 for each additional video tape. ______

Sub-Total ______

Illinois Residents add 6.75% sales tax ______

TOTAL ______

Payment to be made in U.S. funds. Prices and availability are subject to change without notice.

❏ Check or money order enclosed.

I would like to charge to: ❏ MasterCard ❏ Visa

Acct.#: ______________________________

Exp. Date: ______________________________

Signature: ______________________________

Send this order form with your check, money order, or charge information to:

Yoyoga, Inc.
P.O. Box 5013
Oak Brook, IL 60522
FAX (630) 963-4001

Allow 4 to 6 weeks for delivery

Ship to:

Name: ______________________________

Address: ______________________________

City, State, Zip: ______________________________

Telephone: ______________________________